THE HANDY
HOME MEDICAL ADVISER
and Concise Medical Encyclopedia

NEW, REVISED EDITION

THE HANDY
HOME MEDICAL ADVISER

and Concise Medical Encyclopedia

NEW, REVISED EDITION

Combining Good Housekeeping's Pocket Medical
Encyclopedia and The Handy Home Medical Adviser

by MORRIS FISHBEIN, M.D.

DOUBLEDAY & COMPANY, INC.
Garden City, New York

DEDICATED TO
MY GRANDCHILDREN
Morris Fishbein, Merriel Anna, Peter Emil and Rosemary Friedell
AND TO
*Georgia Emily, Laurence Victor, Michael Morris
and the twins—Barbara Ann and Wendy Jo Marks*
AND TO
Amy Louise, Morris Daniel and Ann Marie Fishbein

PREFACE

MANY NEW DISCOVERIES have been developed in medical science with relationship to some of the diseases that are discussed in this book. Some subjects insufficiently discussed in previous issues have been given more complete consideration.

When people come to a doctor, they usually come because they have had pain or some other symptom which has continued to disturb them, or which has not been explained. The pain may be headache, stomach-ache, or pain elsewhere in the body like the pains of rheumatoid arthritis. People consult the doctor because of sudden or extreme loss of weight, or unexplained fever, or similar conditions. For any unexplainable condition, the person should consult the doctor at the earliest sign. The modern doctor will attempt to solve the condition through a complete examination which will include not only attention to the special pain or symptom or disturbance, but also tests to detect any condition in the body that needs attention. Regardless of what he himself may know of disease or disability, the patient should consult the doctor at the earliest sign, and he should be prepared to have his condition approached from the point of view of his whole body. This may necessitate a study which requires the use of the X-ray, or a variety of laboratory examinations, of a record of all of his previous diseases, and a most intimate search into the condition for which he consults the physician.

This book, it is hoped, will give the reader a better understanding of his own medical troubles and thereby make him a better patient for his doctor.

MORRIS FISHBEIN, M.D.

Chicago

CONTENTS

CONTENTS

INTRODUCTION

THE RULES OF HEALTH

HEALTH, according to the dictionaries, is a feeling of well-being. That was the old definition! The modern definition of health says that you must not only feel all right but also that you must not be aware of any pain or irritation anywhere in your body. Moreover, you must have what the quacks used to call vim, vigor and vitality—a feeling of positive health. You must have the desire to be up and doing. You must be free from fatigue. You must not get tired easily.

Once we thought that we could give people a lot of simple rules for keeping their bodies in health. Now we have learned so much more about the nature of disease that the rules have become complicated. Doctors used to say that you could take three or four meals a day and that this would take care of your needs as far as health was concerned. The list included breakfast at 8 o'clock, dinner or lunch at noon, perhaps a supplement in the form of tea or a little snack around 4:30 in the afternoon, and then supper or dinner about 7:30. Nowadays we know that some people do even better on six small meals a day; others seem to be quite healthful with just a light lunch but with a fairly good breakfast and not too large a dinner. We are so individual in our construction and in our constitutions that it is impossible to put down a rule for positive patterns of eating or amounts of eating that will apply to all people.

The same considerations apply to rest and sleep. Some people need more rest and more sleep than do others. Some are able to get along quite satisfactorily on six hours; others seem to require as much as ten or twelve hours of sleep to be at their best during the waking hours. Eight hours of sleep might be put down as an average, with recognition, however, that some are above and others below the average.

The hygienists used to say that everyone ought to have at least a quart of water a day, recommending eight glasses—one before breakfast, one between each meal, one at each meal and one before going to bed. Nowadays we know that our appetites and our sense of thirst may be a reasonable indication of what we ought to have in the way of fluids. One health expert recommended three pints of water daily, indicating, however, that it could be taken in tea, coffee, cocoa, milk, soup or some other liquid. Pure water is an excellent drink, as is milk. When you take a beverage that is rich in nourishment as, for instance, beer, the nourishment must be counted in the daily intake as well as the fluid.

Food is not just bulk but includes also such specific constituents as protein, carbohydrates and fats, mineral salts and vitamins. The National Research Council, through its Food and Nutrition Board, has compiled a list of seven basic foods that everyone ought to have every day and on which he may build the remainder of his diet. These will be discussed later.

Why do we exercise? Among other reasons, exercise improves the power and tone of the muscles. It helps the blood by increasing the amount of oxygen that is carried by the coloring matter of the red blood cells. It stimulates the circulation, thus making certain that all of the tissues receive the proper amounts of oxygen and also that waste products are carried away. Exercise also provides relaxation because it is a pleasant undertaking if performed under proper circumstances. People who take competition too seriously and who disturb their nervous systems and fail to relax during exercise are not helped, but may well be injured by the wrong kind of exercise. Finally, those who exercise to the point of exhaustion find that recovery is somewhat slow; for them, overexercise has proved just as harmful or perhaps more harmful than would be no exercise at all.

The human body is a self-regulating mechanism. Ordinarily, elimination of waste material from the bowel and the bladder goes on without much attention from the person concerned. There is no absolute rule about elimination from the bowel. Doctors say once daily is average but some people go much longer and others go much more frequently, and both may be quite within the range of what is normal for them.

Even bathing may be carried to excess. Some people develop an absolute obsession about cleanliness. They will rush to wash their hands at the slightest sign of soiling. These people, in many instances, need examination from a psychological point of view. Some people indulge in bathing to a point at which they become a nuisance not only to themselves but to the rest of the family. They soak long hours in the tub, and end with fatigue. A bath that is too hot leaves a person gasping; a bath that is too cold may shock the entire heat-regulating mechansim of the body. All sorts of specialized baths, such as steam baths, salt-water baths, carbon-dioxide baths and similar ablutions are recommended for special purposes; but like every other specialty they need to be prescribed for the individual for certain specific purposes and when not so regulated may do harm.

One of the first books on hygiene designed to keep people in health was the Bible. The rules there set forth as to rest and relaxation and mental attitude and diet were all designed for people of a certain period. Modern conditions have brought new points of view. Thus the day of rest varies among different races of people and among various religions. Similarly attitudes toward food vary with various races and religions. Scientific study has shown that it is not so much exactly what you do in this regard as observance of the need for regular periods of rest to permit recovery of the tired tissues. The diet should be free from infectious material and visible dirt. The point of view toward life must be moderate and temperate.

In the Middle Ages the School of Salerno developed a book called *The Regimen of the School of Salerno*. The chief emphasis in that guide to health and hygiene was moderation in all things. Any modern book of advice on health has to begin with the same general admonition: Be moderate in everything—moderate in food, in drink, in work, in thought and, particularly, in temper.

Nowadays we give much more consideration to the way in which anger, agitation, worry or excitement may seriously damage the functioning of various portions of the body. A contented mind is an essential to a healthful body.

In the early 1900s life expectancy at birth in the United States was about 45 years. In the 1960s it is 70.2 for men and 75 for women. Many people now reach the eighties and nineties. This creates new problems in the medical care of the aged. Research here may yet develop methods for growing old healthfully.

PART ONE

THE HANDY
HOME MEDICAL ADVISER

CHAPTER I

WHEN YOU SEE THE DOCTOR

ONCE PEOPLE CALLED THE DOCTOR only when they were sick—weak, disabled, troubled by pain or suffering. Now the doctor's functions include not only relief from symptoms, but the prevention of disease and its cure when possible. Moreover, modern medicine realizes that the whole human being is always involved—not just one spot of pain or disability. The doctor studies the patient as a complete unit, including both mind and body and the effects on mind and body of the patient's surroundings or environment.

The doctor sees people nowadays for periodic physical and mental examinations, for study before the insurance company grants insurance, and for a survey before the person undertakes any employment or enters on any new activity. The doctor has to know why the patient wants an examination. Is he or she contemplating marriage or giving birth to a child? Does the young man or woman want to engage in sports that carry with them hazards to life and health? Is the young man trying to get into the armed services, or is he trying to get out of them? Is the woman trying to find an alibi for avoiding some unpleasant duty or relationship? The doctor must evaluate the situation, because the nature of the patient's symptoms and his method of description may be greatly influenced by his reasons for being examined.

When you see the doctor, he will be interested first in relieving you of the distress which in most instances caused you to seek his advice. In connection with this immediate problem he will want to find out about your background—the family, social, or business situation in which you live, and how that relates to your trouble. Then too, the doctor has the responsibility of protecting others from hazards that arise out of your condition.

DIAGNOSIS

Proper treatment of any condition depends on a knowledge of its causes. The process of finding out the cause of a condition is called diagnosis. Most conditions have not only immediate causes but also contributing causes. A man may have a broken arm from getting hit by a motorcar; perhaps he was blind in one eye and would not have been hit by the car had he been able to see it. A person gets tuberculosis when invaded by the germ of tuberculosis if his body is such as to be unable to overcome the germ. His body may have been weakened by undernutrition and exposure to cold and damp. Moreover, his germs may have come in overwhelming numbers from a boarder who had the disease, and who lived closely crowded with the family and did not know how to dispose properly of his sputum.

One of the first steps in making a diagnosis of a disease is to get a record of the patient's life and environment related to his trouble. This the doctors call a "history." Some remote fact in the patient's past may carry the chief responsibility for his condition. If a prospective mother has German measles during the first three months of pregnancy, the child when born may be damaged in the eyes, the hearing or the heart. A difficult childbirth may be responsible for cerebral palsy in the child. A man may get ulcers in the nose from inhaling chromium substances at his work. A woman may have a swollen eye because she touched it with a finger contaminated by some substance to which she is especially sensitive. A baby may have eczema because of sensitivity to milk. An executive may have high blood pressure because he is constantly at war with his employees and the board of directors. These are contributing causes with direct manifestations in body disturbances. Sometimes, however, the causes are remote. The mind seems to play a part in affecting the part of the body that may succumb to disease.

THE EXAMINATION

After the doctor has inquired carefully into the life history of the patient as related to his symptoms or his disease, a physical and laboratory examination may follow. A physical examination may vary from a casual use of inspection, palpation, auscultation, percussion and testing of reflexes, to the use of a great variety of instruments which now extend the senses of the doctor.

Inspection involves use of the eyes. The doctor can see eruptions on the skin, bumps below the surface which stretch the skin, ulcers, bruises, swellings, loss of hair or nails, redness of the throat, fluids coming from the eyes or nose or nipples of the breasts.

With his trained fingers he can feel the margin of the liver, lumps on the smooth surfaces of inner organs, organs out of place, areas of tenderness, broken bones or other disturbances.

He can hear, with his ear alone or with the aid of a stethoscope, changes in the sounds of the lungs and heart and intestines. He can thump the chest and abdomen and detect areas of fluid or solidity.

The reflexes, like the knee jerk, and reactions in the skin tell him about the integrity of the nervous system.

With a variety of instruments, he can look into the eye with the ophthalmoscope, the ear with the otoscope, the nose with the rhinoscope, the throat with the laryngoscope and the pharyngoscope, the lungs with the bronchoscope, the stomach with the gastroscope, the bladder with the cystoscope, and the rectum with the proctoscope. With the sphygmomanometer he measures the blood pressure; with the electrocardiograph he records the motions of the heart; with the basal metabolic tests he determines the rate of the body chemistry. The X-ray shows changes in organs and tissues far below the surface of the body. A spirometer may be used to determine the amount of air taken in by the lungs during respiration.

THE X-RAY

One of the most important devices ever invented to help doctors in diagnosis of disease is the X-ray. By the use of this equipment, accompanied by various substances taken by mouth or injected into various cavities, all sorts of changes can be detected in their earliest stages. Your dentist uses X-ray to find cavities in teeth or abscesses at the roots of teeth. The brain specialist is helped in finding tumors or abscesses in the brain and spinal cord. The nose and throat specialist uses X-ray, particularly for finding trouble in the sinuses. The earliest signs of tuberculosis or silicosis in the lungs may be seen in X-ray pictures. The gastroenterologist who specializes in conditions of the stomach and intestines uses X-ray to locate ulcers or tumors in the stomach and duodenum, or in other portions of the thirty feet of intestines. Indeed, every specialty in medicine has been so greatly helped by X-ray that it must be considered one of the greatest discoveries ever made in medical science.

TEST	PURPOSE OF TEST	HOW TEST IS MADE
Schick	To determine if person tested is susceptible to diphtheria.	Minute amount (1/10 cc.) of diluted diphtheria toxin is injected into skin on front surface of forearm with hypodermic syringe and needle.
Dick	To determine if person tested is immune to scarlet fever.	By injecting 1/10 cc. of diluted scarlet-fever toxin into skin on front surface of forearm with hypodermic syringe and needle.
Widal	To determine if person tested has typhoid or paratyphoid fever.	The finger is pricked, and about 1 cc. of blood is collected. Several dilutions of the blood serum are made with salt solution; it is then added to cultures of typhoid bacilli and paratyphoid bacilli. These mixtures are placed in an incubator at about 98°F. for an hour, then are examined to determine if the germs have been clumped by the serum.
Tuberculin	To aid in determining presence of tuberculosis infection.	Diluted solution of tuberculin is injected into the skin, usually on front surface of forearm. Tuberculin is prepared from culture of tubercle bacilli. Test is examined after forty-eight hours.
Sedimentation	To aid in diagnosing tuberculosis and acute infections such as rheumatic fever.	Five to 10 cc. of blood are drawn from patient's vein and mixed with one drop of a potassium-oxalate solution. Special tube is then used to determine amount of settling of red blood cells. Speed of settling is called sedimentation rate.
Complement Fixation	To aid in diagnosing syphilis. (Also called Wassermann, Kahn test, etc.)	To blood serum or spinal fluid from patient are added various extracts and serums.
Aschheim-Zondek	To determine if pregnancy has occurred.	Specimen of urine from the patient is made slightly acid, filtered, and then injected into number of young, normal mice. (In Friedman modification, rabbits are used.)
Basal Metabolism	To aid in diagnosing thyroid and other glandular disturbances.	Patient breathes into and out of container of oxygen. His heat-production rate is determined by his rate of oxygen consumption. Percentage of variation from normal heat-production rate is called his basal-metabolic rate. Or it may be measured by examining the blood for protein-bound iodine, called the PBI test.
Hemoglobin Determination	To determine amount of hemoglobin in blood.	Patient's fingertip or ear lobe is punctured, and a measured amount of blood is drawn into a pipette. Prior to further laboratory test, blood is placed in tube containing hydrochloric acid.
Red Blood Cell Determination	To determine presence of anemia or polycythemia.	A drop of patient's blood is diluted in a special pipette, and after proper preparation, the red blood cells are counted.
White Blood Cell Determination	To aid in determining presence of infections or leukemia.	Blood from patient is diluted with a special fluid that destroys the red blood cells but does not injure the white cells. After proper preparation, the white cells are counted.
Urine	To determine presence of kidney disease or diabetes.	Urine specimen is examined for presence of albumin, red and white blood cells, and sugar.
Clotting Time	To test clotting ability of blood.	Skin is punctured and time estimated before bleeding stops.
Prothrombin Time	To determine vitamin-K deficiency.	Test to determine adequacy of a substance in blood necessary for clotting.
Blood Pressure	To detect high or low blood pressure.	Measured with mercury column or spring instrument by putting cuff around patient's arm and getting record at contraction (systolic) and relaxation (diastolic) of heart.

TESTS

INTERPRETATION OF TEST	REMARKS
Positive reaction shown by red area at point where toxin was injected. Negative reaction indicates person is immune to diphtheria.	Schick testing of children about every two or three years is advised by many physicians; also testing of adults before inoculation during epidemics.
Positive reaction consists of red area one centimeter or more in diameter, occurring eighteen to twenty-four hours after injection. No reaction indicates immunity to scarlet fever.	Some physicians do not consider the Dick-test results comparable in dependability with those of the Schick test.
Clumping of germs brought about by this serum indicates that patient has typhoid fever.	Test is of no value if person has had typhoid fever previously, or if he has been vaccinated against the disease.
Positive reaction is a red area above the point of injection after forty-eight hours.	Tuberculin test should always be considered in conjunction with other examinations.
Speeded-up sedimentation rate is evidence of the presence of some infection.	Many factors influence sedimentation rate, such as room temperature, concentration of red blood cells, length of sedimentation tube.
Reactions are judged by degree to which destruction of red blood cells is prevented.	Some doctors now deem it advisable to report the complement-fixation reactions only as positive, doubtful, or negative.
If the mice's ovaries are enlarged, test is positive for pregnancy.	Test stated to be reliable after tenth day following first missed menstrual period. Test remains positive until seven days after the birth of a full-term baby. Other new tests involve use of frogs, rabbits, etc.
Ten percent or more above or below normal—between plus or minus seven—indicates an abnormal condition. Above is a sign of hyperthyroidism.	Useful only in conjunction with physical examination and study of patient's symptoms. For accurate results in test, patient must be completely relaxed. Test is made after patient has fasted for twelve hours and has rested thirty minutes just before test.
Decrease in hemoglobin means anemia.	Sahli's method is briefly described here. There are other methods, but none is absolutely accurate.
Decrease of red blood cells below 4,500,000 to 6,000,000 per cubic millimeter indicates anemia.	When normal care is taken in this test, results are invariably reliable.
Above normal usually indicates infection.	Same as above.
Albumin may indicate acute or chronic kidney inflammation or infection of kidney. Red blood cells may be present in acute nephritis and in tumors or stones of the kidney. Large numbers of white blood cells indicate a bladder infection or infection of the kidney pelvis. Sugar usually means diabetes.	Color and odor of urine, presence of sediment, its reaction—that is, whether alkaline or acid—its specific gravity, are all important in diagnosing kidney and related disorders.
Usual time is one to three minutes.	Used in purpura and hemophilia.
Test shows insufficient amount of substance necessary for clotting blood.	Technique used before gall-bladder operations and in liver inflammation.
Normal rate is approximately 120 plus years over twenty to thirty.	Routine in life-insurance examination.

LABORATORY STUDIES

Every fluid, tissue, secretion or excretion of the body is now submitted to examinations for the detection of disease. Our knowledge of disturbances of the blood is quite recent, because the microscope is used to count the red cells and the white cells of different varieties and also the blood platelets. The blood is examined as to its content of sugar, protein, various salts and vitamins, drugs and bacteria. The urine gives early hints of trouble with the kidneys and the beginnings of diabetes. The excretion from the bowel shows the presence of worms and of the parasites that cause dysentery and diarrhea, blood may be due to cancers or even to bleeding piles.

With a stomach pump the doctor obtains material from the stomach and the upper portion of the intestines. He can tell whether or not there is excess of acid or absence of acid in the gastric juice. Recently the test called the Papanicalaou test has been applied to find cancer of the lungs, uterus or elsewhere.

Your doctor will not use every test that has been mentioned every time you see him or even any one time. A wise doctor is guided by his knowledge and experience as to the tests he wants to use, and he lowers the cost of medical service by having only those tests that may be really helpful in the individual case. However, many tests are so simple and inexpensive that they are simply routine.

With a watch the doctor can count the pulse and feel its volume and regularity. Estimation of the blood pressure is a simple office procedure now often carried out by technicians. Determination of the red blood cells and the amount of red coloring matter can be done in the patient's home or elsewhere.

Here are some normal or average values from which the doctor may get a clue of importance:

Red blood cells—4.2 to 5.5 million per cubic millimeter
White blood cells—5 to 10 thousand per cubic millimeter
Blood platelets—200 to 500 thousand per cubic millimeter
Bleeding before blood clots—1 to 5 minutes
Hemoglobin or red coloring matter in blood—13 to 16 grams per 100 milliliter
Blood sugar—70 to 100 milligrams per 100 milliliters
Urine is tested for presence or absence of albumen, sugar or blood or pus; also as to quantity, density, color, etc.
Spinal fluid is examined as to presence of protein and sugar and as to number of cells
Circulation time—23 seconds during 27 beats of the heart

Heart rate—measured by pulse—

        Men .... 65 to 72 beats per minute
        Women .... 70 to 80 beats per minute
        Children .... 72 to 92 beats per minute
        Infants .... 110 to 130 beats per minute

Blood pressure—Systolic above 140 considered abnormal
                Below 100 considered abnormal

Calories needed per day—From 2,400 for a sedentary person to 6,000 or 8,000 for a heavy worker

Duration of pregnancy—About 280 days

Temperature—By mouth ......98.6° Fahrenheit ......37.0° Centigrade
             By rectum ......99.6° Fahrenheit ......37.5° Centigrade

Highly technical are new procedures which depend on the use of radioactive isotopes.

HOW TO CHOOSE A DOCTOR

Now how do you get a doctor to consult? You can call the medical society and ask them for a list of reputable licensed doctors. A qualified man will be a graduate of a qualified medical school and will probably have had an internship. He will probably be on the staff of a hospital. He will be licensed as a doctor by the state in which you live.

An ethical doctor does not send out or publish advertisements about himself and his competence. He usually has an established place of residence and an office in a building or in his home. He will be well and favorably known in the community, including his church, lodge, and service club groups.

A competent doctor will take an interest in you as a person as well as an interest as a patient. A good doctor is not reluctant to request another opinion if it seems to be needed in any case, nor does he object to being dismissed and having another doctor summoned if for any reason the patient has lost confidence.

The decision as to what and how much a doctor should tell the patient or the family about an illness must rest with the doctor. He will make his decision on the basis of his knowledge of the person and of the family. Most doctors are unwilling to lie to patients or their families to serve some doubtful psychological purpose. Yet circumstances may arise when the patient's fears are such as to demand that the doctor dissemble in giving his verdicts.

You, as a patient, owe your doctor your confidence and all the help that you can give him in finding out what is wrong. You owe him compliance in following his instructions, if you want to get the maximum benefit of his knowledge and experience.

CHAPTER II

SYMPTOMS OF DISEASE

PEOPLE CONSULT THE DOCTOR because they have had feelings and sensations that are disturbing and uncomfortable. Perhaps they have had reactions in various portions of the body which are quite different from the usual. For instance, symptoms may include pain, weakness, shortness of breath, cough, or itching. One may notice a sudden increase of weight, or loss of weight. The hands and feet may seem to be cold and numb. Indigestion may occur, with dizziness or vomiting or diarrhea. Because of jaundice the skin may develop a yellow appearance. These are signs and symptoms of disease; they are a warning that an investigation of the cause is needed.

People who are emotionally disturbed are likely to feel pain sooner and more intensely than are people in general. With the reaction to pain may come other changes, brought about through functioning of the sympathetic nervous system. These include rapid beating of the heart, sweating, rise in the blood pressure and disturbances of digestion.

PAIN

Pain is described as burning, sticking or pricking, sharp, dull, throbbing or knifing. Different parts of the body feel pain in different ways. The skin reacts easily. Muscles may not feel puncture by a needle, but ache when they are in spasm or suffer cramp. Compact bone may be cut without pain but porous bone may be painful when injured. The brain tissue may not be sensitive, but the blood vessels have nerve connections and anything that pulls or stretches the blood vessels in the brain will give a pain in the head. Pain from the intestines may be due to injury of the intestinal wall, stretching of the muscles in the wall or pulling on the tissues that hold the intestines in place.

HEADACHE

When you have a headache the doctor will want to know about the location of the pain, its quality, its intensity, the time when it comes on, and the way it is influenced by moving, reading, noise, and other factors. Usually a headache is a dull, aching pain, that arises from the structures within the skull. Sometimes a headache may be associated with a disturbance in the sinuses, or the eyes, or in the bones in the upper part of the spine.

Sensitivity to pain in the head varies in different people and in the same person at different times. The worst headaches are those associated with inflammations or infections of the meninges, which are the tissues that cover the brain. When a sudden, sharp pain affects the head the sensation may be due to a branch of the facial nerve. Usually headaches last longer, for minutes or even hours. When the headache is described as "throbbing" the effect comes from transmission of the pulse in the blood vessels.

A headache may be associated with exposure to cold. Other headaches may develop in healthy people during periods of great fatigue or emotional stress. Such headaches occur toward the end of the day; they begin as a dull ache in the forehead and spread toward the temples or toward the back. These headaches disappear when the person concerned has some good rest or sleep. Fear and worry seem to make headaches worse. Some headaches come from tenseness of the facial muscles, which in turn may be caused by pain or anxiety or strain. Tenseness of the muscles at the back of the neck is a cause of headaches in some people. Such headaches may be relieved by warmth or mild massage.

Psychologic disorders or mental disturbances may also be reflected in pains which are referred to the head. Such people complain of pressure on the head, of a tight-fitting band which squeezes the head, or of a pain that presses on the very top of the head.

PAIN IN THE CHEST

Pain in the chest may come from the ribs and the tissues related to the ribs; from organs in the abdomen; from the heart or from other organs in the chest.

The muscle of the heart has to have oxygen, and when this essential is not provided the muscle responds with pain. Angina pectoris is a pain of this type which is usually continuous and which is provoked by walking, or an emotional strain, or any other factor that increases the work of the heart. The pain tends to be relieved when the burden is removed. Interference with the flow of blood carrying oxygen through the coronary arteries into the heart will bring on an attack of pain. The pain of angina pectoris and that of coronary thrombosis are about the same. Usually that of coronary thrombosis is more severe and lasts longer. Occasionally, however, thrombosis may occur with little or less severe pain.

I should like to caution about jumping to conclusions relative to pain in the heart. Some people complain of pain over the heart, or the heart area, who do not have the slightest sign of any real disturbance of the heart. Doctors call this a cardiac neurosis, and credit it to abnormal anxiety about the heart. Such pains are not related to effort or work of the heart. They are usually accentuated by fatigue and emotional stresses.

Other pains in the chest may come from disturbances of the large blood vessels, from the nerves that reach the linings of the chest cavity, and from growths or abscesses behind the breastbone.

Heartburn probably arises from constriction at the bottom of the esophagus or swallowing tube, because material has been regurgitated from the stomach into this tube.

Rheumatism may attack the tissues associated with the ribs and cause pains in the chest.

ABDOMINAL PAIN

Abdominal pain is usually lumped by most people into the common term "stomach-ache." Just as the organs in the abdomen may transmit pain to the chest, so also may chest organs transmit pain to the abdominal area. As a result of pain in the abdomen, a person will have a look of pain on his face, walk slightly bent over and avoid motion when possible. Many people try to overcome abdominal pains by putting a finger down the throat to provoke vomiting; go repeatedly to the toilet and strain to empty the bowel; take enemas or purges; they will lie with the knees drawn up. Abdominal pains are described as colicky, sharp or knifing, continuous or steady.

The doctor inquires particularly about abdominal pains to find out when the pain began in relation to the taking of food. Then the doctor will try to locate the exact spot or the diffuse area where the pain appears.

One of the most important pains is that which follows the sudden rupture of any of the organs in the abdomen, like the gall bladder, the spleen, the liver, the uterus or the appendix. This is a sudden, sharp, terrifying pain, that seems to disappear soon; nevertheless it is a warning of extreme danger, and the doctor should be called immediately to make certain what is wrong. Pain associated with inflammation is made worse by pressure on the abdomen.

"Ileus" is a name given by doctors to obstruction of the passage of material through the gastrointestinal tract. Such obstruction is a source of great danger to life itself. The blocking may come from many causes. The doctor gets important clues from the location of the pain, its waxing and waning, its frequency or continuity, and the amount of distention associated with the trouble.

PAIN IN THE BACK

Strangely, one of the most difficult of all the diagnoses that a doctor has to make concerns the cause of a pain in the back. Excluding the pain that comes with breaking the bones of the spine or twisting the spine completely out of line, a number of different conditions may be responsible for different kinds of pains in the back.

Infections may attack the tissues of the back as they do other parts of the body. Rheumatoid arthritis may select the many joints of the backbone as a place in which to locate. The little cartilages or discs that act as cushions between the bones may be crushed or slip out of place. The ligaments which attach to the bones of the spine may be pulled to the point where they are painful with every movement.

Careful study by an experienced physician reveals the cause of pain in the back and indicates the type of treatment to be followed. This may vary from changing the shoes and wearing a specially designed brace or corset, to instructions for reducing weight, improving the posture or even a surgical operation. A recent postural instruction sheet designed by Dr. Paul C. Williams says:

When standing or walking, toe straight ahead and take most of your weight on the heels.

Sit with the buttocks tucked under so that the hollow in the low back is eradicated.

When possible elevate the knees higher than the hips while sitting.

Sleep on your back with your knees propped up or on your side with one or both knees drawn up. Bed should be firm.

Never bend backwards.

Avoid standing as much as possible.

Learn to live 24 hours a day without a hollow in the lower part of your back.

Avoid sleeping on the abdomen.

PAINFUL ARMS AND LEGS

Burns, frostbite, and cutting of the arms and legs may be painful. Similarly arthritis, abscesses in the bones and soft tissues, tumors and damage to the nerves may result in severe pain.

From the limbs of the body the nerves pass along until they connect with the roots in the spinal cord. Pressure, irritation or damage to these nerves at any point along their course may result in pain that is felt in the limb itself.

Pain may also be transmitted to the limbs from impulses arising elsewhere in the body. For instance, pain from the hip may be transmitted to the knee. Pain from the deep muscles of the back or from the small bones of the spinal column may be felt in the legs. Pain from angina pectoris or coronary thrombosis of the heart may be felt along the inner sides of the arms.

Various disturbances of the blood supply to the limbs may result in pain. This applies particularly to blocking of the circulation so that the tissues do not receive a proper amount of oxygen. As the blood supply becomes blocked there is a feeling of numbness and finally difficulty of movement. You say "My leg has gone to sleep." Blocking the blood to the arm causes the fingers to get quite numb in about twelve minutes, and then they are painful when touched. As the blood returns a sensation of tingling is felt, which is due to renewed activity of the nerves of the arm. If an arm or leg is moved while the circulation is blocked severe pain may be felt. This may be called a cramp, although actually the muscles are not in spasm but flaccid.

After a limb has been amputated pain may be felt as if it were in the limb. This is called "phantom limb" pain.

In diagnosing the causes of pain in the extremities the character and location of the pain are most significant.

CHAPTER III

UNDERSTANDING SYMPTOMS

WEAKNESS

PEOPLE come to the doctor saying, "I'm weak." Or they may say "I get tired easily." People who are healthy have vim and vigor. Ben Hecht once said: "They have bounce." Elasticity in both mind and body is a sign of health. Those who lack energy and who are listless usually have something wrong. Such symptoms may be quite different from the loss of power in the muscles, which may be due to other causes. Just being unduly fatigued is also different from being faint or slightly dizzy.

Any physical or emotional disorder can be accompanied by lack of energy or listlessness. After an acute infection, following hemorrhage whether sudden or prolonged, or following long-continued subjection to cancer, this lack of energy may be a prominent symptom.

A severe emotional outbreak or upset leaves people weak, exhausted. Such outbreaks can also lead to depression or neurosis accompanied by anxiety.

Lassitude or languor may also be noted frequently as the result of insufficient action of the thyroid gland or from deficiency of secretion in the adrenal glands. However, excessive action of the glands can also lead to overstimulation and ultimate exhaustion.

Lassitude is often observed by the doctor in cases of chronic disease of the liver; in the old days people called this "debility." Shakespeare says in *As You Like It,* "I did not woo the means of weakness and debility."

Various drugs, by their effects or actions on the body can bring about lassitude, among these particularly bromides, alcohol, and the barbituric acid derivatives.

13

ASTHENIA AND FEEBLENESS

People who are old and those who have been confined in bed for a long time get weak. Their muscles seem to lose the power to act. In a disease called *myasthenia gravis* the muscles get weak but seem to recover strength after rest, becoming weak again almost immediately after the least exertion. During their action the muscles use up certain materials. Through actions of the nervous system the use of this material, called cholinesterase, is inhibited. The giving of drugs like neostigmine prevents the destruction of cholinesterase and thus helps these patients.

As in the case of lassitude a number of conditions can also produce asthenia. A long-continued infection, an excessive action of the thyroid with too-rapid beating of the heart, severe anemia, nutritional deficiencies, or habitual taking of drugs or poisons may be responsible. The doctor has to make a thorough study using many laboratory tests to determine the cause with certainty.

Dr. Tinsley Harrison has said that nearly all patients with true asthenia have lassitude but the majority of patients with lassitude do not have asthenia.

When people are troubled by faintness, lightheadedness or dizziness a great variety of conditions must be investigated. Usually this symptom results from disturbance of the supply of blood to the brain. The difficulty may be in the blood vessels of the brain, in the power of action of the heart or in the quality of the blood. The symptom can occur also in epilepsy and in hysterical conditions. Sudden drop in the sugar in the blood also causes this symptom. This symptom makes people anxious, although the conditions causing it are seldom fatal.

COMA OR UNCONSCIOUSNESS

Persistent unconsciousness or coma is quite different from recurrent or repeated attacks of sudden fainting. The coma may be preceded by stupor or may alternate with delirium. Among the common causes of coma are serious deficiencies of oxygen, sugar or vitamins; excessive amounts of sedative or hypnotic or narcotic drugs. Coma occurs from intoxications associated with diabetes, uremia or liver disturbances. Heat stroke or freezing may result in long periods of unconsciousness. Damage to the circulation of the blood and excessive pressure on the brain, such as that which follows fractured skull or concussion, may be the cause of loss of consciousness that persists.

14

When the doctor examines a patient who has been long in coma he must find out first and as soon as possible the cause of the condition. The prompt application of treatment frequently means the difference between life and death, but proper treatment cannot be given unless the cause is known. Frequently unconscious people have been thrown into jail with a charge of drunkenness, when the cause of their stupor was not alcohol but a skull fracture. The same thing has happened to people who have had too much insulin. A person intoxicated by alcohol has the odor of alcohol on the breath; diabetic coma carries with it an odor like that of spoiled fruit and uremia gives an odor to the breath like that of urine. An exceedingly high temperature may mean heat stroke.

The doctor may measure the patient's blood pressure as a clue to the cause of unconsciousness. An exceedingly high blood pressure may mean a stroke, or apoplexy, or uremia. An exceedingly low pressure may mean diabetes, drugs, drunkenness, or a hemorrhage.

CONVULSIONS

Strangely, almost any condition that can cause coma or persistent unconsciousness can also cause convulsions. No single mechanism is known that is responsible for all kinds of convulsions. Changes in the supply of oxygen reaching the brain, in the relationship between acid and alkali—called the acid-base balance; changes in the amount of calcium, sugar or chlorides in the blood; disturbance of the fluid balance or equilibrium between salt and water in the body and associated changes in the pressure on the brain have all been related to convulsions. A great variety of conditions may develop in which these chemical changes in the tissues of the body occur.

By a series of careful examinations the doctor can often classify convulsions in relationship to a definite cause, but there still remain great numbers of cases for which no specific cause can be determined. Where some positive factor is established—for instance, pressure on the brain from a growth, a gunshot wound or a fracture—some positive measures may be taken to control the spasms. Convulsions in young children are often epilepsy. In older people a definite cause may be found as a tumor, or a change in pressure on the brain from some other cause.

When a person has convulsions, help should be given to keep him from injuring himself by falling against hard or sharp objects. A soft gag in the mouth will prevent biting or injuring the mouth and tongue. Doctors can prescribe or give by injection drugs that serve to induce quiet. However, any attack of convulsions should always be an indication or a warning that steps must be taken immediately to determine what is wrong.

PARALYSIS

Startling and frightening to any person is sudden loss of ability to move any portion of the body that one moves voluntarily. The anxiety associated with sudden loss of ability to see, or hear, or taste, or feel heat or pain, strikes terrible dismay. Yet these conditions are frequent enough to warrant the assurance that good medical care can do much to alleviate the difficulties and benefit people who have been stricken with paralysis.

The term "plegia" means a paralysis. If one leg or an arm is paralyzed the condition is called monoplegia. If one side of the body is paralyzed the term is hemiplegia. If both legs are paralyzed, most frequently as a result of spinal cord disease, the condition is paraplegia. Weakness of all four extremities which occurs in a few severe and long standing conditions is a quadriplegia or four-way paralysis. Such diseases as infantile paralysis or meningitis or encephalitis may damage only certain groups of muscles.

From the area involved and the symptoms associated the doctor may be able to tell the portion of the spinal cord or brain that is damaged. Much depends on whether there is just failure of movement, or whether this is accompanied by wasting of the tissues, difficulty in circulation of the blood or other significant factors.

Harm may come to the nervous system from hemorrhages, infections, blows or injuries, tearing or breaking of the nerves. A nerve can be injured in an arm or a leg, which then affects only the muscles reached by that nerve. A knowledge of just where each nerve originates and goes is needed for a diagnosis. Specialists with such knowledge are called neurologists.

SHORTNESS OF BREATH CALLED DYSPNEA

When people get so short of breath that the very effort of breathing is difficult and when breathing is harsh and labored, anyone can tell that something is wrong. Since respiration is necessary to life, difficult breathing creates serious anxiety. Usually people breathe eighteen to twenty times a minute, and regularly. The breathing is effortless and without any special sensation. If breathing becomes irregular or if a severe effort has to be made to get enough breath, pain may appear.

Anyone can get short of breath after severe work or exhaustive exercise. Shortness of breath occurs more often in fat people than in thin ones, in old people than in young ones, and in women than in men. The response of the heart and the breathing to a measured physical effort may be used as an indication of physical fitness.

When shortness of breath is not accompanied by extra effort, the trouble may be more mental than physical. Anyone can imitate shortness of breath. Allergic conditions and asthma which narrow the bronchial tubes bring on "wheezing." Damage to the diaphragm, the lining of the chest cavity or the lungs may bring about trouble in breathing. In pneumonia when a portion of the lung is inflamed and congested, the breathing is labored. Severe anemia, which lessens the supply of blood able to carry oxygen, may result in quickened breathing to get the necessary oxygen to the tissues.

The most important causes of shortness of breath are diseases of the heart and lung, and disorders which in any way prevent air from getting into the lungs. As with every other part of the body, damage to the nervous system can also be reflected in serious difficulties with breathing.

WHEN YOU COUGH

Anything that irritates the surface of your breathing tract between the throat and the secondary branches of the bronchial tubes can make you cough. A cough has three stages: first you draw in air; then you compress the chest; then you expel the air. In order to expel the air with force you draw up your diaphragm while your chest cavity elongates, and then by pressure of the abdominal muscles you drive the diaphragm up toward the chest like a piston.

In many common diseases cough is an outstanding symptom. In acute bronchitis one begins with a dry cough, which becomes moist as secretion develops. In this condition the chest X-ray will not usually reveal any altered condition.

In chronic bronchitis cough and expectoration, usually much worse in the morning, are the chief symptoms.

Chronic bronchiectasis has symptoms like chronic bronchitis, but the volume of sputum is large. Some patients produce as much as a quart a day. The breath and the sputum usually have an offensive odor.

Tuberculosis is associated with cough, and for this condition examina-

17

tion of the chest with X-ray is of utmost importance. The doctor makes a physical examination of the chest and may also send a specimen of sputum to the laboratory to search for germs of tuberculosis.

Heart failure, cancer, abscesses, embolus in the lung due to a clot that has broken loose somewhere in the circulation, and infection with parasites may be causes of cough. Some people develop a cough habit and then keep it up without any physical cause for the cough.

BLEEDING FROM THE LUNGS—HEMOPTYSIS

Blood coming from the lungs is usually bright red and frothy whereas that from the stomach may be dark red, brown or black and mixed with scraps of food. Vomiting is usually preceded by retching and nausea, but a hemorrhage from the lung may come quietly and without warning. Blood in the lung may be associated with severe coughing and occasionally severe coughing may tear tissue so as to produce bleeding.

In the early stages of pneumonia a severe cough may bring up blood, because the lungs are at that time heavily congested. Such blood has a rusty or prune-juice color, but may be bright red.

Among the commonest causes of blood from the lungs, in the absence of tuberculosis, is the passing of a clot elsewhere in the body into the pulmonary artery, the large blood vessel that supplies the lung with blood. The small blood vessels around the area become congested and the irritation causes a cough which may bring up blood.

In chronic bronchiectasis the surface tissue of the bronchial tubes may be torn with severe coughing so that blood appears in the sputum.

The hemorrhage from the lungs in tuberculosis is due to actual erosion or destruction of blood vessels by the disease. Cavities form in the lung in tuberculosis due to destructive action by the germs. The blood vessels in the walls of these cavities may be eroded. One of the dangers is spread of the infection by inhaling and by forcible expulsion of germs in severe coughing.

Among young people with hearts that have been damaged by disease, especially with narrowing of the mitral valve of the heart, the backing up of blood into the lungs causes swelling of the large and small blood vessels with occasional breaking and therefore a hemorrhage from the lungs.

Any time blood comes from the lungs the symptom should be taken as a warning that something serious has occurred.

PALPITATION OF THE HEART

Ordinarily we are not aware of the beating of our hearts. If you do become conscious of the heart's beating, the symptom may have significance but often is unimportant. Many letters come to doctors who write health columns from people who say they have noticed that their hearts were flopping, skipping, pounding, bumping or fluttering.

If you run too hard or engage in too much muscular activity an extra burden is put on your heart, and you may feel it pounding. As soon as you have "caught your breath," the sensation disappears. When the heart beats too rapidly, as it does in excessive action of the thyroid or in other disturbances, you become aware of it. People seem to be conscious of sudden alterations in the heart rate. Different people respond differently to various conditions that affect the body. Those who are placid may pass without noticing a situation that will seriously disturb a person who is sensitive to minor stimulations.

Palpitation may be due to sudden alterations of the heart rate, particularly in cases when the heart beats too rapidly; this condition in turn may be due to excessive action of the thyroid gland. Anemia, hemorrhage, fever, and a lessened amount of sugar in the blood are other conditions in which palpitations occur. In such instances an excess of epinephrine secreted by the adrenal gland may be basically responsible. Many people who complain of palpitation constantly swallow air while eating too rapidly; when the stomach is distended they become conscious of the beating of the heart.

Many people described as nervous and who have nothing physically wrong complain of palpitations. These people have a cardiac neurosis in which their minds are centered on their heart action. The suspicion that one has heart disease may set up or intensify such a neurosis. A doctor can find out the facts, and thus cure both the neurosis and the palpitation which arises from it.

CHAPTER IV

OXYGEN IN THE BODY

THE TISSUES OF THE BODY have to have oxygen to live. When the supply of oxygen is inadequate the condition is called "anoxia." The shortage of oxygen may be apparent in the circulating blood. The red cells of the blood may be inadequate in amount or in the red coloring matter necessary to carry oxygen. Anything that blocks the circulation will also block the oxygen supply. Sometimes the cells of the body are unable, because of changes, to take up the oxygen that reaches them.

Since all parts of the body must have oxygen, a shortage will affect all of them. However, some tissues of the body are much more dependent on oxygen than are others. Most sensitive of all are the tissues of the nervous system. Sudden lack of oxygen to the nervous system results in impairment of judgment, lack of co-ordination of movements, and a condition which, in general, resembles that of a person who is drunk. After the lack of oxygen has persisted the person becomes fatigued, drowsy, inattentive, and unable to respond to ordinary stimuli.

If lack of oxygen to the brain persists, death will result from inability to breathe.

A failure of sufficient oxygen to reach the liver and the muscles where foods are broken down to their ultimate condition for use by the body, results in acidosis and is therefore also incompatible with life. The body tries to meet the threat of anoxia by increasing the breathing rate, by increasing the number of red blood cells, and the amount of red coloring matter. The heart and the kidneys are likewise affected unfavorably if oxygen is not supplied to their cells. The increase in red blood cells and hemoglobin in response to anoxia may begin gradually and continue for weeks. At high altitudes the total increase may reach 40 per cent above the usual.

CYANOSIS AND ARGYRIA

The word "cyanosis" means blueness, but in medicine it is restricted to the kind of blueness that follows a reduction in the amount of hemoglobin or red coloring matter in the blood. A condition called "argyria" which is due to deposit of silver in the skin gives a silvery-blue appearance. Blueness due to lack of oxygen in the blood is best seen in the lips, the white of the eye, the fingernail beds, the ears and the area over the cheekbones.

Certain poisonous substances including drugs may lead to cyanosis, by changing the nature of the hemoglobin or red coloring matter of the blood. Among these drugs are the nitrates which are sometimes used to dilate blood vessels and lower blood pressure. Also hydrogen sulfide and acetanilide may have this effect. When people are poisoned by carbon monoxide gas, the blood develops a cherry-red color rather than blue. Occasionally people who take sulfonamide drugs get bluish blood due to a chemical change.

When there is any interference with the flow of blood through the skin the color may seem blue or a pale bluish-gray. Such difficulty may come from a weak heart, an obstruction of the flow of blood or simple exposure of the skin to severe cold. Some people suffer constantly with cold and bluish hands and feet because of poor circulation in the extremities.

Obviously the determination as to just which mechanism is responsible for the blue appearance of the body is highly important in relationship to what will be done about it. The doctor must determine whether the difficulty is due to the heart, or the lungs or some trouble in the blood itself. By special signs such as clubbing of the fingers, the duration of the condition in relationship to employment, examinations of the heart and lungs, and chemical and physical studies of the blood, he can make the distinction.

TOO MANY RED CELLS—POLYCYTHEMIA

Doctors put together names of diseases frequently out of portions of words. "Poly" means multiple or too many; "cyth" refers to cells; "emia" means the blood. An alarming increase in the number of red blood cells might also be called an erythrocytosis, which merely means a condition of the red blood cells. An excess number of the cells may develop as a result of an insufficient oxygen supply, such as occurs at high altitudes, or as a result of an excess manufacture, producing a dis-

21

ease the cause of which is not known. This true polycythemia is also called Osler's disease and Vaquez's disease after physicians who first noticed it.

Polycythemia comes on gradually and persists for ten or twenty years. The person with this condition has constantly a deep red flush which may have a bluish appearance. Usually the spleen and the liver are enlarged. The blood clots easily. Hemorrhages in various parts of the body are not uncommon. Whereas the blood count ordinarily is around five to six million, the count rises in this condition to nine to twelve million cells in each cubic millimeter of blood.

Among unusual causes of secondary polycythemia, in addition to residence at high altitude, are disturbances such as silicosis, which interfere with receipt of oxygen by the lungs; abnormalities of circulation of the blood through the lungs; cases which occur in infants that have been unable to get a good oxygen supply before birth; and even certain tumors of the brain and failure of the adrenal glands. Among methods of treatment now used to control excess production of the cells are X-ray of the bone marrow, giving of radioactive phosphorus and use of the nitrogen mustards.

CHAPTER V

BLOOD PRESSURE

YOUR BLOOD PRESSURE is a measure of the activity of your heart in pumping, and of the resistance created by the size and the hardness of the walls of the blood vessels. When the doctor measures your blood pressure he puts an inflatable cuff around your arm, then stops the blood flow by pumping air into the cuff; then he listens with a stethoscope to get the pressure at the time when the heart was contracted—systolic pressure—and when it has dilated or relaxed—diastolic pressure. The pressure is taken by a column of mercury measured in millimeters or by a spring device calibrated to the mercury column.

Normal or average blood pressure may range from 95 to 160 systolic and 65 to 90 diastolic. There may be a range in the systolic pressure from 85 to 300 and in the diastolic pressure from 40 to 160. The pressure may vary with sleeping or waking, sitting or standing, with exercise, lack of oxygen or anemia; with chilling, anger, anxiety, frustration or the height of pleasure.

LOW BLOOD PRESSURE—HYPOTENSION

People with blood pressure somewhat below the average used to be said to suffer from low blood pressure. The condition was called hypotension. Now records are available of great numbers of people with somewhat lower blood pressures who nevertheless feel quite well, and who seem to be likely to live long. Hypotension is recognized as a condition in which the systolic pressure is under 80 mm. of mercury or 20 mm. below the usual average of the person concerned. The blood pressure may be quite low after prolonged rest in bed or with malnutrition. The blood pressure may also be lowered by conditions affecting the spinal cord or by the operation which cuts off the sympathetic nervous system.

A feeling of faintness or weakness may be the only indication that the blood pressure is lower than it should be.

HIGH BLOOD PRESSURE—HYPERTENSION

High blood pressure, or hypertension, is diagnosed by the doctor when, after repeated examination, the pressure is found to be above the average for healthy young people in the area in which the person lives. In the United States, levels are around 120 to 140 systolic and 80 to 90 diastolic. The pressure may reach 180 systolic and 100 diastolic without the appearance of any symptoms.

If the person suffers with acute hypertension, such symptoms as convulsions, loss of vision, severe headaches and kidney inflammations may be indications. In chronic high blood pressure dizziness, headaches, hemorrhages in the eye or the brain, heart failure and uremia may be present. Still, cases are known in which people with definitely high blood pressures on measurement have failed to manifest any of these symptoms.

Associated with high blood pressure the doctor may find disturbances of the function of the kidneys; disturbances of function of the adrenal glands; or in some instances, apparently no immediate cause except some psychologic problem. When a cause cannot be found the case is called "essential hypertension." Often the first indication of the condition may be changes in the blood vessels at the back of the eye, which the doctor sees with an ophthalmoscope. Definite relationships have been established between the blood-flow through the kidneys and the pressure of high blood pressure. A high salt or sodium chloride intake may set up high blood pressure. The kidney condition is believed to indicate some substances are elaborated by the kidney which may establish high blood pressure. The pressure with high salt intake is associated with the functioning of the adrenal glands.

In an examination of the patient with high blood pressure study of the urine, which indicates the condition of the kidneys, is important. A low specific gravity—under 1020—and the presence of albumin or pus may show that the kidney condition is responsible. If the kidney function, as determined by a variety of tests, is normal, the doctor then sees if the adrenal activity is proper. A number of laboratory and functional tests are available which the doctor can use.

24

Wise physicians recommend that patients be reassured and do not disturb themselves about the pressure, in the absence of severe symptoms and in failure to find anything wrong about the blood vessels of the retina of the eye, the heart size and action and the kidney function. If the patient has vague symptoms and sound organs, suggests Dr. William Dock, search should be made for sources of anxiety and frustration. The facts ascertained by the doctor in his study determine the nature of the treatment that may be prescribed.

The suggestion has been made that the first steps are: reassurance of the patient, sedation with the appropriate drugs and restricted use of salt. Rigid elimination of salt from the diet is recommended when there is headache, dizziness, and heart failure. Several drugs are known which will lower blood pressure but all are difficult to use and must be prescribed by the doctor for the individual patient. The operation called "sympathectomy" is tried when the condition cannot be controlled, but always with a recognition that it may have aftereffects with annoying symptoms and disability.

Weight reduction, adequate rest, suitable mental hygiene, are among the best measures that can be recommended in a majority of cases of high blood pressure.

ESSENTIAL HYPERTENSION

The most common form of consistently elevated blood pressure. The cause is unknown.

CHAPTER VI

YOUR HEART AND CIRCULATION

TROUBLE WITH THE HUMAN BODY may be approached from the point of view of its structure or its function. The heart may be enlarged, or its valves may leak or be narrowed, or its blood supply may be inadequate because of blocking. The changes in structure produce changes in function which are reflected in symptoms. From the functional point of view the heart may beat too fast or too slowly, or irregularly. Its beat may be weak or strong. The heart may be overactive or underactive.

When the heart is overactive people complain of palpitation. The heart sounds are loud and the pulse is full and bounding. Signs of an overactive heart may be seen when one has had severe exercise or emotional stress. With excessive action of the thyroid gland the heart beats more rapidly, as it does also with severe anemia. Whenever there is fever or lack of oxygen the heart becomes overly active.

When the circulation of blood through the blood vessels is insufficient because of failure of the heart, which means underactivity, the symptoms include apathy and lassitude, sometimes faintness, and collapse. If a sudden hemorrhage occurs the circulation fails. With failure of the heart the blood pressure falls and the skin becomes cold, clammy, dry, and inelastic.

In heart failure congestion of the lungs follows, with shortness of breath and the difficulty with breathing that occurs because of fluid. The doctor can hear with his stethoscope sounds in the lung that show the congestion. The patient coughs to get rid of the congestion.

THE OVERACTIVE HEART

After severe muscular exercise the amount of blood returned by the veins to the heart increases. Something similar occurs when there is anemia, lack of oxygen, overactivity of the thyroid gland or fever. Increase in materials carried in the blood occurs also in the toxemia of pregnancy, in dropsy, or with disturbances in the way in which the body uses salt and water.

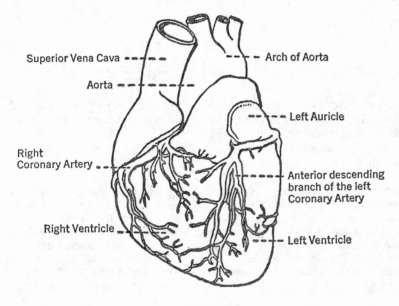

Superior Vena Cava — Arch of Aorta
Aorta
Left Auricle
Right Coronary Artery
Anterior descending branch of the left Coronary Artery
Right Ventricle
Left Ventricle

THE HEART

As the inflow increases, the pressure in the blood vessels into which blood is pumped lessens. The heart beats more rapidly and strongly. As long as the heart can handle the change in its load of work, the patient may not be too much disturbed. When the load gets too big and the reserve power of the heart is damaged, emptying of the heart will fail to keep up with the inflow of blood. This may cause beginning failure of the heart.

If the flow of blood into the heart is inadequate, the tissues of the body will not get the blood and oxygen that they need. If this occurs suddenly, as it may do from a variety of causes, the brain does not get the blood and oxygen that it needs and the person faints or collapses. If

27

the onset is gradual the blood vessels may accommodate themselves by contracting in less vital areas.

A sudden, severe lessening of inflow may occur after a large hemorrhage, by loss of fluid into the tissues as occurs in shock and burns, or as a result of insufficient water intake, or large loss of water as takes place in diarrhea. Pouring of much blood into the legs with large, dilated veins will lessen heart inflow, as will also some disturbances of the nervous system. Some drugs that greatly dilate veins or permit pouring of fluid into the tissues have a similar effect.

HEART FAILURE

More people die from heart failure than from any other cause, and probably conditions affecting the heart will continue from now on to be the leading cause of death.

The chief manifestations of heart failure are seen in the difficulties of breathing. Dr. Harold Hyman describes this graphically:

"The person notes that his 'wind is failing' and he becomes breathless as the result of any unusual effort. Once the breath is lost, it takes an unaccustomed span of time for recovery. The sufferer is compelled to sit down and 'rest a bit' and, when activity is resumed, it is not with accustomed vigor and elasticity; an extra pillow is required at night and then another until the most comfortable position for sleep is semi-recumbent. Members of the family and co-workers note that the now potentially cardiac invalid pants a bit even at rest, and that the chest heaves more than has been its custom."

Failure of the heart is usually associated with high blood pressure, and with extreme narrowing of the valves that carry the blood from the heart into the large blood vessel called the aorta into which the heart empties.

The heart always makes an effort to handle its increasing burden. It does this by enlarging the muscle fibers and dilating to increase the size of its cavities. When the load gets too heavy the rhythm of the heart becomes irregular. There may be pain like that of angina pectoris. The cough that occurs is due to the congestion in the lungs. With heart failure digestive symptoms may be prominent, including nausea, vomiting and loss of appetite, and sensations of fullness in the middle of the abdomen. A heart that has been damaged by disease such as rheumatic fever or other infections is more likely to fail than a healthy heart.

28

CARE OF THE FAILING HEART

The doctor's treatment of a failing heart is designed to take work off the heart, help to get rid of excess fluid, and improve the heart's action. The person with congestive failure of the heart is like a man who is going bankrupt because his income and assets have been sharply reduced. He has to cut down immediately on expenditures, and maintain a rigid conservation of what he has. Several new drugs—Diamox, Diuril—and similar remedies help to eliminate excess fluid.

In this condition the patient must depend on the doctor to outline his conduct for him. If the man must earn his living, he should get home after work as soon as possible and spend every moment he can actually resting; this applies equally to the use of the weekend. The person with a weak heart must avoid climbing stairs; must never lift heavy objects or carry packages. Every source of tension, including family disagreements and arguments, must be eliminated. In this condition, above every other, *moderation* is the key word. Excess of tea, coffee, tobacco, and alcohol is a serious misdemeanor for the patient with congestive heart failure.

While rest must be the objective, enough movement must be employed to keep muscles alive. The simplest kind of household activity or, for some, a few holes of golf on a flat course may be desirable.

With this routine the weight must be kept down by a low-calorie, principally protein, diet. Infections must be prevented and promptly cared for if they occur. For those who can afford it, visits to resorts or spas, quiet ocean voyages, and residence in warm dry climates are recommended.

BYPASS SURGERY

For hearts damaged by coronary disease, an operation has been devised in which a portion of the saphenous vein taken from the leg is transplanted. One end attaches to the aorta and the other to the coronary circulation of the heart. X-ray pictures show that the new circulation thus established has been effective in cases for several years.

CORONARY THROMBOSIS

Blocking of the coronary arteries, which supply blood to the heart itself, may damage the muscle of the heart. Immediate treatment includes rest, oxygen, and prescription by the doctor, if he thinks desirable, of drugs to prevent further clotting. Most patients who survive the initial shock recover and may live quite normally thereafter. If the causes such as high blood pressure, hardening of the arteries, bad habits of work and leisure persist, the mechanism for further obstructions may result in subsequent heart attacks.

CHAPTER VII

DIGESTIVE DISTURBANCES

INDIGESTION

FOR MANY YEARS indigestion has been considered the number one disturbance of American businessmen. Irvin Cobb told the story of the dyspeptic who hears the noon whistle: "Twelve o'clock," he says. "I'm going home. If lunch isn't ready, I'm going to raise Cain. If it is ready, I won't eat a bite." Heartburn, the belching of sour material, nausea, vomiting, a feeling of fullness or pressure, are the symptoms that trouble most.

While the symptoms listed may be relatively insignificant as far as any serious disease is concerned, the difficulty for both doctor and patient lies in the fact that the same symptoms in varying degree may be associated with exceedingly serious disorders. The severity of pain varies from one person to another, and the agony of the pain is not really a measure of the condition that is wrong. Most people digest their food and move the residue along toward elimination without much attention to what is going on. If the symptoms that have been mentioned come on one or two hours after eating, they may be due to uncomplicated ulcer of the stomach or duodenum, and the doctor will have to make extra studies, including use of the X-ray to be sure of the diagnosis. Similar symptoms may occur in conditions related to the appendix or the gall bladder, or to blocking of the passage of the food, or to a weakness in the diaphragm, the large muscle of breathing which separates the abdomen from the chest.

Indigestion may, moreover, be associated with psychologic problems, excessive use or abuse of tobacco, coffee, or alcohol, rapid eating with insufficient chewing, constipation with the cathartic habit, and many other errors of digestive hygiene.

When there is sensitivity or allergy to certain food substances, eating of such foods may arouse gastrointestinal distress.

NAUSEA AND VOMITING

Usually nausea, or a feeling of sickness, precedes vomiting. Vast amounts of research have been devoted to study of the mechanism of vomiting. We know now that it is intimately connected with the whole nervous system. Any severe pain can bring on these symptoms, such as a sharp blow in the center of the abdomen, or bruising of the male sex glands. Disagreeable sights, odors or tastes, or, in sensitive people, even thinking of disagreeable incidents may set up the reaction. The old novels about delicate young ladies tell of the girl who comes home after a disagreeable social evening and gets quite sick thinking about it. Vomiting can result from the action of drugs. Painful sensations coming from the urinary tract, as by the passing of a stone, can set up this series of reactions.

Sometimes vomiting occurs without any preliminary warning of nausea, particularly when there is increased pressure inside the skull. Vomiting occurs in diabetic acidosis, in congestive heart failure, in cases of insufficient oxygen to the brain, in airsickness and seasickness or other conditions that disturb the sense of balance or equilibrium.

The doctor has to find out promptly why anyone vomits. He has to rule out the beginning of acute infectious diseases, and then make sure there is no acute surgical emergency like an inflamed appendix or gall bladder or peritonitis or obstruction of the bowel.

Severe indigestion, high blood pressure, pregnancy in women, disorders of the nervous system, drugs and poisons are other possible sources of difficulty in holding down food and water. Severe emotional upsets must be investigated. Finally come such rare and extraordinary problems as cancer, uremia, diabetes, and many more.

CONSTIPATION

When the bowels do not move with their accustomed frequency or when waste material is passed in small, hard masses, sometimes with pain, the symptom is called constipation. Accompanying the condition one may have a sense of fullness or tightness in the abdomen, and sometimes pain. Other associated symptoms include headache, weakness, indigestion, belching, aching muscles, and even painful urination.

Constipation is not a disease—it is a symptom indicating that the fundamental difficulty lies in improper diet, wrong eating habits, a variety of diseases or abnormalities of structure, and, quite frequently, emotional difficulties or disorders of personality.

Most people have one or two actions of the bowel daily, usually after breakfast or after the largest meal of the day. Irregularity of eating or sleeping brings on irregularity of bowel action. Travel, stress, complete changes in nature of food, also disturb regularity of bowel action.

In old people blocking of the lower bowel may occur, due to inefficiency of the bowel musculature and lessened sensitivity of the nervous system. Exceedingly old people, who spend much of their time in bed, note particularly the tendency to less frequent action of the bowel. Most people under sixty years of age may be trained to proper rhythm by teaching good habits aided by a carefully selected diet.

The simplest materials for use in ordinary cases are the lubricants such as paraffin oil or mineral oil, which must not be used routinely because it picks up vitamin A; also useful are bulk materials, such as agar or cellulose, which are available in special preparations.

Spasticity of the colon and sensitivity to various foods such as chocolate, onions, garlic, cabbage, or other common sensitizers must be investigated.

The frequently used laxatives contain phenolphthalein, or senna, or magnesia; stronger are salts and castor oil.

DIARRHEA

When the actions of the bowel are too frequent, the amount of material large, loose, frequently foamy and full of mucus, the condition is diarrhea. Abdominal discomfort and pain at the end of the bowel are often associated with severe diarrhea. Constipation is the predominant digestive order of the city dwellers in the temperate zone, and diarrhea is common among primitive peoples in tropical areas and in men living under military conditions.

TRAVELERS' DIARRHEA

So common is the diarrhea that develops among people who travel to tropical and semitropical areas and who eat strange foods that many

33

slang terms have been developed for this reaction. Among the most amusing are "Montezuma's Revenge" and the "Turkey Trot." Acute diarrhea may be the result of an infection with either a germ or a virus. Severe diarrhea within 24 hours after eating may be due to a toxin in the food. The one due to Salmonella comes on from 48 to 72 hours after eating. The physician diagnoses the cause not only from the record, but also from the examination of the material that is passed. In the prevention of such diarrhea the traveler should be advised to eat only what can be peeled or has been cooked; drink only boiled or bottled water, or bottled carbonated drinks, beer, or wine. Remember that the ice in many instances comes from contaminated water, and therefore one should avoid water from the tap for brushing teeth and putting ice in drinks.

In most instances the condition clears up in two or three days. For the immediate care drink lots of fluids, take any pain-killing drug that is available. If there is fever, or if the material from the bowel is heavy with mucus or blood, call a doctor. One of the drugs most generally used in such conditions is a product called Entero-Vioform.

BLEEDING FROM THE STOMACH AND BOWEL

Bleeding is frightening. Bleeding from the nose is fairly frequent, as is bleeding from a tooth socket or a cut. But a sudden hemorrhage from the lungs or the vomiting of fresh blood or the passing of blood in the urine or in the bowel movements is a cause of anxiety. Because the appearance of blood from the interior of the body is shocking, the statements of people as to the amount of blood lost are seldom dependable. A teaspoonful may seem like a pint. Blood in the stomach or intestines when it appears in the stools has a black or tarry appearance, but it takes at least an eighth of a pint to make the coloration visible.

The severity of the shock that may come from internal bleeding depends on the amount lost and the suddenness with which it occurs. Fever may occur after a hemorrhage, particularly a large one.

The most common cause of vomiting of blood—in 40 to 80 per cent of cases—is ulcer of the stomach, or duodenum. Usually the person concerned will have had a previous diagnosis of ulcer. The bleeding usually comes from erosion of a blood vessel in the ulcer. In about 5 per cent of the cases the cause of vomiting of blood is cancer; that is the reason for having a complete and scientific diagnosis as promptly as possible when this symptom occurs. Hardening of the liver and enlargement of the spleen may back up the circulation so that there are varicose veins in the esophagus or swallowing tube; like other varicose veins these may break and cause the person afflicted to vomit blood. Among miscellaneous and less frequent causes are diseases of the blood like hemophilia and thrombocytopenia in which bleeding is easy.

The first step after vomiting of blood or large hemorrhage from the bowl is to control shock and save life; then comes a careful scientific study to determine the cause and prevent additional bleeding.

JAUNDICE

In jaundice the skin and the whites of the eyes and, in fact, even the mucous membranes have a slightly yellowish tinge due to discoloration from bile. The amount of jaundice may vary from a deep yellow color to such slight staining that only blood tests will reveal the abnormality. Jaundice develops when the bile passages are blocked. Since the bile comes from destruction of red blood cells, jaundice also appears when there is excessive breakdown of those cells, or when the function of the liver which takes part in the process is impaired by disease or other damage.

Naturally, wear and tear of the blood vessels goes on all the time. About $\frac{1}{120}$ of them are destroyed every day. This means that the life of a red blood cell is about 120 days. When an ordinary bruise turns black and blue the change in color is due to breakdown of the red cells to bile salts. The liver usually disposes of this material.

As I have already said, jaundice is a sign that the liver is not functioning as it should. Scientists recognize at least six different activities for which the liver is responsible:

The liver ges rid of bile pigments from destroyed blood cells.
The liver helps to get rid of toxic and waste materials.
The liver participates in using protein material for growth and repair of body tissue.
The liver is important in the digestion and utilization of sugars or carbohydrates by the body.
The liver has a vital role in the metabolism of fats and the part played by cholesterol in the chemistry of the body.
The liver is concerned in the mechanism of blood clotting and the development of prothrombin in the blood which needs vitamin K for proper functioning.

The liver has been called the warehouse, the chemical factory, the unit for controlling waste, and other titles. It is a vital organ and we are fortunate that we were created with seven times more than we usually need.

HEPATITIS

Inflammation of the liver may follow infection by a virus called the virus of hepatitis. The condition used to be called "catarrhal jaundice." This infection is becoming more frequent. A specific treatment is not yet available. People with hepatitis should be at rest while there are acute symptoms. They should take enough calories and protein to overcome too great loss of weight. In severe cases doctors use some antibiotics and Cortisone derivatives. By far the majority of patients recover but sometimes convalescence is slow, lasting even a year.

In the prevention of hepatitis, gamma globulin taken from the blood is injected. The gamma globulin contains the anti-substances which are frequently effective in preventing hepatitis. The incubation period in this disease varies between 15 to 60 days. Therefore, early use of gamma globulin in the presence of an epidemic may prevent infection. There is no specific treatment for viral hepatitis. Rigid isolation of patients with this condition is not usually practiced.

Practice has shown that 0.01 mil. of gamma globulin per pound of body weight given intramuscularly in the incubation period will prevent symptoms and jaundice in people who have been exposed by contact with patients who have infectious hepatitis. Pregnant women and elderly people in whom the disease may be more severe are also given gamma globulin prophylaxis.

CHAPTER VIII

THE KIDNEYS

MOST PEOPLE THINK OF THE KIDNEYS as organs concerned only with getting rid of waste material, but they have the double function of keeping back what should not go out in water. The composition of the body is stable, and the kidney helps to keep it so. In each kidney there are about 1,300,000 nephron units into which the blood comes. Here water and the dissolved material to be excreted are picked out and the blood returned to the stream.

One of the most significant tasks of the kidney is to retain sodium or salt while sending out acid material. The kidneys have a vital task; when they are damaged or find it impossible to handle their duties the whole human being suffers, sometimes to the point of death.

Due to the intimate knowledge of the working of the kidney assembled by physiologists, doctors now make a much more accurate diagnosis of what is wrong with the kidney than was possible formerly. There are many highly technical tests which are used on special occasions, but in the majority of instances the doctor can diagnose kidney troubles from the history of the patient and the examination of the urine. First he makes sure there is no albumin or protein in the urine which cannot be accounted for by known conditions. He looks for blood cells which may be related to disease of the kidneys or other portions of the renal tract. If there are elements in the urine called "casts," he relates these to the progress of the disease. There are functional tests which measure the capacity of the kidneys to do their work.

Urination should be free from pain; the urine should come easily and regularly. Failure to hold the urine is abnormal, as is also the necessity to get up to urinate at night.

URINATION

Ancient doctors used to attach even greater significance to examination of the urine than do moderns, but actually they knew very little about it. They based their judgments largely on color, odor, and quantity, which were easily determined.

Painful urination is usually associated with infection, irritation, or inflammation in the lower part of the urinary tract and to the passages of stones. Any obstruction to the flow of urine may be painful. Such conditions may also cause frequent urination, but that may be due as well to excitement or anxiety. Hesitancy in urination may also be due to psychological causes. Failure to control the flow of the urine, which is called incontinence, may come in times of great fright or during unconsciousness, but children may fail to control the urine for a variety of both physical and mental causes.

Increase in the amount of urine associated with frequent urination may be due to increased intake of fluids, or to failure of sweating. A sudden change from warm to cold weather causes a rise in the volume because of lessened perspiration.

Certain diseases that affect the urinary mechanism, including conditions affecting the pituitary gland and diabetes, cause an increase in amount of urine. People with dropsy or collection of fluid in the body may respond to rest, or treatment with certain drugs that rid the body of large amounts of fluid through the urine. Similarly a diminished output may result from failure of the heart to put enough blood through the kidney and from collection of fluid in the tissues and cavities of the body.

Usually the quantity of urine is diminished during sleep. Anything that disturbs sleep may result in urination at night. Irritations along the tract may also cause awakening and urination at night.

FLUID RETAINED IN THE BODY

Ordinarily the body contains a certain amount of water which is distributed in the cells of the different structures that make up the body. Extra water is a problem. It may collect in or around the cells in small amounts, or it may collect in large amounts in the different body cavities. The word "edema" is used to describe extra fluid in the tissues beneath the skin; its presence is determined simply by pressing with the finger, in which case the indentation or pit remains. Fluid in the abdomen is called "ascites" and fluid in the chest is known as "hydrothorax." When there is excess fluid everywhere in the body the term "anasarca" is used. One sign of excess fluid accumulation may be rapid gain in weight.

A variety of conditions may be responsible for these disturbances of handling of water by the body. The trouble may be with the blood, or the blood vessels, or the blood pressure. The difficulty may be in the composition of the tissues themselves. There may be blocking of the flow of lymph. Finally, the kidneys play an important part in the elimination of fluid.

Actually the taking of an excess of water as fluids or in food is not the chief or important factor in water accumulation. Ordinarily the excess of fluid is simply eliminated by the kidneys, which can get rid of twenty times as much fluid as they usually eliminate. An excess of sodium or salt is more likely to cause accumulation of water in the body since the ability of the kidneys and sweat to get rid of excess salt is much less than for water. Since the adrenal glands are important in controlling the salt-water balance, disturbances of the action of these glands may be responsible for excess fluid in the tissues.

Swelling of one leg or arm is likely due to an obstruction of circulation affecting that organ. When both swell the difficulty is probably a general one. Swelling of eyelids and face in the morning is associated with insufficient protein intake.

KIDNEY STONES

The technical term for this condition is nephrolithiasis, which simply means kidney stones. People who have kidney stones (which may vary in size from tiny particles to large, irregularly shaped masses) occasionally suffer severe pain when such stones pass down from the kidney to the bladder and out through the urethra. The pain of the kidney stone is usually a cramp that begins in the side or back and radiates down to the genitalia and the inner thigh. The attack may last for several hours or disappear in a few minutes, depending on how rapidly the stone passes. Some blood may appear afterward in the urine. The condition is sometimes confused with appendicitis, inflammation of the gall bladder, or other diseases. The formation of kidney stones is believed to be related to excessive drinking of milk and excessive action of the parathyroid glands, causing calcium in the urine to be increased. The physician must decide after study, involving especially the use of the X-ray, whether or not the condition is to be treated with medical methods or by surgery. People who have this condition should increase the amount of water that they drink. Urinary calcium is decreased by taking phosphates which the physician prescribes.

CHAPTER IX

INHERITANCE OF DISEASE

CUSTOMARILY WE SAY THAT DISEASE is not inherited by people, but that the body constitution which makes people susceptible is inherited. Structural disturbances may be inherited. Red-green color blindness affects males, who transmit the condition only to their daughters—who do not have it—but transmit it to their sons in about half the births. The response of our bodies to any infection or other trauma or stress depends to a large extent on the nature of our constitution.

Many disease conditions seem to occur more often in some families than in others. Hardening of the arteries, diabetes, rheumatic diseases, and some forms of cancer are conspicuous examples. Tuberculosis, goiter, ulcers of the stomach, and even appendicitis seem to be related to body structure in ways that make a hereditary factor a possibility.

In addition to red-green color blindness, hemophilia—the tendency to bleed—is passed from males through females. Baldness is another condition which is related to the genes that determine characteristics. Strangely the experts in genetics are now convinced that a large amount of head hair is not correlated with virility. Instead, once the baldness gene is present, the excess of male hormone associated with virility is the likely additional factor for baldness. Degrees of baldness and the pattern of distribution are also regulated by hereditary factors.

Absence of certain teeth, deformities in the growth of the jaws, sweat gland deficiencies, albinism—or lack of pigment in the eyes, skin and hair—and extra breasts or nipples as well as extra fingers and toes may also be inherited. Difficulties of vision, and of hearing, taste, and smell occur in families. Finally, heredity also plays a part in determining intelligence or the lack of it.

DEFECTS AT BIRTH

A number of serious defects at birth have been related to inheritance. Such conditions as Mongolism, Tay-Sachs disease, sickle-cell anemia, and phenylketonuria called "PKU," and also structural disorders like hare-lip, cleft palate, congenital dislocation of the hip and even baldness are included. New knowledge is being developed about lack of enzymes, blood diseases, and many other conditions. Defects may be due to infections of the mother during pregnancy as with German measles, or toxic effects of drugs as happened with thalidomide which resulted in babies born with deformed arms and legs.

SICKLE-CELL ANEMIA

In this condition the red blood cells appear sickle-shaped instead of round. The condition is related to abnormal genes. If both parents have the condition, the child is most certain to show it. In the United States, the disorder is almost entirely one affecting the Blacks. These people develop an anemia associated with the sickle cell. Those afflicted are often poorly developed. Their hands and feet are disproportionately long and thin. The eyes appear to be jaundiced. When sickle-cell anemia develops, it may be mistaken for other conditions like rheumatic fever or various neurologic disorders. The person with sickle-cell anemia may also develop iron-deficiency anemia. There are several varieties of the condition, varying from person to person. Thus far no method has been found for controlling the condition although recent experiments have involved treatment with derivatives of urea and cyanates. In the most severe cases, blood transfusions may be used.

MONGOLISM

About 250,000 Americans have Mongolism or Down's syndrome, a form of mental retardation. In this condition, investigators found on examination of the cells of the body an extra chromosome. Most people have 46 chromosomes; those with Mongolism have an extra one in the twenty-first set. The condition is sometimes called trisomy 21.

The frequency of Mongoloid births increases with the age of the mother at the time of conception. The child with this condition may have somewhat slanting eyes, a broad nose, a large tongue and a protruding lower lip. However, the chief symptom is mental retardation. Children with this condition do not talk until about six years of age and often do not advance beyond six years of age in mentality.

41

CHAPTER X

AGING AND BREAKDOWN
OF THE BODY

MANY OF THE COMMON SAYINGS and beliefs about growing old have had to be revised in the light of new information that has been developed by medical science in the last twenty years. We used to say that a man is as old as his arteries. Now we realize that changes in the arteries may go on without aging of all the rest of the body. A man is as old as his skin, his adrenal glands and his nervous system, even more than his arteries. Aging shows up most definitely in the skin and in the brain.

Changes go on in the tissues of the human body at varying rates. Some require a long time and others occur rapidly. Hardening of the arteries is a slow process and is therefore seen most frequently in the aged. Actually, the human being has a life cycle of about seventy years and, barring accident or other stresses, will probably live that long. During his seventy years the human being is subjected to a good deal of wear and tear. This may include excesses of food, drink, or narcotic substances. The wear and tear may include infections, bad weather, accidents while at work, overwork, boredom, or emotional upsets. Even without excessive wear and tear, however, the tissues gradually lose their ability for growth and repair, and we grow old. Pathologists talk about the atrophy of disuse. At certain ages both women and men lose their ability to reproduce, which is a function of youth and middle age.

Actually the blood vessels carry on longer than most other tissues of the body. Operations are done on very old people and they recover, with blood supply flowing into the area that has been shut off by the operative procedure. Dr. William Dock mentions some signs of aging and the way we meet them. Gray hair can be dyed, the long hairs in the nose and ears clipped, and baldness covered by a wig.

Aging and Breakdown of the Body

For the aging process doctors use the word "involution." The loss of ability to read small type as one grows older is associated with changes in the tissues of the eye. As our tissues age they tend to recover less rapidly from disease or injury. The aging heart beats with a little more trouble than does the young heart. Modern medicine has learned to substitute for some of the disappearances of tissues and their secretions. We give liver extract for forms of anemia, insulin for diabetes, eye glasses for visual disturbances, and canes or crutches for weakening muscles.

Disappearance of neurons or nerve cells in the nervous system come on with age. This helps to make old people less agile than the young and less capable to carry on hard work for a long time. The tremors of old age are accredited to similar loss of neurons.

Old people do not observe as acutely as do the young. They do not remember recent events. Eventually the loss of tissue from the aging brain may reveal itself in apathy, irritability, or stolidity. Many old people talk and talk and talk. This garrulousness may be accompanied by too great a concern over little, unimportant things and less concern about essential problems.

Doctors have learned that the accounts old people give of their symptoms, the trials and tribulations, neglects and concerns of their families, are not quite as dependable as were accounts by these same people given when they were younger.

Actually, old age needs lots of sympathetic consideration from the young. Read the ages at death of the people in your community. You will discover great numbers over sixty-five, with only here and there one from fifteen to fifty. The span of life has changed and we must learn to accommodate ourselves to it.

CHAPTER XI

EMOTIONAL DEVELOPMENT AND MENTAL STRESS

DURING THE LAST FIFTY YEARS much attention has been given by physicians to the manner in which emotional development affects the general health of people. Almost from the moment of birth a child begins having emotional experiences. Among the first of the child's relationships is that with his mother. From her he gets his food; therefore his early emotions are related to eating and elimination of waste material. Later in life his emotional relationship to his mother may be reflected in gastrointestinal disturbances.

Practically all little children suck their thumbs. I asked one of my little grandchildren why he liked his thumb. "Is it salty?" "Is it sweet?" "Are you hungry?" He said, "I suck my thumb 'cause it's mine."

Among primitive people much symbolic magic is associated with eating. People devoured their enemies or portions of the bodies of their enemies to gain strength. They would choose the heart of the lion as a special prize. The most intelligent mother looking at her new baby says: "I would like to eat you." As people grow older these gastrointestinal attitudes are reflected in such conditions as alcoholism, overweight, inability to keep food down, loss of appetite, and ulcers. People reared with ritualistic taboos in their religions against certain foods respond with gastric distress when they violate these taboos after they have become detached from the family shelter.

Babies also react in relation to their habits of elimination and "get even" by refusing to eliminate or by doing so too often. Doctors have related colitis, constipation, and diarrhea to emotional factors.

Modern dynamic psychology also makes much of the family relationships of the older child, including envy of father, mother, brothers, and sisters. Frigidity in women or sexual inability in men may be far more mental than physical.

From the moment of birth the child, who has been warm and almost completely protected in the body of its mother, becomes subjected to great numbers of new sensations. These may include noises, lights, bruises, hunger, infections, smells, and irritations. While no longer a part of his mother, he is still completely dependent on her for food and water and freedom from mental and physical stresses and irritations. Psychologists state that throughout life the individual meets stresses by trying to get back to the security and pleasure of his prenatal and infantile life. If he cannot do it actually in his waking hours, in daydreams, he does it in sleeping and dreaming at night. Some people shut themselves off so completely from reality that they show this in hysterical paralyses like inability to speak, to see, to hear, to eat, or to awaken. Again and again we read of patients, mostly young girls, who have slept for weeks or months. Fainting in the presence of any unwelcome sensation is a similar sort of phenomenon.

As the child grows older he learns to reject or spit out what is bad, to eat or assimilate what he likes. The psychologists use the word projection to indicate the way in which a person will project onto someone else their own unsatisfactory feelings or responses. A jealous husband, one authority suggests, is merely projecting onto his mate his own desire to be unfaithful.

As we grow older we learn by imitating others or identifying ourselves with others or with ideas, to satisfy our cravings for mastery. For that reason generals or leaders who command the admiration of their men get more successful results. We can control feelings of anxiety by translating them into action. Under the threat of bombing in London, those who participated in civilian defense were free from feelings of helpless anxiety. When people become helpless they revert to an infantile state with crying, inability to control elimination and similar phenomena.

CHAPTER XII

ALLERGIC DISORDERS

NOT UNTIL 1915 did bronchial asthma, hay fever, urticaria and certain forms of eczema or inflammation of the skin come to be called allergic disorders. At that time the idea of sensitization and reaction of the body to certain foreign substances was established as a reality. Later other conditions such as serum sickness, reactions to drugs, and some blood vessel disturbances were added to the list.

Allergy today is conceived to be the results of contact of a foreign substance with its specific antibody in the human system. Repeated exposure to the foreign substance or allergen sets up the excess sensitivity. The possibility of autosensitization has been established by new research. People may become sensitized to their own tissues and destroy them. Some disorders of the blood are credited to this mechanism. It is likely that multiple sclerosis occurs because the body destroys its own myelin sheaths of the nerves.

Experts distinguish certain allergic disorders as atopic—meaning a strange disease—because they are largely hereditary, because the allergens which set them up are nontoxic substances like pollens or foods, and because the first manifestation is a swelling with accumulation of water in the tissues. The diagnosis of the condition is made by putting the allergen on the skin, whereupon a blister or wheal forms. This accumulation of fluid is due to the release of a substance called histamine. As a part of our progress we have developed antihistaminic drugs. If these are given before making the skin tests, the wheals do not develop. Substances like ACTH and Cortisone derivatives act against allergic disorders. They may be used in asthma and in thrombocytopenia.

The majority of people who develop atopic conditions do so before they are twenty years old. The real allergic conditions appear usually after the person affected is thirty years of age or older. Dr. Harry Alexander believes that a child who becomes subject to asthma at the age of five almost surely is hypersensitive to a specific allergen which it inhales or swallows.

Because of the reactions that occur in the skin the use of tests for determining the nature of allergic conditions is standard.

BRONCHIAL ASTHMA

When a person has bronchial asthma, the bronchial tubes are narrowed by spasm of the muscles and excess secretion from the mucous glands. As air is forced through these narrowed tubes a wheezing sound

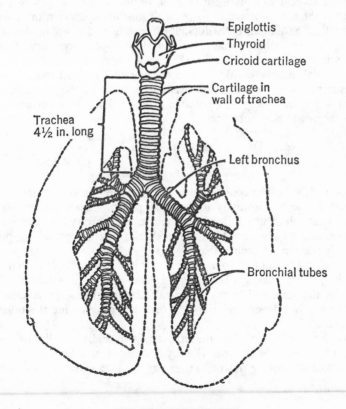

THE BREATHING TRACT

is heard. Air is more easily drawn in than expelled. Since part of the air is trapped, it accumulates and the lungs grow larger. The still air in the lung makes oxygenation more difficult and the blue color that denotes lack of oxygen appears.

This form of asthma runs in families. The patient with bronchial asthma usually reports that he had eczema or hay fever when younger or was sensitive to various substances. The symptoms usually come on and are worse at night. The secretion accumulates at night. Because of the difficulty in breathing, the asthmatic person sits up and bends forward with elbows on the table, in which position he breathes more easily.

The asthmatic attack may last for hours or days. It is relieved by the use of epinephrine or adrenalin. Dr. Harry Alexander distinguishes three types of bronchial asthma. The mild form is limited merely to a persistent cough with a few paroxysms of bronchial spasm and wheezing. The second form is most serious, beginning with sieges of coughing at night and proceeding to severe bronchial spasms with shortness of breath. The patient finds difficulty in eating and sleeping and drinking and loses weight rapidly. In the third type, secondary infection comes in and is responsible for additional symptoms.

Bronchial asthma should be treated promptly and seriously in order to prevent the permanent changes that develop in the lungs in long-continued cases. Everything possible must be done to detect and eliminate the sensitizing substance.

HAY FEVER

About 4,000,000 people in the United States have hay fever. Most cases are due to sensitivity to ragweed pollen. These pollens may be blown as much as fifty miles from their sources. Every area has its own pollens, and charts have been prepared showing the prevailing pollens in each portion of each state.

The allergists say that some time is required to sensitize the individual with hay fever. The antibodies get in the mucous membranes of the nose, in the skin, and in the bronchial tubes so that some asthma may accompany hay fever, and the skin tests are positive for the offending allergens.

For the hay fever patient the first step is to find the pollens to which he is sensitive. This may be done by a series of skin tests. He then has the choice of moving out of the area to a place where he will be free from such contact, or of being desensitized with injections of the offending substance. Usually treatment is begun a few months before the hay fever season begins. Gradually the strength and amount of the injections are increased, so that the patient is receiving large doses by the time the season begins. In some instances treatments are given every two or three weeks all through the year. The use of such methods requires skill and experience, because patients sometimes react most seriously to injections of large doses of the substances to which they are sensitive.

Among other measures used for hay fever is the use of air conditioning, air filters, masks and covering of windows to exclude pollen. Most physicians now supplement the specific treatment with use of the antihistaminic drugs, which are often remarkably effective in stopping the most annoying symptoms.

Vasomotor rhinitis is a condition like hay fever due to sensitivity to dusts or food substances.

OTHER ALLERGIES

In addition to the allergies that localize in the nose and the bronchial tubes, such reactions may come in the stomach and intestines, in the skin and in the joints. They may manifest themselves as headaches and in disturbances of the blood vessels.

The reactions to foods is manifested by swelling, excess secretion, and spasm of the bowel. This is not nearly so frequent as commonly thought. Nevertheless, children react to eggs, milk, or other proteins. Diets from which the offending substances are eliminated stop the symptoms.

Sometimes the taking of foods to which there is sensitivity is followed by headaches due to pressure in the brain from swelling of tissues. Chocolate, nuts, onions and spices, garlic, and similar foods are the most frequent offenders.

Sensitivity to foods may also reveal itself by eruptions on the skin with severe itching and sometimes with wheals or blisters. Similar reactions occur from the taking of glandular substances or, secondarily, from infections. Occasionally sensitivities manifest themselves by inflammation of the eyes, swellings in the internal ear, purpura with blood spots in the skin, inflammations of nerves or eczema. The investigation of such cases, with determination of the factors of importance and elimination of exposure to them, requires patience and intelligence on the part of both physician and patient.

People may be sensitive to the injection of serums and respond excessively to the injection of preventive inoculations.

Allergists describe reactions called "contact dermatitis" from mascara, the material in dress shields or brassieres, the eyes used on furs or shoes, or the filler used in rayon underwear. Sometimes the drug used to relieve a sensitivity creates a sensitivity to itself.

CHAPTER XIII

DISEASES OF CONNECTIVE TISSUE
—COLLAGEN DISEASES

SEVERAL rather unusual and rare diseases are now being grouped together by medical investigators as a result of information derived from recent research. Their names are *polyarteritis nodosa,* diffuse *lupus erythematosus, scleroderma,* and *dermatomyositis.* All of them represent disturbances of connective tissue in the body, in contrast to glandular tissue or surface secreting tissue. The connective tissue of the body includes what is elastic and the material between the cells. Sometimes tumors consist almost wholly of connective or fibrous tissue. The walls of blood vessels contain much tissue of this type.

THE COLLAGEN DISEASES

All of these diseases are benefited at least temporarily by use of ACTH or Cortisone. All of them resemble also the reactions that occur in tissues in response to hypersensitivity or allergy. Arthritis, which also responds to the drugs mentioned, occurs commonly in connection with each of these diseases.

POLYARTERITIS NODOSA

Polyarteritis nodosa (poly-ar-ter-itis) is a disease in which the blood vessels are chiefly affected. Because this disease includes primarily serious damage of blood vessels, it may be reflected in any part of the body. The condition affects men four times as often as women and,

51

mostly, those between twenty and forty years old. Arthritis and many of the reactions associated with hypersensitivity are seen by the doctor in these patients.

LUPUS ERYTHEMATOSUS

Disseminated *lupus erythematosus* (loo-pus er-i-the-ma-to-sus) is a chronic, usually severe disorder occurring mostly in females fifteen to forty years old. A characteristic is a butterfly-shaped inflammation over the nose. Other symptoms involve the joints and the heart. Fever and anemia and a progressive course make the disease fatal.

SCLERODERMA

Scleroderma is a disease that affects the connective tissue of the body and particularly that in the skin where there is hardening. Chiefly women between thirty and fifty years old are affected. The swelling in the skin may be followed by calcification. This disease comes on slowly and insidiously, but as it progresses changes occur in the skin of the face, neck, and arms. The skin looks waxy and tight and loses its color and hair. When the face is involved there may be difficulty in moving the jaw. Fortunately this is not a common disease; certainly it is not as serious as *polyarteritis nodosa* or diffuse *lupus erythematosus,* which are similar. In the older forms of treatment emphasis was placed on the use of thyroid and vitamins. Great care was given to prevent secondary infections.

DERMATOMYOSITIS

Fourth in this group of collagen disorders is one called *dermatomyositis.* This is a common and often fatal disorder involving the skin and the muscles. The exact cause is still unknown. It affects people of all races and colors, both men and women, and in general those between the ages of ten and fifty years.

Characteristic of this condition is the involvement of the muscles. As they deteriorate the organs concerned show effects, as in the eyes, throat, diaphragm, or muscles between the ribs. The symptoms then are difficulties of vision, swallowing, breathing, speech, etc. Naturally such people lose weight and get weak. Unfortunately this condition is progressive and few who have it live long. Until recently little was known about treatment, and vitamins, hormones and physical therapy were tried. Salicylates were thought to be beneficial. Now we know that the salicylates can to a small extent stimulate the condition.

ARTHRITIS

Rheumatism is a word used to describe a number of diseases, acute or chronic, which are accompanied by pain and stiffness of the muscles, the joints and other tissues involved in movement. Arthritis is the term used to describe inflammation of the joints only. So frequent are the conditions grouped under rheumatoid arthritis that cases exceed tuberculosis by ten times, cancer by seven times and diabetes by ten times. One expert says that 150,000 people are made invalids by these conditions every year; others estimate the total number of people in the United States with such conditions as anywhere between eight and ten million.

Joints have to bear weight and at the same time be able to move. So perfectly are they formed for their purpose that the great artist, engineer and anatomist, Leonardo da Vinci, spent much time drawing them and studying their methods of operation. The joint includes the ends of bones, cartilages between the ends, a capsule holding it all together, ligaments which attach the muscles to the bones, membranes and the joint fluid. Nerves accompany the blood vessels into the joints; while the bones and cartilage do not feel pain, inflammation and swelling with the pouring of extra fluid into the joint can produce exquisite pain.

People with arthritis can be quite eloquent about their joints. The pain may be described as excruciating, throbbing, burning, aching, squeezing, or just hurting. The patients also complain of crackling, stiffness, and loss of motion.

The American Rheumatism Association has classified arthritis into seven types: (1) due to infection; (2) due to rheumatic fever; (3) rheumatoid; (4) degenerative; (5) due to injuries; (6) due to gout; (7) arising from the nervous system.

Rheumatoid arthritis is not just a disease of the joints, but a general condition affecting the whole body. While the exact cause or causes may not be known, the discovery of the effects of ACTH and Cortisone have led to new concepts of the nature of the disease. Now rheumatoid arthritis along with a number of other conditions is called a "collagen" disease. In all of these the connective tissue of the body is

53

chiefly concerned. The tendency is to consider rheumatoid arthritis a reaction of the body to sensitivity to certain substances, perhaps coming from bacteria, with the sensitivity affecting the connective tissue chiefly. The suggestion has also been made that rheumatism is not a specific reaction to some single substance but a general reaction of the body resulting from several different stimulations.

Women are affected by rheumatoid arthritis three times as often as men. Frequently several cases appear in one family, which does not mean that the condition is hereditary in the true sense but rather that the group may be exposed to similar detrimental environmental factors such as cold, damp, and infections of the respiratory passages. People in all conditions of life and society get rheumatoid arthritis. More people get it, however, in areas that are poor, overcrowded, and unhygienic. Doctors recognize also an emotional or psychological factor. Perhaps for that reason, arthritis is worse on cold, damp days when people are adversely affected emotionally by the weather. Sometimes arthritis accompanies states of emotional tension, frustrations and anxieties, and such patients do not seem to want to get well. The rheumatism is a crutch, or something on which to lean as an explanation for inadequacies.

Rheumatoid arthritis varies from being an acute disease with fever and sudden disability of many joints to a condition that develops gradually in which the patient may at first notice only stiffness or pain in one joint. Some may have deformity of a joint without ever having felt any pain. Sometimes the first signs of rheumatoid arthritis are fatigue, loss of appetite and loss of weight. Patients complain of numbness and loss of feeling in hands and arms, feet or legs. On getting up in the morning and at the end of the day, the joints feel stiff. When swellings of the joints are noticed the condition is usually well advanced. The knees and the finger joints may be the first to give pain. Practically all the joints may be involved, however, including those of the spine.

Other signs and symptoms of rheumatoid arthritis are known and noticed by many people. The palms and soles are cold and clammy. Sometimes the lymph glands near the joint become swollen. The finger joints nearest to the wrist swell and the fingers pull to the sides in a distortion that gives the hand a "flipper-like" appearance. Because of failure to move and use the muscles around the swollen joint, the tissue breaks down and the area looks thin and wasted.

Rheumatoid arthritis is a condition that comes and goes. Doctors have noticed particularly that it disappears during pregnancy and during jaundice. These facts helped to reveal the specific effects of ACTH and Cortisone upon the disease.

Nodules appear under the skin in about one fifth of the cases of rheumatoid arthritis. These nodules may persist for months or years. Inflammations of the eye and red spots on the skin are also seen often in chronic rheumatoid arthritis.

Since arthritis is now recognized as affecting the body as a whole and not just the joints, the treatment is changed considerably. Nevertheless, the methods that helped when most of the attention was focused on the joints were not lost and are still valuable in a direct approach to the control of the pain and disability which are features of the disease.

The sooner good treatment can be applied to rheumatoid arthritis the better are the results secured in stopping the progress and the damage done by the disease. While the disease is active, rest and freedom from motion are helpful. If there is fever and severe pain certainly confinement to bed is desirable. Then as these troubles subside motion is permitted, but never to the point of fatigue. During the severe stages the patients are anxious and disturbed, often by solicitous people, and the doctor must protect the patient against emotional upsets.

No special diet cures arthritis. Nevertheless the patient with rheumatoid arthritis needs to be sustained with sufficient proteins, vitamins and minerals and enough carbohydrates and fats to provide needed energy and to avoid damage to tissues. Good animal proteins, calcium and iron must be adequate in the diet.

Europeans with arthritis go regularly to spring and mineral-water resorts, but there is no evidence that these are helpful beyond getting the patient away from his usual surroundings and under a well-regulated routine of rest, diet, baths, and physical therapy. Drugs are prescribed to relieve pain and permit rest. Bee stings, snake poison, and similar methods are not proved to have any real curative value beyond their psychological effect.

For many years a mainstay in treating arthritis has been the application of heat. Heat may be applied by hot bricks wrapped in towels, hot water bottles, electric heat pads, infra-red heat lamps, heat cradles containing incandescent bulbs, and other methods. If many joints are involved relief frequently comes from a hot tub bath once or twice a day, but prolonged hot baths are weakening.

Doctors help the patient with painful joints by several devices which require medical knowledge and application. The orthopedic surgeons control movements by splints, braces, and casts. These have to be released several times daily to permit help by rubbing and slight controlled motion. A local anesthetic like procaine may be injected around a joint and relieve pain from the pulling of muscles and ligaments. New drugs are known of the curare type which prevent spasm of muscles and thus relieve pain. While preventing pain, the doctor must be sure there is sufficient motion to prevent wasting of the tissues. After long-continued arthritis, deformity of joints may be so severe that surgical orthopedic procedures may be necessary to relieve crippling.

The innumerable treatments of arthritis over the years have reflected the lack of certain knowledge as to the causes and mechanisms concerned in its development. Iodides, sulfur, salicylates and, more recently, gold have been used. Vaccines, serums, and non-specific proteins have been tried. Antibiotics and sulfonamides have been used but have been unavailing, since the condition is not an infection that could be controlled with these drugs. For many years aspirin has been the main drug for relief of pain in arthritis. Drugs based on quinine derivatives are also reportedly helpful. The greatest promise of any medical treatment thus far known has come from ACTH and Cortisone. A new form called Prednisone sold as Meticorten, Sterane, or Deltra is superior because it does not disturb water and salt balance. The dosage and duration of use must be strictly controlled by the doctor.

People do not die of rheumatoid arthritis but complications may occur which are especially serious for the arthritic patient. Troubles with the lungs including pneumonia, damage to the heart and secondary infections are a threat.

Rheumatoid arthritis may be especially serious for children because of deformities that persist throughout life. A severe form of rheumatoid arthritis in childhood is known as "Still's disease." Another form of rheumatoid arthritis is associated with psoriasis, and there are arthritic manifestations that affect women in the menopause.

Rheumatoid arthritis affecting the spine is a crippling condition responsible for much disability. This condition usually occurs in men rather than in women. Pains in the back, soreness on bending over, painful buttocks, and shooting pains in the sciatic nerve area are accompaniments. With spasms of the spinal muscles comes a tendency to avoid movement and in some instances the stiff-poker spine develops. The X-ray reveals changes in the spine as the condition progresses, but early in the disease nothing significant may be observed. These are the patients who are helped by sleeping in a bed with a firm mattress. Hot, wet packs help to relieve the spasm of the muscles. X-ray treatments may also help these patients.

Degenerative joint disease hits people past middle age. The changes may be part of the aging process and associated with injury. The condition occurs all over the world and particularly in certain occupations such as porters, those who stand long at work, scrub women and janitors. In diagnosis of these cases X-ray is of great importance. Use of salicylates and of aspirin, heat, mild massage and liniments are reported beneficial in securing relief for those with degenerative arthritis.

CHAPTER XIV

LOSS AND GAIN OF WEIGHT

A CAREFUL MEDICAL EXAMINATION always includes a record of the patient's weight and, particularly, information as to whether he has been gaining or losing weight rapidly. Doctors have tabulations which show the average weight for people according to their age, sex, height, and body build. Some people are tall and thin with light bones and light muscles. Others may be stocky, short, muscular.

Water constitutes about 70 per cent of the body weight. About one fifth of all the water is outside the individual cells. This is found in the blood, the spinal fluid, the lymph and a small amount between the cells. The remainder of the body weight is in solid structures like the bones; most of the minerals of the body are in the bones. Sugars are stored in the body—principally in the liver and muscles—as glycogen.

Fat is an inactive material deposited around the body in storage depots.

Proteins are the chief building elements of the cells. The body needs four grams of water for each gram of protein. The amount of calories taken by the body to maintain its weight depends on the rate at which the body uses up material, and this in turn is related to the amount of activity. Growth requires increased calories. When inadequate amounts of calories are taken into the body the deficit is supplied by using up material from the tissues. The fat is drawn upon, but also the carbohydrates. When both fat and carbohydrate are utilized, the protein is taken up. This means the breakdown of some functioning cells.

Conditions in which there is interference with the usual elimination of sodium cause increased water retention and gain in weight. Examples are heart failure, toxemia of pregnancy, hardening or cirrhosis of the liver and congestive heart failure. Elimination of water is improved by stopping salt, improving heart action, or by drugs which increase the action of the kidneys.

Increase of fluid in the body occurs when the protein is inadequate. In such cases restoration of protein results in elimination of water. Excess of sweating or severe diarrhea also draw water from the body and thus lower weight.

The weight of the body is also related to the action of the thyroid gland, which has a part in determining the basal metabolism. Fever will increase the metabolic rate. Excess action of the thyroid will also give a rate over on the plus side whereas deficient action of the thyroid moves the rate to the minus side.

Eating is regulated by many factors. Appetite may be part of a habit of large eating. Many families put overemphasis on eating. Grandmothers offer food as cures for most family disturbances. Sometimes a person who has an active life with heavy eating changes to a sedentary life. The eating habits persist and he puts on weight. Some people eat as a substitute for satisfactions that they do not obtain through other emotional sources. Incidentally, alcoholics frequently drink because they escape other demands in this way. An unusual cause of excessive eating is overactivity of the pancreas gland in developing insulin. An injury to the brain which affects certain portions of a part of the brain called the hypothalamus may be associated with the development of a voracious appetite. But by far the vast majority of cases of obesity are due to taking too much food in relation to the metabolism and activity of the body.

Loss of weight can be produced by lowering the calorie intake to less than the body requirement. Starvation may result from lack of appetite, which is called "anorexia." Loss of appetite occurs in acute and chronic infections, in certain forms of cancer and glandular diseases. Loss of appetite may be wholly psychologic or mental, producing a condition called *anorexia nervosa.*

In the book *Your Weight and How to Control It,* which I edited, leading medical and scientific authorities discuss every aspect of weight gain and loss.

NUTRITIONAL DISORDERS

Great numbers of people believe that most diseases come from wrong food. As a result innumerable dietary fads and fancies attract them. Really, the body is a chemical plant which manufactures some of the substances it absolutely must have to survive. Fundamental mineral substances cannot be manufactured by the body. Vitamins cannot be manufactured by the body and must be taken in food or otherwise, since the body depends on them for health and growth.

Dietary deficiencies naturally occur most often among people who get insufficient food but also among those who get the wrong foods. The most common dietary disorder is overweight or obesity.

At present the vitamins which human beings must have for health include vitamin A and carotene, which is its precursor; thiamin and riboflavin and niacin which are parts of the vitamin B complex; also vitamin C and vitamin D, vitamin K, folic acid and vitamin B_{12}.

The Food and Nutrition Board of the National Research Council has prepared a table of recommended daily dietary allowances for persons of both sexes, various ages, during pregnancy and nursing, for sedentary persons, physically active persons, and for heavy workers. Calorie intake varies from 2,000 daily for sedentary women to 4,500 daily for male heavy workers. Women's needs increase during pregnancy and nursing of their babies. Children's needs vary with their ages, weight, sex and activity also.

The lists of substances to be assured in the diet include good proteins, calcium, iron, the vitamins. Also needs must be met for water, salt, iodine, phosphorus, copper, vitamin K and folic acid. Simple tables can be secured from the United States Public Health Service and other governmental agencies.

UNDERNUTRITION

Throughout the world, elsewhere much more than in the United States, people suffer from inadequate nourishment. These inadequacies may involve the total intake, the proteins and amino acids, the vitamins and the minerals.

Loss of weight is not necessarily an indication of undernutrition nor is maintenance of weight assurance that the intake is proper. Troubles of salt and water balance such as occur in a variety of conditions affecting the heart, kidneys, liver and glandular organs may greatly affect the body weight. Starvation due to loss of appetite or profound neuropsychiatric disturbances produces nutritional disorders. While the human body can build up reserves of some substances, others are used up daily and must be regularly replenished. The effects of undernutrition may be aggravated by excessive action of the thyroid, by heat and by cold.

59

The regulatory mechanism of the body provides for using up fat to provide energy, before drawing on the vital protein. A gram of fat provides nine calories. A gram of protein or carbohydrate yields four calories. The body conserves its protein, and for that reason a fat person can stand starvation much better than a thin one. The carbohydrate is stored in the liver as glycogen, and this is used up in a day or two of starvation.

Carbohydrate and fat conserve protein. The protein consists of amino acids, of which ten are essential. Twelve other amino acids are classified as nonessential. People on a high carbohydrate diet can develop protein deficiency because they have not had enough protein or because they have not had the essential amino acids in their protein. Eggs, meat, and milk best supply the essential amino acids. Growing children and pregnant women and nursing mothers need excess protein.

OVERWEIGHT

Since 1950 people have been especially conscious of the relation of overweight to life and health. Weird diets and reducing fads have their day or month and disappear. Formerly just the women were interested, but the weight of men also receives much consideration.

Obesity is a disorder of the body's functioning which results in deposits of excess fat throughout the tissues. Doctors take special note of obesity because of the relationship between overweight and disorders of the heart, high blood pressure, diabetes, and joint disturbances.

Most experts are now agreed that by far the most frequent cause of obesity is the taking of too much food in proportion to the amount of energy that the person uses. Most people eat without too much attention to the weight problem, and yet the body can adjust itself reasonably well to getting rid of what is not used.

Some families consistently overeat, and therefore the children, imitating their parents, become overweight. Occasionally executives find that a snack enables them to carry on at their desks beyond the onset of fatigue; eating becomes a substitute for needed rest. As we get older we tend to walk and climb and move about less than previously. Unless we reduce the food intake overweight appears. Occasionally an illness stops physical activity, and obesity may result.

OBESITY

The person who habitually overeats is always looking for an alibi. He points to someone else who eats a great deal and doesn't get fat;

then he argues that his own body is different and that he absorbs where the other does not. I have seen a fat woman eating one chocolate cream after another while complaining sadly: "Everything I eat turns to fat." People do differ as to the extent to which their bodies will take up fat stores, and people also differ in their basal metabolic rates. Rarely however is overweight due to glandular deficiencies. The glands are more concerned with the areas of the body in which the fat is deposited—for instance, female hips, breasts and buttocks—the male jowls and paunch —than with overweight as a whole. Certain diseases with degeneration of important glands may be accompanied by weight increase. However, Dr. George Thorn says: "Many endocrine disturbances result from rather than cause obesity."

Everybody knows the obvious difficulties of the body associated with overweight. Fat people get out of breath, get tired easily and have pain in the joints of the knees, hips, and lower back. Fat people can't stand hot weather, they get more headaches, irritations of the skin and digestive disturbances. Fat women have more trouble with gall-bladder difficulties, diabetes, blood pressure and disturbances of their periodic functions than do thin women. The gall-bladder patient is frequently the fat woman who is fair, over forty, and who has had four pregnancies.

The proper way to reduce weight is to lessen the intake of food below the amount needed for the individual's energy. However, any person must still get the essential protein, vitamin and mineral substances necessary to maintain health.

WEIGHT REDUCTION

Anyone who is much overweight and who is serious about reducing should begin with a thorough examination by the doctor which will cover heart, lungs, glands, height, weight, blood pressure, condition of the blood and similar factors. A careful study of the urine should be made for presence of albumin and sugar, to rule out nephritis or diabetes. The doctor will want to get at the patient's emotional condition and any psychologic conditions that may be responsible for the overeating. Dr. Edward Rynearson says a "will-power-pill" is needed, by which he means to emphasize the necessity that the person really wants to reduce. By wise counsel, the doctor can support the patient's motivation.

At first cutting down the calories results in some loss of energy and drive, but this is less noticeable as the program continues. The loss of weight is most noticeable during the first few weeks when the basal metabolic rate of the patient readjusts itself to the lessened food intake and when there may be quite a reduction in water that is held in the body. Because of the depression and fatigue first noticed, some physicians recommend that the patient on a dietary reduction regime have some Benzedrine, not only to help his spirits but also because such drugs tend to diminish appetite.

Reduction in the intake of salt results in a prompt loss of water from the body and therefore rapid loss of weight, but this is not significant as far as fat is concerned. Actually the body gets rid of water beyond that needed for its proper functioning, and the patient on weight reduction should not unduly restrict his intake of water.

Young people can reduce more easily than older ones. Because patients may be depressed by failure to observe large reductions, some physicians recommend that the patient be weighed only once each week.

PSYCHOLOGY OF WEIGHT REDUCTION

When an underlying psychologic reason for overeating is absent, and the patient's overweight is merely the result of a long-continued habit of excess nibbling, reduction of weight is easy. When overeating is mixed with emotional satisfactions, removal of the overeating may be associated with disturbing mental reactions. The doctor has to find the mental conflicts that are the real basis of the overweight. Dr. George Thorn has called attention to the difference in care of the fat girl led into the doctor's office by an anxious and yet domineering mother from that of the girl who wants to increase her personal attractiveness in order to achieve certain social relationships. For that reason, control of overeating is much easier with a sixteen-year-old girl than with one approaching thirteen.

With older people, fear of such conditions as diabetes, high blood pressure, arthritis or heart failure may be the reason for weight reduction. Nevertheless, older people have established habits of life including regular meetings of luncheon clubs, banquets, parties and what-not which make dieting difficult. For such people a trip away from their accustomed surroundings to a health resort is advantageous, because the environment is more conducive to restricted eating.

In recent years weight-watcher groups have been successful, for people benefit when their own will power is reinforced by others with similar problems. Weight-reduction classes are successful because of the factor of competition, of exchange of ideas, joint participation in exercises, group walking, dancing, and similar activities.

At the appearance of any sign of distress associated with a weight-reduction program, the patient should consult his doctor. If the program needs to be modified, the earlier it is done the better.

DIETS

WELL-BALANCED NORMAL DIET

Eat These Foods Each Day	*Number of Servings*	*Size of Servings*
1. Cereals	1	½ to ¾ cup cooked, 1 to 1¼ cup ready-to-eat
2. Bread, whole-grain or enriched	2 to 3	1 to 2 slices
3. Milk—to drink or in cooking	3 to 4	1 cup
4. Orange, grapefruit, or tomato	1	½ to ¾ cup of juice, or ½ to 1 fruit
5. Other fruits	1	1, or ½ to ¾ cup
6. Green or yellow vegetables	1	¾ to 1 cup raw, or ½ to ¾ cup cooked
7. Potato and other vegetables	2 to 3	1, or ½ to ¾ cup
8. Meat and other protein foods	2	¼ to ⅓ lb. or ½ to ¾ cup
9. Butter or margarine—as spread or seasoning	3	1 pat ¼ inch thick or 1 tablespoon
10. Other fats, sweets, and beverages as desired.		

THESE FOODS CAN BE INCLUDED IN 3 MEALS A DAY

Breakfast: Orange, grapefruit, or tomato. Cereal, sugar, milk or cream. Bread, butter. Milk, coffee, or tea.

Lunch or Supper: Meat or other protein food. Vegetable. Bread, butter. Milk-drink or soup. Fruit dessert.

Dinner: Meat or other protein food. Potato or other vegetable. Green or yellow vegetable. Bread, butter. Milk-drink. Milk or other dessert.

Important:
Eat fruits and vegetables raw frequently. Choose a dark-green, leafy vegetable two or three times a week. Have a variety of different vegetables from day to day. Include a serving of liver about once a week.

Use at least four eggs each week—in cooking, at lunch, or for breakfast if a first meal larger than suggested is desired.

LOW-CALORIE DIET PLAN

Being on a low-calorie diet means that the energy required above the calories supplied by the diet must come from the stored body fat. The result is loss of weight.

Essential nutrients must be supplied daily by your diet. This is why your choice of foods is as important as the amount you eat. An extreme or one-sided diet is not wise.

LOW-CALORIE DIET

Don't try to lose more than two pounds a week. Faster weight loss is not advised by medical authorities.

Don't give up if no weight is lost the first week or ten days. There are often adjustments in body fluids during this time.

Cut down on salt if you are now a generous user.

Exercise moderately if you sit most of the day; it helps replace lost fat with firm muscle tissue.

Remember that alcoholic beverages add calories and whet the appetite so that it's more difficult to stay on the diet.

Eat slowly, and make your mealtimes pleasant.

SUGGESTED DAILY MEAL PLAN

(For low-calorie diet)

BREAKFAST

Foods Permitted	Amounts	Calories
Unsweetened Fruit or	(see list)	30–100
Unsweetened Fruit Juice	(see list)	25–75
Ready-to-eat Cereals, whole-grain or restored	½ cup	50
Skim Milk	½ cup	40
Toasted Whole-grain or Enriched	1 thin slice	50
Bread or Small Bran Muffin	1	50
Butter or Margarine	1 teaspoon	35
Coffee or Tea without Cream or Sugar as desired		

NOON MEAL

Cooked Lean Meat, Fish, Turkey, Chicken	1 small serv. (3½ oz).	100–200
or Egg	1	70
Cooked Vegetable	(see list)	15–50
Raw Vegetable	(see list)	5–35
Whole-grain or Enriched Bread *or*	1 thin slice	50
Small Bran Muffin	1	50
Butter or Margarine	1 teaspoon	35
Unsweetened Fruit	(see list)	30–100
Skim Milk	1 cup	80
Coffee or Tea without Cream or Sugar as desired		

EVENING MEAL

Fat-free Soup *or,*	1 cup	40–100
Fruit or Vegetable Juice	(see list)	25–75
Cooked Lean Meat, Fish, Turkey, Chicken	1 small serv. (3½ oz).	100–200
or Egg	1	70
Potato, baked or boiled	1 small	85
Cooked Vegetable	(see list)	15–50
Salad without Dressing (Tomato Juice, Lemon Juice or Vinegar may be used)	(see list)	5–35
Whole-grain or Enriched Bread *or*	1 thin slice	50
Small Bran Muffin	1	50
Butter or Margarine	1 teaspoon	35
Unsweetened Fruit	(see list)	30–100
Skim Milk	1 cup	80
Coffee or Tea without Cream or Sugar as desired		
(Vitamin Supplements only as prescribed.)	*Total Calories*	1,000–1,500

BETWEEN MEALS

Milk or Fruit from meal allowances may be eaten between meals.

PERMITTED VEGETABLES—Prepared Without Fat or Sauce.

COOKED:		CALORIES	RAW:		CALORIES
Asparagus, fresh	6 stalks	15	Cabbage, shredded	¾ cup	15
Bean Sprouts	¾ cup	25	Carrots	1 medium	20
Beans, snap	½ cup	40	Celery	2 stalks	10
Beets, diced	½ cup	35	Cucumber	10 slices	10
Beets, greens	½ cup	30	Lettuce	5 large	
Broccoli	½ cup	35		leaves	10
Cabbage	⅔ cup	30	Onions, young	5	25
Carrots, cubed	½ cup	30	Radishes	2	5
Cauliflower	½ cup	20	Tomatoes	1 medium	35
Chard	½ cup	25	Watercress, Parsley	10 sprigs	5
Collards	½ cup	50			
Egg plant, diced	⅔ cup	15			
Kale	½ cup	50			
Okra	5–6 pods	20			
Onions	2–3 small	50			
Peppers, green	1 medium	30			
Potato	1 small	85			
Pumpkin	½ cup	40			
Rutabagas	½ cup	40			
Sauerkraut	⅔ cup	20			
Spinach, other greens	⅔ cup	25			
Squash, Winter	½ cup	45			
Tomatoes	½ cup	20			
Tomato Juice	½ cup	25			
Vegetable Juice	½ cup	20			

* * * * *

Salads may be dressed with tomato juice, lemon or other fruit juice, or vinegar.

Butter or margarine from daily food allowance may be used with vegetables instead of on bread, if desired.

One small potato is allowed each day. If desired, other vegetables may sometimes be substituted or a larger potato may be eaten and bread omitted.

PERMITTED FRUITS—Prepared Without Added Sugar or Syrup.

COOKED:		CALORIES	RAW:		CALORIES
Apple Sauce	½ cup	45	Apple	1 small	65
Apricots, water pack	3	35	Apricots	2–3 medium	55
Cherries, water pack	½ cup	60	Banana	1 medium	100
Peaches, water pack	2 halves	30	Blackberries	⅔ cup	60
Pears, water pack	2 halves	35	Blueberries	⅔ cup	70
Pineapple, water pack	1 slice	60	Cantaloupe	½ small	35
Plums, water pack	2 medium	30	Cherries	15 large	65
FRUIT JUICES—Unsweetened			Grapefruit	½ medium	45
Apple Juice	½ cup	50	Grapes	24	75
Grape Juice	½ cup	75	Orange	1 medium	50
Grapefruit Juice	½ cup	45	Peaches	1 large	50
Orange Juice	½ cup	50	Pears	1 medium	70
Pineapple Juice	½ cup	55	Pineapple	½ cup	60
Prune Juice	½ cup	75	Plums	2 medium	40
			Raspberries	¾ cup	65
			Strawberries	10 large	40
			Tangerines	1 large	50
			Watermelon	½ slice	50

* * * * * *

Two level teaspoons of sugar may be used occasionally in place of 1 teaspoon butter or margarine from daily food allowance.

GAINING DIET

1. Co-operate with your doctor to eliminate any medical causes of underweight.
2. Have eight to ten hours rest in bed. Try to be in bed by 10 P.M. A lukewarm bath at bedtime may help induce sleep. If possible, have a thirty-minute rest before the evening meal.
3. Have pleasant surroundings and forget troubles while eating.
4. Be sure that food is attractively and palatably served.
5. Try these ways to increase appetite:
    Take a mild exercise on getting out of bed in the morning.
    Have a warm, changing to cool, shower before breakfast.

Loss and Gain of Weight

Cut down on or eliminate the smoking habit.
Eat a little more each meal than is needed to satisfy appetite.

At Breakfast:
1. Double amount of fruit juice.
2. Choose a hot enriched cereal and use a pat of butter on it as well as sugar and cream.
3. Double the amount of butter on bread.
4. Take two eggs.
5. Add a breakfast meat such as ham or bacon.
6. Add cream to milk or milk-cocoa, or use generous amounts of cream and sugar in coffee or tea.

At Lunch or Supper:
1. Increase size of main dish and vegetable servings. Use generous amounts of gravies, sauces, and/or mayonnaise.
2. Use an extra pat of butter on vegetables and bread.
3. Add plain or whipped cream to milk, hot or cold chocolate milk, hot cocoa, or cream soup.
4. Select a dessert such as the following:
   Cooked and sweetened dried fruits.
   Banana with cream and sugar.
   Apple dumpling or baked apple with a sweet sauce or cream.
   Fruit pie—use cheese with apple pie; ice cream on others.

Midafternoon:
Drink one of the following—milk, chocolate milk or cocoa, milk with added cream or ice cream, milk beaten up with a raw egg and flavored with sugar, vanilla, and nutmeg.

At Dinner:
1. Increase size of main dish and vegetable servings. Use generous amounts of gravies, sauces, and/or mayonnaise.
2. Use an extra pat of butter on vegetables and bread.
3. Add cream to milk or have hot or cold chocolate milk or cocoa.

FOOD PERMITTED

BEVERAGE	Milk, milk drinks, sweetened fruit juices, eggnogs, hot chocolate.
BREAD	All kinds in liberal amounts.
CEREALS	Ready-to-eat or home-cooked, whole-grain or restored. (Large servings with cream and sugar.)
CHEESE	All kinds as desired.
DESSERT	All kinds; rich puddings, custards, ice creams, cakes, cookies—generous servings.
EGGS	As desired, prepared with butter when possible.
FATS	All kinds.
FRUIT	All kinds, with added sugar if desired.
MEAT	All kinds, particularly fat meat and fish prepared with sauce, and gravy when possible.
SOUP	All kinds, prepared with butter or added sauce.
SALAD DRESSINGS	Any kind, in quantities desired

4. Select a dessert such as the following:
   Baked custard with caramel sauce or whipped cream.
   Bread, cornstarch, or rice pudding with suitable sauce or cream.
   Cake topped with whipped cream or with a fruit, butterscotch, or chocolate sauce.
   Cream or custard pie topped with whipped cream.
   Ice cream sundae with cake or cookies.

At Bedtime:
1. Eat a bowl of cereal with sugar and cream, OR
2. Drink warm milk, cocoa or chocolate, and take with it a light, digestible snack.

LOW SALT DIET

Pure sodium, which is one of the two elements in sodium chloride, or common salt, is seldom found except in chemical laboratories. Many combinations of sodium with other elements are used in diet and in industry. Table salt is sodium chloride. Baking soda is sodium bicarbonate.

The average man takes in his diet about half an ounce of sodium chloride every day. It is easy, on a low salt diet, to reduce this to about one fifth as much. This is done particularly when excess of fluid accumulates in the tissues, as in dropsy. No one knows exactly the minimum or maximum of sodium chloride that any one person ought to have, but fortunately the human body is equipped with factors of safety, so that it can get rid of excesses of various substances. The average human body contains at all times about three ounces of sodium chloride. The use of salt by the body and its elimination by the kidney are apparently controlled by the cortex or outer layer of the adrenal gland.

Many vegetables contain another salt with an element similar to sodium, namely, potassium. A person who subsists on a vegetable diet craves salt, because vegetables contain less sodium than meat. The moment the salt in the human body falls below the amount necessary, a craving is set up.

Salt is also important for supplying the chlorine element, since hydrochloric acid is secreted by the stomach regularly as an aid to digestion. Pepsin works as a digestive substance only in the presence of hydrochloric acid. However, hydrochloric acid should not be taken by the average person in that form except on the advice of a physician.

Various diets free from large amounts of sodium chloride have been developed. Most physicians are convinced that there is a definite relationship between salt in the diet and the occurrence of various conditions affecting the blood pressure and the kidneys. However, in the presence of unusual craving for salt, or, in fact, in any disease condition, it is well to be guided by competent advice.

RESTRICTED SALT DIET

Use NO SALT *in Food Preparation* — *Use* NO SALT *at* TABLE

Food	Permitted
BEVERAGE	Milk, milk drinks, fruit juices.
BREAD	Salt-free bread or rolls.
CEREALS	Ready-to-eat or home-cooked without salt.
CHEESE	Unsalted cottage cheese.
DESSERT	Puddings, gelatin desserts, fruits.
EGGS	One daily.
FAT	Unsalted butter, other salt-free fats.
FRUIT	Fresh or canned.
MEAT	Fresh meat, fresh-water fish, chicken and turkey. (Exclude salted and smoked meats, salt-water fish.)
SOUP	Cream soups.
VEGETABLES	All kinds, raw and home-cooked. (Avoid all commercially canned vegetables and relishes, unless prepared without salt.)

Food	Permitted
BREAKFAST:	Fruit or Fruit Juice
	Salt-free Cereal with Milk or Cream and Sugar
	Egg, if desired
	Toast, Muffins, or Rolls
	Unsalted Butter or other Spread
	Jam or Marmalade
	Beverage
LUNCH OR	Meat, Fish, or other Main Dish
SUPPER:	Vegetable
	Salad
	Rolls or Bread
	Unsalted Butter or other Spread
	Dessert
	Milk
DINNER:	Fruit Juice or Soup, if desired
	Meat, Fish, or other Main Dish
	Potato
	Vegetable
	Rolls or Bread
	Unsalted Butter or other Spread
	Dessert
	Beverage

SMOOTH DIET, FREE FROM ROUGHAGE

In the majority of cases of irritation of the colon and of associated constipation the most important dietetic consideration is that the diets be free from unnecessary roughage or stimulation. Here are suggestions for a smooth diet:

Avoid sugar in concentrated form, and take no candy or other food between meals. Hot cakes and waffles are satisfactory, but should not be eaten with syrup. Fried foods are not bad if they are properly fried, that is, totally immersed in fat at the right temperature. Avoid eating when in a rush and when mentally upset.

The following are suggestions for breakfast: Orange juice, grapefruit (avoid the fiber in the compartments), cantaloupe and melons are inadvisable. Coffee, if desired, is allowed in moderation, but it sometimes causes flatulence. If you are sensitive to caffeine try a caffeine-free coffee or a coffee substitute. Chocolate, cocoa, or tea; one or two eggs with ham or bacon (avoid the tougher part of the bacon); white bread, toast, or zwieback, with butter; any smooth mush such as farina, germea, Cream of Wheat, cornmeal, or rolled oats; puffed cereals and cornflakes are also allowed. Bran is particularly harmful. Graham bread is permitted, but not the coarser whole-wheat bread.

Suggestions for lunch and dinner: In fruit cocktails, avoid the fibrous pieces of orange and pineapple. Broths, bouillon, cream soups, and chowder are allowed; also meat, fish, chicken, squab, or game, except duck (avoid the fibrous parts and gristle). Veal may be tried; it is not digested well by many persons. Eat no smoked fish or pork. Crab and lobster had better be left alone. Oysters and sausage may be tried later.

Bread and butter are allowed, and hot biscuits if they are made small so as to consist mainly of crust. Rice, potatoes—mashed, hashed-brown, or French fried—are allowed; and later, sweet potatoes, hominy, stewed tomatoes (strained and thickened with cracker or bread crumbs), well-cooked cauliflower tops with cream sauce, asparagus tips, Brussels sprouts, squash, beets, turnips, creamed spinach, Italian pastas, noodles, macaroni, and spaghetti—all cooked soft—purées of peas, beans, lentils, lima beans, or artichoke hearts. All sakins or fiber should be removed by passing the food through a ricer. Sweet corn may be used if passed through a colander. There are almost no other vegetables that can be puréed to advantage. String beans are allowed if they are young and tender. Large, tender string beans, which can be used as a vegetable or salad, can now be obtained in cans.

No salad should be taken at first. Later you may try a little tender lettuce with apples or bananas, tomato jelly or boiled eggs. Mayonnaise and French dressing are allowed. Potato salad without much onion may be tried.

Suggested desserts are: simple puddings, custards, ice cream, jello, plain cake, and canned or stewed fruits, particularly pears and peaches. Cottage cheese is permissible; other cheeses often cause trouble. Apple, peach, apricot, custard, and lemon-cream pie may be tried if only the filling is eaten.

Make no effort to drink excess water. Be guided by your thirst. Avoid excessive use of salt or other seasoning.

ROUGHAGE IN THE DIET

Most domestic animals are capable of eating and digesting roughage in considerable amounts. A horse and cow eat hay and get nourishment from it, but a human being cannot. The cellulose of hay cannot be digested properly by the human digestive tract, and the material is passed rapidly through the intestines.

Most vegetables and fruits and whole-grain cereals contain cellulose, which serves to give bulk to the material in the bowel and in that way to give the intestines something to work on.

Cellulose may be sufficiently tender to be partially digested, as, for example, in the form of lettuce, fruits, and cooked vegetables, but in general it is not digested. Potatoes, beans, nuts, and olives have some cellulose, which may be utilized to a certain extent in the body, but in the majority of instances the cellulose is not properly utilized, except for roughage.

Cellulose is found in paper obtained from wood; cotton is practically pure cellulose, and the substance is also found in large amounts in bran. When water acts on cellulose it may swell it up somewhat, increasing its bulk still further.

Few people realize the danger of a diet containing too much cellulose. Such a diet interferes with digestion of the useful material, and it may irritate a sensitive intestinal tract, to the extent of causing an erosion or inflammation.

The bran of rice and wheat contains vitamins which may be of great value to the human body. The bran contains about 22 per cent of the protein of the wheat kernel. Bran proteins are relatively rich in those nutritionally-essential amino acids that are deficient in the endosperm of wheat. However, nature has seen to it that the vitamins are available in many forms, and it is not necessary to overload the intestines with roughage to secure a sufficient amount of any one vitamin.

The various vitamin B components are found in the bran of cereals, and in the embryo of cereals as well. Incidentally, the fiber of the green and yellow vegetables serves as a cleanser of the bowel and is not harsh enough to irritate. Too much bran can easily irritate the bowel.

LOW CHOLESTEROL DIET

The concept that an excess of cholesterol in the blood may lead to hardening of the arteries has led to use of low cholesterol diets. The eating of saturated animal fats in excess, such as butter, cream, eggs, and similar substances, may result in too much cholesterol in the blood. Particularly important in low cholesterol diets is the substitution for the animal fats of polyunsaturated fats derived from corn, peanuts, cottonseed, coconut oil, and similar sources. Special margarines have been prepared for use instead of butter. In general the recommendation is to reduce weight by lowering the total diet, particularly of fat, and in cases of extraordinarily high cholesterol to take a low cholesterol diet. However, many persons using an ordinary diet do not have high cholesterol levels in the blood and do not show any signs of atherosclerosis.

Loss and Gain of Weight

In each instance the physician, after determining the amount of cholesterol in the blood, will make the decision as to the special diet to be used.

Among recent medical discoveries are several drugs which have the special virtue of being able to lower cholesterol in the body. These, however, must be prescribed by the physician for the individual patient after a thorough study of the patient's condition, including particularly the amounts of cholesterol regularly in the blood and also after eating. Among the drugs most widely known are Atromid-S, Choloxin, Cytellin, Nicalex, and Vastran Forte. Since cholesterol is a normal constituent of the skin and of other tissues of the body, including the brain, the dosage must be carefully controlled. The drug is not prescribed for people who have impaired liver or kidney function. Most doctors are inclined to recommend attempts to control the cholesterol by diet before prescribing these potent remedies.

CHAPTER XV

VITAMIN DEFICIENCIES

VITAMIN C

THE DISCOVERY that the lack of certain essential substances in the body —either because they were not in the diet or failed to be absorbed and utilized—would cause serious disturbances of growth and health, was one of the most startling in all the history of medicine. Now these substances are called "vitamins"—a word coined by Casimir Funk around 1910.

Scurvy—a disease known for centuries—is now definitely established as resulting from a lack of vitamin C, also called ascorbic acid. The chief sources of vitamin C are the citrus fruits, the leafy green vegetables, Irish potatoes, and tomatoes. Milk contains a little vitamin C but even this little is lessened by pasteurization, or boiling, or any form of treatment that results in oxygenation.

Physicians see few cases of scurvy nowadays. Such cases as are reported affect chiefly people who live alone on greatly restricted diets, or people addicted to strange eating habits which interfere with normal nutrition. Sometimes the condition is seen in babies fed artificially, when mothers or nurses have failed to make certain that proper amounts of vitamin C-containing substances are included in the diet.

Among the chief symptoms of scurvy are bleeding from the gums and black and blue spots over the body, showing easy bleeding. Wounds of the skin heal slowly in those with vitamin C deficiency.

Scurvy can be controlled by taking plenty of vitamin C, which is now available in several medicinal forms. The material need not be injected into the blood but can be taken by mouth, after which the condition usually clears up promptly. Much better is the prevention of scurvy by the daily taking of some citrus fruit juice, tomato juice, or by eating leafy green vegetables, which add other important factors to the diet.

NICOTINIC ACID DEFICIENCY—PELLAGRA

The chief symptoms of pellagra, which is associated with a deficiency of niacin or nicotinic acid, include a red inflammation of the skin, a burning red tongue and mouth, diarrhea, and, in late stages, some mental disturbance. Many people in backward areas of the United States live on diets consisting largely of cornmeal, fat meat and molasses. The meat is usually salt pork or side meat. The chief deficiency in such diets is the lack of animal protein such as milk, cheese, lean meat, and eggs, and the failure of the diet in leafy green vegetables. Apparently exposure to sunlight of a person who is deficient in niacin brings out the symptoms.

Almost 7,000 people died of pellagra in the United States in 1928. The educational campaign on proper nutrition has been so effective that few cases or deaths are now reported.

While few cases of the complete development of pellagra are seen nowadays, there may be many instances of beginning symptoms or what doctors call a "subacute condition." First come such symptoms as fatigue and loss of appetite. Then, following exposure to the sun, the burning and stinging of the skin appears and next the soreness of the mouth and tongue. With these symptoms the patient is nervous, irritable, and finds difficulty in sleeping.

Since the condition is a deficiency disease, the treatment is primarily the taking of adequate amounts of niacin, which is now available in several forms. If the condition is severe the doctor will inject the niacin rather than give it by mouth. The diet can be provided with the important niacin-containing foods. The doctor will look after the patient's skin condition and make sure that he gets proper nursing care during the severe symptoms of the disease. Some physicians give large doses of liver extract. With proper treatment patients improve rapidly.

RIBOFLAVIN DEFICIENCY

The vitamin B complex includes not only niacin and thiamin but also riboflavin and other substances. When riboflavin is deficient the symptoms noted include principally fissures and soreness at the corner of the mouth, redness of the white portion, or cornea, of the eye with pain on seeing strong light, and also some changes in the tongue and skin.

Seldom is a deficiency of riboflavin observed alone, since it is so closely associated with other portions of the vitamin B complex. Most of the symptoms are regularly associated with pellagra, which is chiefly the result of lack of niacin.

Dr. William Darby has described the appearances around the corners of the mouth which are typical. First the lips get pale at the corners, then they seem chewed or softened, after which the fissures appear. As these heal, pink scars appear. The sore spots may become covered with crusts. The surface of the tongue gets a mushroom-like appearance and the color has been described as magenta.

Patients with ariboflavinosis complain of a sandy feeling of the eyelids, with blurring of vision and burning on exposure to strong light. As in pellagra these patients have a record of failure to include in their diets such substances as lean meat, green leafy vegetables, milk, eggs or liver.

Once the diet of the patient is supplemented with adequate amounts of the food mentioned, the symptoms disappear. In difficult cases doctors prescribe a normal dosage of riboflavin itself. Since, however, few patients have an uncomplicated shortage of riboflavin, but rather a shortage of all of the vitamin B complex and since B complex is so easy to secure and administer, the whole B complex is given.

THIAMIN DEFICIENCY

The chief symptoms of a disease called "beriberi" are due to a lack of one of the portions of the vitamin B complex called thiamin. Thiamin is soluble in water, damaged by heat and found chiefly in whole cereals, peas, beans, lean meats, nuts and yeast. Refined sugar, milled rice and low-extraction flour have lost most of their thiamin.

People whose diets are low in protein and high in carbohydrates are likely to show symptoms of thiamin deficiency. In the United States the condition is seen often among chronic alcoholics who get insufficient amounts of the right foods because of their displacement by alcohol.

The chief damages to tissues of the body seen in thiamin deficiency are found in the nerves and in the heart and blood vessels. Often these tissues become swollen with water. After about three months on a diet really deficient in thiamin the symptoms begin to appear. Gradually the person becomes tired and irritable and the muscles, particularly those of the calf of the leg, become painful. Later serious inflammations of the nerves appear, and these may go on to the point of loss of sensation and paralysis. When neuritis becomes so prominent, the doctor must make sure that it does not result from some other cause, since lead or arsenic poisoning or various infections may also cause neuritis.

As soon as a sufficient intake of thiamin is assured the patient begins to improve. Thiamin is now available in the form of tablets or capsules that can be taken internally, and also in forms that can be injected into the body when prompt action is desired. If treatment is begun sufficiently early most patients recover rapidly and completely. If treatment is delayed until actual destruction of nerve tissue has occurred, results are doubtful.

VITAMIN A DEFICIENCY

The most prominent manifestations of a deficiency of vitamin A include difficulty in adapting to the dark, followed by night blindness and a serious inflammation of the eyes that may end with loss of sight. Other important changes affect the skin. The deficiency may be due to an insufficient intake of vitamin A or carotene, from which it is formed in the body, or in failure of the body to absorb and utilize these materials. We know now that inflammations of the liver may interfere with the body's use of vitamin A. Mineral oil taken in large amounts prevents the absorption of vitamin A. The condition affects infants more often than adults, since infants require the vitamin both for growth and maintenance of certain structures. The liver can store enough vitamin A to carry the body along for six to ten months.

The changes in the skin associated with a deficiency of vitamin A include a generalized dryness and the growth of horny plugs called "hyperkeratoses" over the extensor surfaces of the limbs, the back, and the buttocks. Another manifestation is the appearance of grayish-white spots on the white portion of the surface of the eye.

When a shortage of vitamin A is noted, the condition should be corrected immediately by including in the diet such foods as butter, vitamin-enriched margarine and cod liver oil, which provide plenty of vitamin A. If symptoms have occurred, extra vitamin may be given as a capsule containing up to 25,000 units daily, which is about five times the usual required daily intake.

Cases are known in which people have taken tremendous quantities of this vitamin, even up to 250,000 units of vitamin A per day. Large excesses many cause serious changes in the liver, the spleen, the blood and the hair and nails.

VITAMIN D DEFICIENCY

Rickets, due to a deficiency of vitamin D, is far less frequent nowadays than formerly. Vitamin D may be taken into the body as such in foods or cod liver or halibut liver oil, or it may be formed by action of sunlight on the skin. The ultraviolet rays of the sun are important in this respect. In our industrialized cities most children get little direct sunlight. Dark-skinned people get less ultraviolet than blond, thin-skinned people. Heavy clothing and window glass also prevent the passage of ultraviolet rays.

Children with rickets have beading of the ribs. They are irritable, restless, fretful, and pale. Most significant, however, are the failures of growth of bones and teeth. The head begins to appear overlarge, with prominent frontal bones; little soft areas may be felt in the bones of the skull. There appear enlargements in the region of the wrist and ankles and the legs get distorted into bowlegs, knock-knees, and there are pelvic deformities. The X-ray quickly reveals the extent of the deformities.

Rickets can be prevented by exposure to ultraviolet rays from the sun or an artificial source, but the giving of 400 to 800 units of vitamin D per day is much more certain. Nowadays milk containing vitamin D in adequate amounts is generally available in the United States. When a real deficiency is present vitamin D may be given in one of many different forms including fish liver oils, viosterol, tablets or other preparations.

Excessive vitamin D intake results in a condition called hypervitaminosis D, with many distressing symptoms. Excess calcium may be deposited in various tissues of the body. Stopping the vitamin D promptly gets rid of the annoying symptoms.

VITAMIN B_{12} DEFICIENCY

A disease quite recently included among the deficiency diseases is sprue, observed chiefly in the tropics but seen occasionally also in the United States. Most authorities now classify sprue among the conditions associated with the absence of sufficient vitamin B_{12} or the animal protein factor in the diet. Similar conditions to those prevailing in sprue are also seen, however, in a rather unusual condition called celiac disease, which occurs in infants and in idiopathic steatorrhea. In these latter conditions the patient has difficulty in handling fats in the digestive tract. The primary symptom in sprue is difficulty in the formation of the blood, and with it inflammation of the mouth and tongue and difficulty in absorbing fat.

Vitamin Deficiencies

Most frequent among the symptoms of sprue are diarrhea, indigestion, distention of the abdomen, soreness of the mouth and tongue, loss of weight and, with all this, weakness. The condition is likely to come on gradually in people who have been long on a monotonous low-protein diet. The patients are pale, thin, and sometimes have eruptions of the neck, face and hands and extreme redness of the tongue and mouth. Doctors make certain of the diagnosis by using the X-ray and by making studies of the blood and the bone marrow, where the red blood cells are formed.

Fortunately such preparations as liver extract, folic acid, vitamin B_{12}, vitamin K, and a good diet high in protein bring prompt relief to patients with sprue. The symptoms begin to disappear in a few days and in a few weeks, unless there has been too much damage to the tissues, the patient is well on the way to complete recovery.

A deficiency of vitamin B_{12} is observed also in pernicious anemia and this vitamin is used to produce prompt recovery in this condition.

CHAPTER XVI

THE INTERNAL SECRETING
OR ENDOCRINE GLANDS

ABOUT ONE HUNDRED YEARS have passed since a scientist who removed the sex glands of a rooster found that the animal could be restored to its masculine vigor by transplanting into its tissue the glands of another rooster. Later a British doctor named Addison described a disease due to insufficiency of action of the adrenal glands which is now known as "Addison's disease." In 1889 a French scientist named Brown-Séquard attracted world attention by the claim that the injection into his own body of male sex hormone had produced a rejuvenating effect. It didn't work with him, and it still doesn't work to produce rejuvenation or restore lost sex power, notwithstanding the imaginative and emotional claims of a few too-credulous scientists. Nevertheless, the new knowledge of the glands, most of which has developed since 1900, is one of the greatest contributions ever made to human health and happiness.

From the point of view of chemical study four types of hormones are known, including those, like insulin, which have large protein molecules, those, like ACTH, which are called polypeptides, those, like thyroxin and adrenalin, which are aromatic derivatives, and the steroid hormones which include Cortisone and the sex hormones.

Much has been learned about hormones from the study of animals in which the glands can be removed and in which other glands can be transplanted to determine the effects. Similarly glandular materials may be given to human beings and the effects then studied. Sometimes a tumor will cause overgrowth and overactivity of a gland. The results are reflected by various changes in the body and in its functions.

THE PITUITARY GLAND

Perhaps the most important of the glands is the pituitary, although disturbance of any of the glands of internal secretion is serious. The

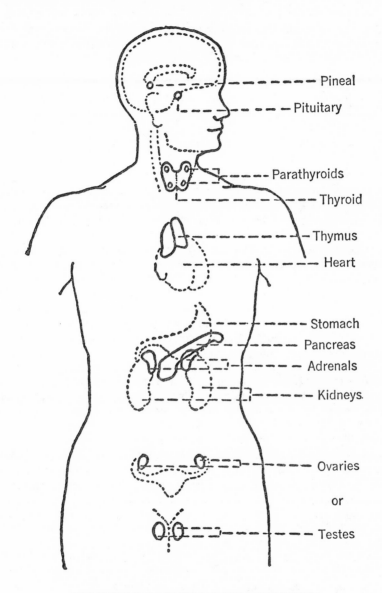

Pineal

Pituitary

Parathyroids

Thyroid

Thymus

Heart

Stomach

Pancreas

Adrenals

Kidneys.

Ovaries

or

Testes

THE IMPORTANT GLANDS IN THE HUMAN BODY

glands include the anterior and posterior pituitary, the thyroid, the pancreas, the thymus, the adrenals and the sex glands. Among the hormones that have been identified in the anterior pituitary are a growth hormone which can increase height and raise body weight.

The anterior pituitary also develops substances which pass by way of the blood to the adrenal gland, the thyroid, the sex glands and the milk-producing glands and influence their function. Recent studies have shown that the pituitary itself may be stimulated to act by adrenalin coming from the adrenal glands and by nervous stimuli coming from the emotional center in the brain. Since so many differently acting substances are developed in the pituitary, disturbances of this gland may be reflected in the body in many different ways.

Lessened activity of the pituitary gland before a child reaches adolescence may be observed as dwarfism and subnormal mentality and sexual development. However, deficiencies of growth also result from deficient action of the thyroid gland, and instances are known in which dwarfism is hereditary. The failure of the pituitary gland may be due to deficient development or to infection or to the presence of tumors which may damage the gland. While substitute materials for the whole anterior pituitary have not yet been developed satisfactorily, some of the deficiencies can be corrected by giving thyroid, or sex gland, or adrenal cortex materials. Research has been given such a tremendous push by the discovery of Cortisone and ACTH that the outlook is more bright now than ever previously.

In the pituitary gland lies the function of creating a substance which is known as the growth hormone. This acts directly on the growth of body tissues. A dwarf is a person who is conspicuously smaller than other people of the same age and species. For normal growth a person must have proper amounts of the necessary food substances. The body takes this material and puts it into proper places as new tissue. People may be stunted in their growth from lack of essential foods or lack of oxygen. In addition, the body must develop for itself the growth hormone, thyroid hormone and sex hormone. Among other causes of dwarfism are diseases or failure of growth of bones, such as may occur with rickets.

Often children have been much smaller than others all through the period of childhood. When they pass into adolescence the body fails to make the spurt that is usual. Not only do they fail to grow in height but also they remain mentally and sexually immature. In some instances this is just a delay in action of the interlocking chain of glands that includes the pituitary, adrenal and sex glands.

The treatment of dwarfism depends on the cause. If a deficiency of essential proteins and vitamins is responsible, supply of these substances will bring about growth. Similarly, thyroid deficiency can be met by giving thyroid extract. Pituitary growth hormone has not yet been developed for general use. In many cases of delayed adolescence doctors can now prescribe certain of the sex hormones with excellent results. The determination of which to give and the time and duration of treatment must be decided for each patient according to the conditions found when the patient is studied. Startling results have been secured by injecting human growth hormones in cases of delayed growth.

If an excess of growth hormone develops in childhood before the centers from which bones grow have ceased to function, the child becomes a giant. If the excess of growth hormone comes after this time, the condition called acromegaly develops. At the beginning the giant may be strong, alert, and intelligent, but in most cases as the giant growth continues the pituitary functions lessen; then the giant becomes weak and slow. Giants naturally attract much attention. Several cases have been recorded of growth over eight feet.

Usually in acromegaly excessive glandular tissue is found in the anterior pituitary gland. Such people may have enlargements of the lungs and liver and other organs as well as general increase in growth. Acromegaly is a relatively rare condition. Attention is called to it first by the increased size of the head, hands and feet. Fatigue, headache, and muscle pain may be noticed. Among the most observed signs is the enlargement of the lower jaw. The features become larger and coarsened, the skin becomes rough and the ridges above the eyes become prominent. A voracious appetite is often noticed and sometimes is blamed for the growth changes.

Acromegaly is not a fatal condition, and many of these patients live to advanced years. Some of the people develop diabetes because of changes in the glands. Formerly, operation on the pituitary gland was recommended for most of these patients but more recently the overgrowth of glandular tissue has been found to be susceptible to the X-ray. Often exposure of the tissue to X-ray will stop the progress of the acromegaly.

Since sex-gland disturbances are frequently associated with acromegaly the provision of male or female sex hormones as needed may be most helpful. Altogether, much more may now be done for such people by giving proper amounts of the glandular substances available.

While the front portion of the pituitary gland provides a number of hormones—substances circulating in the blood—which stimulate the thyroid, the adrenals and other glands to perform their functions, the posterior or back portion of the pituitary gland has quite different effects. When injected into the body, extracts similar to those provided by the back portion of the gland act to stimulate the muscle in the walls of the intestine, the muscle of the uterus and that in the walls of the blood vessels. Hence the bowel is made active, and the blood vessels contract. Thus this substance is used to stop hemorrhages after childbirth. The substance also has a profound effect on the action of the kidneys, controlling the way in which they eliminate water. If, therefore, there is a deficiency of the substance that comes from the posterior portion of the pituitary gland, people develop a condition called *diabetes insipidus* in which large amounts of fluid are poured out of the body. This condition is rare; in fact, a large clinic found only about twelve such cases in 100,000 patients.

The chief symptoms of *diabetes insipidus* are the pouring out of great amounts of water from the body and, naturally associated with it, the taking in of tremendous quantities of water. The amounts may reach fifteen to twenty quarts a day. Because of the excess elimination of fluid, these people have a dry skin and an insatiable thirst. Under the circumstances, the condition is usually treated by giving the substance which is known as "pitressin." Two different substances have been isolated, one of which has the power of contracting the muscle of the intestines and uterus as its chief function, and the other of which controls the elimination of fluid.

THYROID

The activity of the thyroid gland is apparently controlled by the hormone that comes from the pituitary gland. For a variety of reasons, the thyroid gland may be inactive or excessively active. Inactivity of the thyroid may result in the condition called cretinism which is associated with a deficiency of the thyroid gland in early childhood, and the condition called myxedema which comes on later in life. The person with myxedema has a typical face with puffy eyelids, and an apparent lack of interest in what is going on. The skin is dry and rough, the hair coarse, brittle and dry. Because the tongue and throat are swollen, the speech is slow and slurred. With this there is a tendency to slowing of all of the functions of the body and, because of the deficiencies of the blood and the circulation, the person with myxedema is sensitive to cold.

Since the condition is so certainly due to a lack of thyroid material, the treatment includes the giving of thyroid, and the dosage is adjusted according to the need of the patient and his response to the drug. Customarily doctors will begin with exceedingly small doses, because the thyroid is a potent material and overdosage may result in a rapid heart, sweating, loss of weight, and diarrhea. The maximum effect from any dose is not apparent until seven to ten days after the use of the drug is first begun, and the action will persist for one to three weeks after the drug is discontinued. The dosage of thyroid needs to be taken only once a day since, usually, nothing is gained by dividing it over the day.

As people grow old the thyroid function may lessen and many elderly people benefit by taking thyroid substance.

CRETINISM

The lack of sufficient secretion from the thyroid gland during early life, as mentioned previously, results in delayed development which is called cretinism. If a child develops normally and then begins to show evidences of lack of thyroid the case is called "acquired hypothyroidism." The condition may appear as a failure of the thyroid gland to grow or as a result of failure of the pituitary gland to stimulate the thyroid by sending the pituitary secretion necessary for this purpose. The latter failure is rare.

No one sign is typical of cretinism or insufficient thyroid, but a combination is well-nigh unmistakable. The child has physical and mental torpor. The circulation of the blood is poor. In fact, all the activities of the body are under par, including the muscle tone, sweating, and the activity of the bowel. The growth, including bones and teeth, hair and brain, is stunted. The skin is thickened and coarse and fluid accumulates under the skin. The cretin is sluggish and shows little interest in what goes on around him.

The child with deficient action of the thyroid responds rapidly to treatment with thyroid extract. Almost immediately there is improvement in color and warmth of the skin. Within a few weeks there is a loss of weight as the body gets rid of the extra fluid. Almost immediately, growth begins again. Because of this prompt benefit there may be a tendency to give more and more thyroid, and this will have bad results as shown in heightened excitability, nervousness and a rise in the blood pressure.

The earlier a diagnosis can be made and the sooner treatment can be begun the better. Sometimes the damage to the brain by just a few months deficiency may be so severe that it is difficult if not impossible to overcome. Such children may become irritable and unmanageable after treatment, and the doctor must determine the amount of thyroid necessary to keep the child under control.

EXCESS ACTION OF THE THYROID

Although the condition called hyperthyroidism, which is due to excessive action of the thyroid gland, was first observed around 1830, a really complete understanding of the condition did not develop until 1890. Excessive action of the thyroid may occur at any age. The condition is much more frequent in women than in men. In areas in which goiter is infrequent, women may have excessive action of the thyroid gland in a proportion of four women to one man.

The exact cause of excessive action of the thyroid gland is not known, but the most frequently accepted view at this time is that the body responds to stress, either emotional, physical, or infectious, by excessive action of the pituitary gland which in turn overstimulates the thyroid gland. If this condition goes on, such symptoms may develop as bulging of the eyes, which is a part of exophthalmic goiter; and there may be enlargement of the thyroid gland, although there are cases in which the thyroid gland is enlarged without other symptoms. The person who is overstimulated by thyroid is nervous, irritable and emotionally unstable. He perspires a great deal. Frequently shortness of breath and palpitation occur because of overstimulation of the heart. In every such case the doctor will want to watch the heart carefully. The basal metabolism test usually shows excess consumption of oxygen and is not specifically a test of the function of the thyroid gland. There are other conditions which can cause excess consumption of oxygen besides overactivity of the thyroid. The doctor who finds that a patient has a large excess of thyroid action will want therefore to make other tests, as of the pulse and the temperature, the manner in which the body uses iodine, and the response of the body to the taking of iodine.

Since excessive action of the thyroid is due to secretion of too much hormone or glandular substance, treatment of the condition includes a number of different procedures. The certain method is removal of a portion of the thyroid gland by surgery, with or without the use of such drugs as propylthiouracil which diminish thyroid activity. In some cases, combined with the propylthiouracil is the giving of iodine, which has an antithyroid action.

Radioiodine, which is a radioactive form of this substance, is now used to treat excessive action of the thyroid gland. Formerly similar effects were secured by the use of the X-ray but the use of radioactive iodine is now considered to be far preferable by most experts.

In some cases excessive action of the thyroid may be so great that serious symptoms develop, including fever, an exceedingly rapid beating of the heart and even prostration. Obviously, this condition is so serious that the patient should be under the immediate care of a doctor, since he may require oxygen and prompt treatment to control the heart and the fever.

The bulging of the eye in exophthalmic goiter, or as it is now preferably called, *thyrotoxic exophthalmos,* is a condition which can be controlled somewhat if recognized promptly, but not so much can be done if the person waits until permanent changes have taken place in the tissue around the eye. The bulging may disappear promptly following treatment of the excessive action of the thyroid. In other instances, the condition may be so severe that surgery is necessary to decompress the tissue around the eye.

SIMPLE GOITER

The bulging in the throat that is due to enlargement of the thyroid gland was apparently recognized by the Chinese at least as early as 1500 B.C. Such is indicated by drawings and other historical records. Indeed, the people used to overcome the condition in the Middle Ages by eating burned sponge and seaweed which are rich in iodine. Not until 1916, however, was the evidence accumulated that made it certain that small doses of iodine taken frequently by the patient living in areas in which there are small amounts of iodine in the soil and in the water will prevent simple goiter.

Certain substances have been recognized as having the power to stimulate goiter, but goiter caused by these substances—like thiocyanates or cabbage, which cause a lessening of thyroid hormone—is infrequent.

The chief symptoms of goiter are, of course, the enlargement and bulging in the throat due to the large size of the gland. There are cases, however, in which the enlargement becomes so great that it may even interfere with breathing or injure the voice by pressure on the nerves that go to the larynx. The prevention of such enlargement of the gland by the taking of small doses of iodine regularly during the period of childhood and adolescence is now well established. Iodized salt is now commonly used, so that the iodine is taken regularly in this manner. In cases of severe enlargement of the gland obviously removal by surgery is desirable.

PARATHYROID GLANDS

Behind and near to the thyroid gland are other glands which are known as parathyroid glands, their chief function being control of the use of calcium and phosphorus by the body. Apparently this gland responds with secretion of its hormone when the amounts of calcium and phosphorus in the serum of the blood become insufficient. However, extracts of the parathyroid gland have been prepared and are used in cases where people apparently suffer from a lack of parathyroid hormone. The lack of this hormone is made evident by such symptoms as tremors of the body, called "tetany," which occurs also with insufficiency of calcium. The tetany or tremors, which are like muscle spasms or cramps, are due to extra excitability of the nerves controlling the muscles.

Obviously the condition may be controlled by giving extra calcium directly into the blood or by taking large amounts of calcium by mouth. The condition may also be controlled by direct injection of the parathyroid hormone. Calcium is also controllable through the use of vitamin D or of a substance like vitamin D called dihydrotachysterol. The action of this substance is more like the action of the parathyroid hormone than is vitamin D itself.

In the treatment of this condition, the diet should be one which contains much calcium and relatively little phosphorus. The foods which are rich in calcium are milk and cheese products and the leafy green vegetables. Milk also, however, includes phosphorus, as does egg yolk, cauliflower and molasses.

As might be expected, excessive action of the parathyroid glands results in changes of the bones of the body, because the bones are largely made up of calcium. Since the parathyroid glands so definitely control the use of calcium by the body, some have thought that kidney stones might be due to some action of the parathyroid glands. This has not, however, been established with certainty. Cases of excessive action of the parathyroid gland can occur without any evident changes in the bones and, in fact, the condition may be more frequent than is now suspected. There may be excessive growth of the tissues of the parathyroid glands which can result in excessive activity.

When large amounts of extra calcium are found in the blood and with that muscular weakness, loss of appetite, and pain in the bones, and, not infrequently, excessive elimination of fluid through the kidneys, the physician suspects excessive action of the parathyroid glands. There are many different conditions which can interfere with the growth of bones, so that studies of the blood as to the amount of calcium and the manner in which the body handles calcium are fundamental in discovering whether or not disturbance of the bone growth is due to excessive action of the parathyroid gland, or to some other cause.

Since vitamin D has become available as a concentrate, and since people have been taking exceedingly large doses of vitamin D to treat a variety of conditions, difficulty has occurred in recognizing the difference between excessive vitamin D in the body and excessive action of the parathyroid glands.

In every case of hyperparathyroidism the possibility of surgical removal of excess tissue of the parathyroids must be considered as primary in the treatment.

THE ADRENAL GLANDS

Just above the kidneys lie glands which in recent years have assumed so much significance that the knowledge concerning them has created a new era in medicine.

The adrenal glands contain two portions, known as inner and outer, or medulla and cortex. The inner portion of the adrenal glands is related to the sympathetic nervous system and provides the body with a substance that people call "adrenalin." This substance has other names, like epinephrine and suprarenin. There is no disease associated with insufficient action of the inner portion of the adrenal gland, because the body can compensate through other mechanisms for lessening secretion. Excessive functioning of the medulla of the adrenal gland is associated with paroxysmal periods of high blood pressure and other signs of excessive stimulation of the sympathetic nervous system, including dizziness, sweating, a rapid pulse, palpitation, and changes in the blood. Since tumors may occur in the adrenal gland as well as elsewhere in the body, a tumor of the inner portion of the adrenal gland is accompanied by all of these symptoms. This indicates surgical removal of such tumors as soon as their presence is determined.

The outer portion of the adrenal gland is a shell made up of cells which create hormones called "steroid hormones." At present, physiologists believe that there are as many as twenty-six different hormones developed by the cortex of the adrenal gland. Six of these have been isolated and two of them are known as Compounds E and F or Cortisone and Cortone. The cortex of the adrenal gland is stimulated to give off these hormones by a substance coming from the pituitary gland called ACTH or adrenal cortex *trophic hormone.*

Among other functions, the hormones from the cortex of the adrenal gland can regulate the distribution and secretion of sodium, potassium and chlorides by the body; they can regulate the water balance; they are concerned with the quantities of carbohydrates, protein, and fat used in the chemistry of the body; increasing particularly the use of protein and fat, and lessening the use of carbohydrates. They are concerned with the development of certain types of cells in the blood. They are also related to the keeping of nitrogen in the body, and they are related to the action of the sex hormones. Failure of the cortex of the adrenal gland to supply its hormones may create a variety of conditions, as will also excessive action.

When there is an insufficiency of the adrenal cortical material, the person suffers from insufficient sugar in the blood and from a variety of symptoms such as pain, lassitude, nausea, and circulatory collapse. A brown pigmentation of the skin appears which is typical of the disease known as "Addison's disease," named after the British physician who first recognized this condition. An extract of the adrenal cortex called *desoxycorticosterone acetate* has been prepared, which can be used to overcome the condition of disturbance of the handling of salts and water by the body.

Many tests have been devised which laboratories can perform to show the extent to which the cortex of the adrenal gland is doing its work. Excessive functioning of the gland may result in the development of conditions such as serious changes in the bones, swellings of the face and trunk, weakness and wasting of the muscles, thinning of the skin and difficulty in healing of wounds. Apparently the body must maintain a balance between the action of the various hormones coming from the pituitary and adrenal glands, because imbalance may result in serious changes in growth. In women, for instance, a condition called virilism may develop, with appearance of hair on the chest and face, rapid growth, and interference with usual functions.

CORTISONE

From the adrenal cortex come hormones now called Cortisone and many derivatives such as Meticortin[R], Kenacort[R] and Prednisone or Prednisolone are available. This hormone has a definite relationship to many different conditions, some of which have already been mentioned in previous chapters.

Both the cortex and the medulla of the adrenal gland are important in enabling the human being to adapt himself to conditions of stress. The adrenalin, as has been mentioned, is closely associated with the sympathetic nervous system. The hormones of the cortex help the body build resistance to all sorts of damaging influences, such as cold, heat, burns, exhaustion, fasting, chemical agents, and even bruises. The hormones help the body to maintain adequate amounts of sugar in the blood. Among the conditions that have been treated successfully with Cortisone and with ACTH—which stimulates the production of Cortisone—are the allergic reactions such as asthma, hay fever, and serum sickness. Remarkable results have been achieved in treatment of acute rheumatic fever with termination of the attack and apparently, in some cases, complete control. Rheumatoid arthritis, *lupus erythematosus* and *polyarteritis nodosa* are conditions now believed to result from sensitivities of the tissues to certain substances and which have responded favorably to treatment with Cortisone. Even certain infections and some serious conditions affecting the blood have responded favorably. Apparently the conditions are not a result of a deficiency of the hormones, but rather that these hormones in some way alter the reactions of the tissues in the body.

Again one should realize that ACTH and Cortisone are not identical. ACTH can stimulate the secretion of all types of hormones of the adrenal, including those concerned with water and salt, sugars, and the sex hormones.

Aldosterone is another adrenocortical hormone concerned particularly with metabolism of salts and water in the body.

THE PANCREAS—DIABETES

The pancreas is a gland which lies near the liver, stomach, and duodenum. It has a number of secretions, some of which go directly into the intestine and are concerned with digestion. One secretion goes instead into the blood and is intimately concerned with the way in which the body uses sugars. This substance is called insulin. A deficiency of insulin in the body results in a chronic disease called diabetes mellitus. Diabetes has been known for thousands of years and was described by ancient Greek and Chinese writers, who were principally concerned with the large amounts of fluids excreted by the body in this condition. The fact that the urine contained sugar was first noted in the seventeenth century. Not until 1889 was it proved that diabetes results from failure of the pancreas. In 1921 Banting prepared an extract of the pancreas which is now called insulin. At least a million people now in the United States have diabetes, and the number increases, because the condition tends to come on with advanced years. More than half the people with diabetes develop the condition before they are fifty years old. Women are affected more frequently than men, particularly in diabetes in advanced years.

Studies of diabetes show that heredity plays an important part. This relationship is becoming more and more clear as people with diabetes tend to live longer and have more children. Once diabetes in childhood was considered invariably fatal. Now these children grow up, marry, and have families. We now know that if both parents are diabetic, the children will most certainly inherit the disease. Overweight is also important in relationship to diabetes. Not everyone who is overweight develops the disease. In fact, diabetes is seen in only a small proportion of the people who are overweight. However, nine out of ten people who develop diabetes are overweight. Among those who are overweight and who develop diabetes, dieting and restoration to normal weight lessens the severity of the symptoms and sometimes controls the condition. The person who is overweight, however, can produce more and more insulin and this may be a factor in exhausting the function of the pancreas. As I have mentioned in previous articles, both the pituitary gland and the adrenal glands are also related in their functions to the use of sugar by the body. Excessive action of the pituitary gland may result in the appearance of sugar in the urine. Excessive action of the thyroid gland may make diabetes worse by increasing the work of the gland, through the fact that the person is taking in large amounts of food.

SYMPTOMS OF DIABETES

Chief among the symptoms of diabetes are general weakness, loss of weight, excessive appetite, thirst, and excessive flow of urine. Itching is a much noticed symptom. The first sign of severe diabetes may be loss of consciousness, which is called diabetic coma.

Children have the disease more severely than do adults, and doctors believe that the greater the age when diabetes begins the less severe is the disease.

Nowadays diabetes is usually discovered by an examination of the urine, and sugar is likely to be found most often if the test is made immediately after a meal. When sugar is found in the urine, studies must also be made of the amount of sugar in the blood, particularly after the person has been fasting. A normal person has a blood sugar level when fasting of approximately 70 milligrams per 100 milliliters of whole blood, whereas if the person has diabetes, the figure is nearer 150.

Simple tests have now been developed which people use themselves to get an indication as to whether or not there is sugar in the urine. When this is found, the physician should be asked to make all of the necessary studies to determine the severity of the condition and to prescribe treatment promptly in order to control the disease.

Diet and the use of insulin are the basic steps in controlling diabetes.

Since infections are exceedingly serious for persons who are diabetic, a complete study of the body should be made to eliminate any infections in the teeth, the sinuses, the chest, the gall bladder or elsewhere.

The diet is designed to bring the person to his ideal weight and to lessen the total amount of sugar taken into the body. Many persons do not require insulin immediately or when they are on the reduction diet. When insulin is required, the amount is given in relationship to the diet and the maintenance of normal weight. Patients must co-operate with the doctor in regulating the control of sugar in relation to insulin intake. Emotional stresses are serious. Infection may be severe, if not fatal. The diabetic patient must be kept clean. Immediate attention is given to all bruises and cuts of the skin. In caring for the nails the diabetic should avoid cutting or pushing of the cuticle. Most important is proper attention to the feet. These should be washed with warm water and a bland soap every day. They should be dried thoroughly but gently. Injuries to the feet must be avoided, and particularly injuries from the cutting of toenails or corns. Stockings should be clean, and loose-fitting but without wrinkles.

EXCESSIVE INSULIN

While deficiency of insulin, resulting in diabetes mellitus, is far more serious and more common than excessive action of the pancreas, cases do occur in which there is too much insulin, with a resulting low blood sugar. The sugar level of the blood is maintained by the body's use of glucose in the muscle, liver, brain, and other organs, and by the way in which the glucose is brought back into the blood from the liver and the muscles, and the secretion of insulin, which makes possible the use of sugars by the body.

Following meals or periods of excitement there may be excess sugar in the blood, so that the body puts out extra insulin tending then to lower the sugar below normal. In other instances there may be low blood sugar because of a deficiency of the liver in storing sugar. Other cases are known in which tumors affecting the cells of the pancreas may produce excess insulin and with that a low blood sugar.

Overactivity of the nervous system can cause excessive flow of insulin into the blood. In all these conditions the blood sugar becomes low; as a result, there is weakness and faintness, a rapid heart, anxiety and palpitation. When the person takes sugar or carbohydrates the symptoms are relieved.

A highly concentrated carbohydrate called Glucagon[R] is available for injection in cases of "too much insulin."

In general, people who have low blood sugar do well on diets that are high in protein and fats and low in sugar. When a high sugar diet is taken, the body reacts by putting out excessive insulin, which tends to lower the sugar below normal. Excessive secretion of insulin can be controlled by the taking of certain drugs such as derivatives of belladonna and atropine, but control of the emotional and dietary factors is considered a more satisfactory method of treating the condition.

THE SEX GLANDS

The glands of sex serve a double function: they provide the necessary materials for reproduction of the human being, the male sex cell uniting with the female sex cell; they also provide material which goes directly from the glands into the blood, and which determines the nature of the growth of the body. If the amount of the material secreted by the gland into the blood is insufficient, definite changes will take place in the body inclining toward the female side if the male sex tissue is insufficient, and to the masculine side in the woman if the female sex tissue is insufficient.

A deficiency of the male sex material may result from absence or destruction of the gland or from failure to function, in cases where the pituitary gland does not produce the trophic hormone that stimulates the male sex gland. Again, there may be disturbance of the function of the cells within the gland, without actual destruction of the tissue.

A deficiency of male glandular material varies in its effects according to the age at which it occurred. If the material is completely absent, the condition called "eunuchism" is developed; this usually refers to a complete loss. When the loss of sexual gland function takes place before the time of maturation into an adolescent, a deficiency is shown in growth. The skin is delicate; the hair that ordinarily covers the surface of the body of the male is absent; there also may be exaggerated length of the arms and legs with broad hips and a tendency toward the development of a "pot belly"; sometimes also the breast of the male will enlarge.

SEX GLAND DEFICIENCY

If a deficiency of sex gland hormone takes place after adolescence, the changes include a retardation of the growth of the beard and thinning of the skin with lessened pigmentation, and perhaps also a diminution or complete absence of hair under the arms and around the sex organs. Interestingly there is also a failure to grow hairs on the ear, which is rather typical of men past twenty-five or thirty years of age.

After men have matured and have reached the age of forty-five or fifty, they do not usually suffer the changes that come on in women about the same time and which are known as the "climacteric." The specialists believe that this is due to the fact that the sexual function of men declines gradually, rather than abruptly as occurs with women. The changes that occur in men are not visible in any way in the structure of the body, since this has been well established by the age of forty-five, but are more definitely related to the functions of the body and to symptoms that manifest themselves often in the nervous system.

When there is an absence of sex gland material, as is determined by some of the signs that have been described, administration of the artificially prepared material is now possible by the development of the glandular material called testosterone. The amount of the material to be given and the duration of the time over which it is to be given depends, of course, on the condition of the patient, whom the doctor watches carefully. Actually there may be the growth of pimples, and in the case of women a tendency toward a masculine appearance from too much sex gland material. There are also effects on the handling of salt and water by the body. It has been established that excesses of testosterone, particularly in young boys, may result in difficulty in the development of sperm cells necessary for reproduction.

EXCESSIVE MALE SEX GLAND ACTION

Excessive production of male sex hormones is observed in men particularly when there are tumors of the male sex glands. Such tumors have been observed by physicians in many cases. Occasionally excessive growth of tissue of the anterior pituitary gland or in other portions of the brain may stimulate the sex glands excessively, so that large amounts of male sex hormones are thrown into the circulation. The manifestations of excessive secretion vary with the time when the condition occurs. If it comes on before the young boy has reached puberty, the excessive gland material may cause puberty to come on much sooner than normally. Associated with this precocious pseudopuberty is a too-early development of all of the male sex characteristics, including excessive growth of the sex organs, the development of a large amount of hair around the sex organs and under the arms, and, even in little boys, the development of a beard and a mustache, a deep voice and similar conditions. Physicians have observed that excessive amounts of male sex gland material will cause increased secretion of the oil glands in the skin, and associated acne is not uncommon. There may often also be changes in the growth of the skeleton. In this instance, the trunk, the arms and legs are found to be short due to too-early closure of the points from which the bones grow. Associated also with these developments may be excessive and definitely increased muscular development and strength; the so-called "infant Hercules."

If the excessive secretion of glandular material comes on after the body has passed puberty, the condition manifests itself by accentuation of the masculine character. Obviously, the skeleton has already developed so that there cannot be effects on the skeleton.

The only known treatment for excessive activity is removal of the tumor which is responsible. Removal of portions of the tumor or of all of the tumor would naturally result in lessening the amount of sex gland material. This can be measured by chemical study so that the return to normal can be definitely known. If, however, the tumor material should return and grow again, the excess of glandular secretion can be determined through examination of the urine. In this way the physician can trace the progress of the tumor growth.

Fortunately tumors of the male sex gland are relatively rare. Doctors believe that these tumors occur more often when there has been failure of the male sex gland to descend into the sac, which it normally does before ten or eleven years of age, if not sooner. Experience has shown that the best thing to do whenever there is any tumor of this area is to have it removed by surgery as soon as possible. If the tumor is not a malignant tumor, it is in any event a threat. If, however, it is a malignant tumor, the growth quite certainly threatens life itself. In fact, so definitely is that threat known that it has become customary to use the X-ray to irradiate the area from which the tumor has been removed, to make certain that all excessive action has been stopped.

If the male sex gland is retained and fails to descend into the sac, its function may be destroyed by the heat to which it is subjected in the body.

Failure of sexual gland function causes psychosexual changes in the males, including loss of initiative and drive. Some psychiatrists feel this effect is wholly mental and results from a feeling of inferiority because the person knows of his deficiency.

Sexual precocity associated with excess of testosterone or androsterone has also been noted with adrenal and pituitary gland tumors.

OVARIES—FEMALE SEX GLANDS

The ovary, which is the female sex gland, has the function of preparing an egg cell called the "ovum." This is involved in reproduction. Following the development of this egg cell, the ovary prepares hormones or glandular materials which go into the blood and which are significant in the functioning of a woman's body. Menstruation of women periodically is largely regulated by these hormones from the ovary. The ovary, in turn, is regulated by hormones which come from the pituitary gland and which are necessary in order for ovulation to occur. Following ovulation the ovary develops a substance called the *corpus luteum* which provides a hormone called progesterone. Progesterone is responsible for the preparation of the uterus to receive the egg cell. When the egg cell fails to be fertilized, the uterus gets rid of the material by the usual flow.

The follicle which prepares the ovum or egg cell also is important in the formation of estrogen which is known as the female sex hormone. Although the function of the ovary was recognized as far back as 1673, only within recent years has this understanding of the glandular materials developed by the ovary come to light.

When a girl matures the flow occurs, which is usually seen between the ages of twelve and sixteen. This is a rhythmical or periodic function, taking place generally about every twenty-eight days although many cases are known in which the flow occurs at shorter or longer periods. Usually ovulation discontinues at the time of the menopause which generally takes place between forty-five and fifty-five years of age, the average being forty-eight. Estimates indicate that at the time when the girl matures there are approximately 300,000 possible egg cells ready for development. Only a few of these mature and eventually come to the surface.

After an ovum has been developed each month the follicle ruptures and the ovum travels by way of the Fallopian tubes into the uterus. If a male sex cell reaches the ovum and fertilizes it, the ovum remains in the uterus and pregnancy occurs.

In the absence of the female sex hormones, changes occur in the body of a woman which reflect the lack of these chemical regulators of the body.

OVARIAN DEFICIENCY

If the ovary is not adequate, or if it is absent following surgical

97

removal, an insufficient secretion of the female sex hormones occurs. Absence of such hormones is associated with a disappearance of the usual menstrual flow. Development of the body is complete and the characteristics of women which are peculiar to the sex disappear.

As with a deficiency of the male sex hormone, absence of ovarian secretion results in overgrowth of the long bones, which fail to close their points of growth during adolescence. An insufficiency of ovarian secretion may lead to failure of the sexual organs to develop, so that they appear infantile in type. Associated is a lack of development of the breast and a lack of the usual growth of hair under the arms and around the sex organs.

If there is an adequate amount of female sex hormone up to the time of puberty and a failure to secrete thereafter, the symptoms are different, because the child will have achieved rather full growth by the time it comes to adolescence.

Fortunately, substitutes for the usual hormones have been found. These can be prescribed by the doctor in amounts as needed, and thus cause a return to normal conditions.

As with the male sex hormone, the function of the ovary is dependent on the hormones that come from the pituitary or master gland in the brain. Failure of the pituitary gland to send its hormones will result in failure of the ovary to develop normally. With this comes lack of menstruation, lack of development of the breasts and delay in appearance of the other secondary female characteristics.

FAILING OVARIAN FUNCTION

If the ovary is not functioning following the time when the girl reaches adolescence, as may occur when there is a necessity for surgical removal or when cysts form in the ovary and destroy the ovarian tissue, a number of significant conditions may appear. One of the most important is development of irregularity of the usual rhythmic flow, sometimes culminating in complete absence of the flow. With this there is a tendency to put on too much weight, to grow extra hair and to develop a pasty skin.

Occasionally the menopause comes on in a woman long before she is forty-eight years of age. This is definitely abnormal. Such an occurrence should lead to an immediate medical examination because it may be associated with social and psychological difficulties. The doctor who is called to study such a patient can bring relief in many instances by prescribing the necessary hormones, according to the condition in each patient.

The menopause may occur quite suddenly. When it does, a number of serious symptoms may develop, including excessive flow and what are commonly called "hot flashes" with drenching sweats, the development of a ravenous appetite and a rapid gain in weight. There are also sometimes changes in the bones and joints, giving rise to the condition known as "menopausal arthritis." Obviously such symptoms are serious, affecting the entire life of the women concerned. They should be an indication for a complete and careful study of the case and for the administration of such hormones as might be considered by the physician to be desirable.

For the arthritis of the menopause, the use of Cortisone or ACTH has already been shown to be helpful in bringing about relief.

The physician always remembers that the glands are an interlocking chain and the source for disturbance may be not only the sex gland itself, but quite as often the pituitary gland or, occasionally, the thyroid gland. In any event, the psychologic aspects must be studied. It is impossible for anyone to treat himself successfully for disorders of glandular functions such as I have described.

EXCESSIVE OVARIAN ACTION

Excessive secretion of glandular materials from the ovary is manifested most often by disturbances of the usual rhythmical functions of women. The disturbance may be reflected in abnormal bleeding, frequent bleeding, excessive bleeding, or similar symptoms. Whenever there is irregularity in the duration or frequency of flow, a careful examination should be made to find out the cause.

Bleeding is a serious symptom whenever it occurs from any portion of the body. Any bleeding before the child has matured or after the cessation of the regular flow is an indication which demands immediate study. In over half of such cases the necessity for determining the presence of any serious growth is obvious.

Excessive action of the ovary before the time of maturation into adolescence is manifested by bleeding, associated with excessive development of the breasts and premature establishment of growth of hair under the arms and on the sex organs. Rapid growth of the skeleton and, occasionally, an interest in the opposite sex which is far above the normal may occur. All this is called "precocious puberty."

Any time the rhythmical flow is established before the age of ten, an investigation should be made. As in the case of men, the presence of tumors can cause excessive activity of any glandular organ, including the female sex glands.

As was previously mentioned, the mechanism for the process of reproduction is in women quite complicated. It begins with the coming of glandular materials from the pituitary gland which, in turn, stimulate the ovary to produce its egg cell regularly every twenty-eight days. Following the production of this cell, the ovary produces another hormone. This, in turn, is associated with the activity of the uterus. Hence any excessive activity of any portion of the glandular chain will bring about definite changes in the body of the woman concerned. The conditions are now known to be reflected in changes in the temperature of the woman and also in such changes as the pigmentation of the skin, the growth of hair on various portions of the body, irregular bleeding and many other symptoms. The one which concerns women most is, of course, bleeding. In the treatment of such bleeding a variety of hormones are used, depending on the nature of the condition, the time when it occurs, and the facts that are determined by the doctor following his examination.

THE THYMUS

Innumerable experiments have been made, both on human beings and on animals, to determine the exact functions of the thymus gland. Does it give off some substance directly into the blood—commonly called an internal secretion—which would affect the growth of the body?

When a child is born, the thymus is found as a closely packed mass of cells. This gland is large enough in many instances to occupy much of the space directly under the breastbone. Later in life the size of this glandular material decreases in relationship to the size of the body. Finally the gland disappears and is replaced by fat.

When there is a deficiency of material coming from the cortex of the adrenal gland the thymus is likely to enlarge, as well as the lymph glands elsewhere in the body. This has been called *status thymicolymphaticus*. Sometimes these patients die suddenly; death has been attributed to the enlargement of the thymus, whereas it was actually due to the deficiency of the secretion of the important material from the cortex of the adrenal gland.

Sometimes people who have a condition called *myasthenia gravis*, in which there is the development of serious weakness and incapacity, have been found to have enlargements of the thymus gland.

It has been thought that removal of this gland surgically or breakdown of the gland by exposing it to X-ray would be helpful in such cases. While some of the patients seem to improve, others do not.

One is not quite certain whether the improvement was merely a coincidence and would have occured anyway, or is in some way related to the treatment. Recently attempts have been made to treat this condition with ACTH. Some have said that great benefit has been brought about, but others indicate that cases have become worse. This would indicate that ACTH does have an effect in changing both the mental attitude of these patients and also perhaps the general constitution. The drug does not appear to be a specific drug for the treatment of *myasthenia gravis.*

Physicians now believe that the thymus, being composed of lymphoid tissue and containing a high concentration of essential substances, is a storehouse for aid of the body which is directly under control of other glands and a part of the interlocking gland system of the body. Research in 1962 establishes the great importance of the thymus in the ability of the body to form antibodies against infections and foreign proteins.

INFERTILITY

Infertility means inability of any species to conceive and to reproduce its kind. In general, the words infertility and sterility are used interchangeably. Estimates indicate that approximately 10 per cent of married couples are unable to reproduce or have children. The reasons vary according to the many different aspects of the problem.

The difficulty may be due to inability of the sperm cells of the male to travel into the female tract because of some obstruction in either the male or the female. Obviously studies must be made as to this condition on both husband and wife, before any positive decision is reached. Difficulties with glands are relatively insignificant because they are exceedingly uncommon. Psychologic and emotional disturbances may lead to complete disorganization of both the male and female sexual activities. Certainly emotional causes may make it impossible for a man to be potent sexually.

There are of course cases in which either the male or female sex glands may be deficient in their reproduction of the necessary cells. Before a doctor will give a definite diagnosis he must make extensive and careful studies as to the marriage relationship and the general physical and mental conditions of both husband and wife, with particular attention to the sex organs and glands. He will have to study the question of dietary, glandular, or other disturbances. He may find it

101

necessary to call in psychiatric consultation when the preliminary studies indicate the difficulties are chiefly mental or emotional.

In many instances physicians have found that detailed sex education is all that is necessary, because of some wrong sexual pattern that a married couple may have adopted. In the treatment of such conditions the use of both male and female sex glandular materials has been helpful in a few instances. Sometimes the difficulty is in the pituitary gland or in the ovary or in the male sex gland. In some instances, even, the giving of thyroid extract has been helpful as a sort of general glandular stimulation. Study of the sex cycle is also important, since there are certain periods when the woman is much more fertile than others, and the intensive efforts toward having a child may be concentrated in this period.

CHAPTER XVII

DISORDERS OF BONES

THE SKELETON WHICH SUPPORTS THE STRUCTURE of the human body is composed of bone; this consists of protein materials in which a calcium phosphate and carbonate combination constitutes the hard material. The bone is naturally fed with blood, and the blood removes material from the bony skeleton.

Various diseases may seriously damage the system by which the bone is formed and may also bring about destruction of bone. I have already mentioned the importance of the hormones that come from the parathyroid glands in their relationship to the growth of bone. Certain general disturbances of the body chemistry may also influence the bones unfavorably. People who have remained long infirm will have changes in the bone structure of lower parts of the body, whereas the bones of the jaw and other bones which are active will not degenerate. The bones of the spine are the ones chiefly affected.

There are other diseases of bones, such as "Paget's" (see page following) in which 95 per cent of the skeleton of the body may be involved.

Bone disorders in adult human beings are divided into two main groups in relationship to whether there is too much calcified bone or too little calcified bone. Since the discovery of the X-ray it has become possible to study the bones much more carefully than previously. Frequently, conditions are detected which formerly were passed unnoticed.

In cases of loss of calcium from the bones, they may become porous. If the loss affects the bones during the growing period, they may bend,

103

so that bowlegs will occur. Softening of the bones by the condition called osteoporosis may occur also, from disuse of the body generally. This happens sometimes following the long retention of a plaster cast. Frequently osteoporosis is found in cases of excessive action of the thyroid and in other instances in which nutrition has been inadequate, particularly when the diet is deficient in calcium and in phosphorus. Osteoporosis has been found when there is deficiency of vitamin C—particularly in growing children. Finally, osteoporosis is seen in old age when all of the tissues of the body begin to lose their ability to function in a normal manner. No one knows just how much of the breakdown in old age is due to lack of function of the sex glands. Senile osteoporosis is more common in women than in men.

PAGET'S DISEASE

Paget's disease of the bone is a rather unusual condition in which calcium disappears from the structure. The exact cause of the condition is not known. The parathyroid glands have been studied, but cases of Paget's disease have been found in which the parathyroid glands were entirely normal. Questions have also been raised as to whether the condition may be associated with some difficulty of the blood, or of the blood vessels, including hardening of the arteries. Several cases have been reported in which Paget's disease of the bone was related to extraordinary stresses or strain placed on the bones of the body. In Paget's disease the bones most frequently involved in the destruction are those subjected to the greatest stress or strain, including the bones of the lower portion of the spine.

While the description refers to the most common condition called Paget's disease, the name is also used to describe an inflammatory condition, sometimes cancerous, of the nipple of the breast and the areola which surrounds it.

OTHER BONE DISEASES

Like other tissues bones may become infected—osteomyelitis—or develop cysts or tumors. The bone-producing cells may become subject to an extremely malignant form of cancer called sarcoma. Early diagnosis and prompt surgery are the only hope in such cases.

CHAPTER XVIII

POISONING

POISONING MAY BE INTENTIONAL or accidental. Most cases of accidental poisoning occur in homes because people are careless about what they put in their mouths. In industry, workers may be poisoned by a variety of vapors, gases, or powders which are inhaled. Intentional poisonings result from suicidal swallowing of drugs or poisons and from purposeful desires to eliminate people who trouble the murderer.

Chemical poisons number in the hundreds, and injure the body according to the organs in which they have their chief effect. They may do their chief damage in the mouth, stomach or intestines; or in other cases they may be absorbed, and act on vital organs or on the nervous system. The diagnosis of poisoning is difficult and demands a knowledge of various drugs and their effects on the body. When a person is found unconscious without any recognizable cause and without the presence of fever or any injury, poisoning is suspected. Some poisons act slowly and others accumulate in the body when small doses are taken over a long time.

The work of the toxicologist who investigates cases of poisoning, is fascinating; it involves all the technics of the detective and research worker. He looks into the job of the person concerned, asks about those with whom he is in contact; studies his habits at home and away from home. Every secretion of the body may need to be studied in the laboratory, particularly material vomited, the urine, the sweat, and material from the bowel. Therefore those who first observe a case of poisoning should save all such materials for the investigator.

First aid in poisoning demands maintenance of life and stopping of the further action of the poison, if possible. Artificial respiration may be needed. The stomach can be washed in various ways.

COMMON POISONS

Phenol—Once phenol, known as carbolic acid, and related material like the cresols were common causes of poisoning. Now other antiseptics have been developed and have replaced phenol as a commonly used germ-destroying material. Phenol is a dangerous caustic substance which damages tissue with which it comes in contact. Moreover, it is absorbed and then injures the body generally. When absorbed it affects the centers in the brain responsible for breathing and for the circulation of blood.

Contamination of the skin or clothing with phenol demands immediate attention. The clothing should be removed and the skin washed as soon as possible with warm water or 50 per cent alcohol. Artificial respiration may be necessary and also rest and warmth.

Wood Alcohol or Methanol—Poisoning with this industrial solvent may lead to blindness and death. Since it has been used as an antifreeze many deaths of drunkards have resulted from drinking antifreeze solution. The symptoms of wood alcohol poisoning are like those of ordinary drunkenness except for the symptoms that include blurring of vision or blindness. In treating wood alcohol poisoning, the stomach is washed out by having the person drink copious amounts of salt solution which is then vomited back. Afterward a saline cathartic is taken to wash out the bowel. Thiamin and nicotinamide and vitamin K are given to protect the nervous system. The pain, restlessness, or delirium should have prompt medical attention. The doctor may provide oxygen for breathing and necessary stimulation.

Benzene—Benzene is cheap and is widely used in industry as a solvent. Acute benzene poisoning is manifested by effects on the nervous system and on the blood. Chronic benzene poisoning, which comes on insidiously, injures the blood-forming organs, with lessening of the number of blood cells.

A person acutely poisoned should be removed immediately from contact with the benzene fumes. Artificial respiration is given, and the patient is put to bed and given the necessary treatment. Rescuers should wear masks to avoid getting poisoned themselves.

When chronic benzene poisoning has seriously damaged the blood-forming organs recovery is difficult. Large doses of vitamin C are given. Liver extract and other aids to blood formation are frequently prescribed. All workers in industry where benzene is much used should have frequent examinations of the blood.

Carbon Tetrachloride Poisoning—Carbon tetrachloride is a clear, colorless liquid, non-inflammable, which is much used as a solvent. It is

106

used in fire extinguishers. Because it is not a fire hazard it is widely used in the cleaning and similar industries. Also it has been used as a treatment for worms. Poisoning may follow swallowing, or breathing the vapors of the drug.

The first signs of poisoning include headache, dizziness, and mental confusion, associated with vomiting and cramping pains. Later damage involves the kidneys, liver, and heart.

The person poisoned should be removed at once to good air and, if necessary, given artificial respiration. The doctor should be called, since every possible step must be taken to overcome the damage to the kidneys, liver, and other vital organs.

Cyanides—These are the most rapid poisons known. They produce death by asphyxia because of their interference with the carrying of oxygen by the iron in the blood. Cyanides are used as a gas to kill insects and rodents, and a few states use cyanide to execute condemned criminals.

All the detective-story writers tell of the bitter almond odor associated with cyanide poisoning. Few criminals use cyanides, because they kill so quickly and are so easily traced and detected. A variety of treatments are used, designed to restore to the blood its ability to carry oxygen.

Bromides—Bromides depress the central nervous system and induce sleep. Excessive doses lead to impairment of memory and depression, and large doses lead to disorientation, delirium, and death.

Treatment includes stimulation and giving salt to aid elimination of the chlorides and bromides in the urine. Aid to breathing is especially important.

ALCOHOLISM

Five to 50 per cent of fatal automobile accidents are due to alcoholism, and 25 per cent of psychiatric patients have some alcoholic background.

About one half of a drink of alcohol is absorbed in the first fifteen minutes and practically all that is taken is absorbed in three hours. The alcohol is picked up from the stomach and bowel and carried by the blood to all portions of the body. Most of the alcohol is oxidized to carbon dioxide and water. Each gram of alcohol burned yields seven calories.

The chief effects of alcohol are on the nervous system. The drug is primarily depressant, the apparent stimulation being due to its removal of inhibitions. The symptoms depend on the amount of alcohol consumed. Small or moderate amounts produce a state of "euphoria," or well-being, with warmth and a feeling of lightness. Judgment and co-ordination are damaged, but the person feels superior and is thereby all the more troublesome. With large doses of alcohol speech becomes thickened, vision is blurred, the sensations are lost in arms and legs. Some drunks are happy and others are sad. Eventually all inhibitions are lost and the intoxicated person becomes overtalkative, excited, abusive, or sullen. Finally there may be tremors, or convulsions or unconsciousness. Conditions may become so severe as to cause death.

When the alcoholic "comes to" he is dull, has a headache, cannot remember what happened, and may be quite sick with the hangover. It doesn't sound worth while—and it isn't.

Most people get over an episode of acute alcoholic intoxication, but severe manifestations may require sustaining of the heart and breathing by artificial respiration and the prescribing of necessary drugs. Doctors give thiamin, because of associated deficiencies.

The results of chronic alcoholism are physical deterioration, mental disintegration and, ultimately, death. The border that separates the social drinker from the chronic alcoholic is not easily defined. Most chronic alcoholics drink to escape mental stresses and unsolved social adjustments. They need the help of psychiatrists—but they need treat-ment also to overcome the nutritional and other physical disturbances that accompany chronic alcoholism.

Persistent drinkers eventually lose their appetite and have stomach troubles, with nausea and vomiting. Ordinary foods do not appeal, and everything has to be highly spiced. The alcohol damages the walls of the stomach and bowels and interferes with absorption of vitamins. Beer drinkers may take such large quantities as to distend the stomach and bowel.

The picture of a chronic drinker is generally well known. The ab-domen is bloated, the eyes and skin reddened with dilated blood ves-sels. The nose becomes bulbous and as red as a tomato. The injury to the nervous system produces shaky hands and an indecisive balance and gait. Because of the lack of thiamin, inflammations of the nerves occur. The emotions hang on a hair trigger. Rage follows giggling and laughter, remorse succeeds a period of exuberance. Judgment disap-pears, and the alcoholic cannot make up his mind to do even things that are important. Finally deterioration becomes complete, and delirium tremens may require hospitalization and emergency care.

Chronic alcoholics are now treated by combined physical and mental treatment. Psychiatrists try to find the underlying stresses. Alcoholics

Anonymous uses the values of group action to get alcoholics to help each other. Antabuse is a new drug which makes drinking so unpleasant as to condition the alcoholic against drinking.

BARBITURATE POISONING

Most sleeping pills to which people become addicted nowadays are modifications of barbituric acid. Some act promptly and shortly; others act slowly and longer. People get used to depending on drugs to get them to sleep. They may take larger and larger doses. The drugs are treacherous. The person becomes stupefied and confused and may take repeated doses without realizing what he is doing.

Excessive doses produce a dull sensation in the head and inability to co-ordinate movements. All the sensations become lessened in sensitivity including hearing, smell, taste, and the sense of touch. Nausea and vomiting may occur. Sleep may ensue, leading on to stupor from which awakening is difficult. Finally the skin gets cold and clammy, the respiration is shallow and slow, the circulation gets weak and, unless aroused and supported, the person poisoned by barbiturates will die.

The patient poisoned by sleeping pills should be taken to a hospital where the necessary supportive measures may be applied. These include oxygen, and stimulants to the brain like caffeine, ephedrine and amphetamine or Benzedrine. An antidote called "picro toxin" is sometimes used as a sudden harsh stimulant, but amphetamine seems to be just as certain and safer.

Some people take barbiturates habitually in small doses and get a form of chronic poisoning like a mild continuous jag. They have hallucinations, poor memory, difficulty with speech, and possible damage to blood and circulation.

Habitual reliance on drugs is a form of psychiatric or mental disturbance which should be studied to see if the difficulties cannot be resolved or removed. In any event, the drug should be stopped and resistance cultivated, at the same time attempting to restore physical health, which is damaged by all drug addictions.

CARBON MONOXIDE INTOXICATION

During the colder months newspapers contain many stories of people poisoned by carbon monoxide, most often from the exhaust gas of a motorcar but sometimes from illuminating gas. Natural gas does not contain carbon monoxide, but carbon monoxide poisoning may occur in homes which are supplied with natural gas, due to incomplete combustion.

Carbon monoxide will poison by excluding oxygen from the tissues. Carbon monoxide has a greater attraction for hemoglobin, the red coloring matter of the blood, than does oxygen. It forms a combination with the red coloring matter, and this prevents the oxygen from being picked up and circulated to the cells of the body. The length of time one is exposed to carbon monoxide is important, as is also the amount of carbon monoxide in the atmosphere. People who are working hard or exercising will succumb more rapidly to carbon monoxide, as will also children or small animals. Canary birds are kept in mines and are used as a warning system to indicate the presence of dangerous conditions before the amount of carbon monoxide reaches the level that would poison a man. As soon as one is removed from the carbon monoxide atmosphere, the blood eliminates it through the lungs. This takes place rather rapidly at first and then more slowly as more oxygen comes in. The exchange can be accelerated by giving pure oxygen for breathing. If the carbon monoxide level is kept low, small amounts are not harmful. This has been proved by studies of the people working in the Holland Tunnel where they are exposed for long periods of time.

The symptoms of carbon monoxide poisoning are, of course, those of asphyxiation. Breathing becomes more rapid, due to the difficulty in securing oxygen. A headache and a feeling of constriction about the temples are warning signs. Mental confusion and hallucinations may occur. Weakness of the muscles and inco-ordination, particularly of the legs, appear as symptoms with greater concentrations of the gas. The person who is inhaling carbon monoxide may at first appear pale, but eventually the skin becomes a cherry-red color which is used by the doctors as one of the important signs in diagnosis. Naturally the color changes back to the normal as oxygen is taken in and the carbon monoxide is eliminated. Sometimes after a poisoning there will be serious changes as a result of damage to the brain, which is quite sensitive to lack of oxygen. The symptoms may be as serious as those associated with Parkinson's syndrome or the shaking palsy or there may be gradual paralyses like those associated with multiple sclerosis.

Carbon monoxide does not accumulate in the blood, but the damages that result over long periods of time are the result of the injury to the blood and to the tissues, particularly to those of the nervous system.

All of the treatment in carbon monoxide poisoning is designed to get the gas out of the blood. For this reason artificial respiration, using oxygen, is important. The first thing to do is to get the person affected out into the air. If he has not lost consciousness, he can be treated with various technics. The headache and other symptoms disappear as soon as sufficient oxygen is taken into the body.

MORPHINE AND OPIUM POISONING

Opium is widespread throughout the world and its many derivatives, including morphine, codeine, heroin and other modifications, have extensive uses in medicine. Heroin is so addictive that its use is forbidden in the United States but heroin peddlers bring the material from abroad.

People acutely poisoned with opium or morphine have giddiness, flushing, a lazy feeling and a sort of feeling of well-being, followed, however, by slowing of the pulse in breathing and, finally, unconsciousness. Nausea and vomiting frequently appear; itching of the skin and nose are so common that frequently actors simulate the heroin or morphine addict by their reactions of this type.

Severe poisoning is marked by such signs as constriction of the pupils to pinpoints, blueness, and convulsions. Some people become nauseated and vomit easily, whereas others become agitated with even small doses of the drug. People who are anemic or who have insufficient action of the thyroid gland or of the adrenals are especially sensitive to morphine, and respond to much smaller doses than do ordinary people.

When anyone has been poisoned by opium or morphine, the first thing to do is to neutralize the drug and to sustain the patient so that he does not completely collapse. A doctor will pump out the stomach and give materials which will oxidize the opium or morphine in the stomach. The respiratory failure is overcome by giving artificial respiration and by administering oxygen with carbon dioxide. The carbon dioxide stimulates the breathing center in the brain; also stimulating drugs are given for getting over the coma and collapse. Benzedrine or amphetamine may also be used to stimulate the high centers in the brain.

Since people poisoned by sedative drugs often get secondary infection from congestion in the lungs, it is customary to give antibiotic drugs to prevent secondary pneumonias.

All drugs of the opium series can cause addiction and once a person is addicted to the drug, control and treatment are exceedingly difficult. The greatest trouble with opium addiction is the moral disintegration that occurs. Everything is subordinated to the desire to obtain

111

the drug. Morphine addicts lie, steal, cheat and do anything necessary, even to occasional violence, in order to secure the supply of drug for which the craving is completely uncontrollable and constant.

There is much discussion among doctors as to why people get addicted to opium, morphine, and especially to heroin. Unquestionably, psychological factors are important. However, there seems to be also something that develops in the body of the person who becomes addicted which continues the desire and even brings about the craving to increase the amount of the drug.

When the drug is withdrawn serious symptoms occur, such as yawning, restlessness and, finally, irritability, loss of appetite, vomiting and diarrhea. Eventually there may be tremors, insomnia and finally prostration and even collapse.

Physicians used to think that the drug could be withdrawn gradually and in that way recovery could ensue. Nowadays the so-called "cold-turkey" treatment is practiced, in which the drug is withdrawn completely and immediately and substitutes in the form of barbiturates or less addictive drugs may be used to tide over the serious symptoms. Patients who are undergoing withdrawal treatment need to be kept in hospitals or sanitariums where they are given all of the benefits of what modern medicine can do to avoid serious symptoms and produce comfort. Many physicians are convinced, however, that permanent cure of addicts is difficult, if not impossible, and only a small percentage remain cured for as long as five years. Obviously those who are mentally disturbed or psychopathic are much less frequently cured than are others.

METALLIC POISONS

All sorts of metal substances may produce serious poisoning of the human body when these poisons are swallowed or inhaled. Among the most serious are arsenic, cadmium, beryllium, mercury, zinc and lead. Cases of gold poisoning are also seen occasionally since the introduction of the gold treatment for arthritis. Fortunately modern medicine has developed a specific drug called BAL or British anti-lewisite which is now considered to be the most effective treatment of poisoning due to arsenic, mercury, and gold. BAL is also helpful in lead poisoning, silver poisoning, and poisoning due to thallium, selenium and tellurium. Indeed it is of some benefit also in poisoning by cadmium, antimony and zinc.

Arsenic—Most metal poisoning occurs in industries in which these metals are used. Arsenic is used in agriculture in sprays to get rid of pests; it is also used in copper refining and chemical industries. Arsenic poisoning sometimes follows the use of large doses of drugs which are tried against parasites of one kind or another that invade the human body. Arsenic has been used at times to commit murder and particularly when small doses are added to food, so that arsenic poisoning is a favorite among the writers of detective stories.

The symptoms of arsenic poisoning resemble those of a severe inflammation of the stomach with great amounts of gastric distress, associated sometimes with damage to the nerves, rashes on the skin, and similar symptoms.

When arsenic poisoning is suspected, it is customary to find amounts of arsenic in the urine, the hair or nails since arsenic is excreted from the human body in this way. This also adds to the value of arsenic poisoning as a favorite in murder stories. Once a person has been exposed to arsenic, the best treatment is to stop the exposure as soon as possible and to give BAL promptly and continuously until recovery has occurred.

Beryllium—Since beryllium is much used in the study of atomic energy and also as a constituent of the materials in fluorescent lamps, cases of poisoning are now seen more frequently than previously. The workers who are exposed to beryllium dust in their work also occasionally become poisoned. When the dust gets into the lungs, it sets up serious inflammations and reactions, sometimes followed by difficulties with breathing. Cases have also been reported in which beryllium has gotten into wounds when a fluorescent lamp broke. A "granuloma" forms, which is overgrowth of the tissues something like a tumor. Therefore special preventive measures are now being taken to get rid of old fluorescent light tubes without exposing anyone to the danger of injury from them.

Cadmium—Cadmium seldom causes poisoning but instances are known, when acid foods are prepared in containers which have cadmium in the lining. Enough cadmium can be absorbed to cause severe inflammation of the stomach, accompanied by nausea, vomiting and, later, diarrhea. Serious poisoning can also follow the breathing of cadmium oxide fumes. This happens when cadmium-plated steel is heated or welded, without adequate ventilation in the room. The inhalation of the fumes is followed by slight irritation of the eyes, dryness of the throat and tightness in the chest. Later the person develops cough, pains in the chest and may ultimately find some blood in the sputum. Cases are reported of fatal poisoning from cadmium. Formerly the only available treatment was rest, oxygen and the usual supportive

113

measures, but now BAL is being tried and presumably is sufficiently effective to warrant its regular use in such instances.

Gold—Gold is now given in the treatment of a number of diseases, and cases have occurred in which poisoning has followed injection of gold salts. The effects are chiefly on the bone marrow, resulting in damage to the blood-forming organs. The lessening of the thrombocytes may cause easy bruising and hemorrhages; there may also be damage to the kidneys. BAL, or British anti-lewisite, has also been shown to be especially effective in poisoning with gold salts.

Lead—Lead has been for many years known to be a dangerous and insidious metallic poison. Lead fumes may be inhaled or finely divided lead dust may be inhaled and produce serious poisoning. Food and drink may become contaminated with lead from containers. Lead salts are stored in the body, and accumulation of small doses may produce serious poisoning. As with other metallic poisons, the first symptoms relate to irritation of the gastrointestinal tract. Later, however, patients develop what is called a "lead line"—a series of bluish dots occurring along the margins of the gums. Examination of the blood shows characteristic damage of the blood cells. The nervous symptoms are especially important since lead poisoning may damage the brain, with mental depression or even severe mental disturbance. Children may develop convulsions. The peripheral nerves—those near the surface of the body—become paralyzed and the characteristic wrist-drop of painters, weakness in the shoulders of laborers who use shovels and paralysis in the legs of tailors are known as occupational injuries due to lead. The red blood cells become fewer in number; examination of the blood, I may repeat, is one of the most important technics in causing a suspicion of lead poisoning in the mind of the doctor. When lead poisoning is diagnosed, the first step is to withdraw the person from all exposure to lead and to promote elimination of lead from the blood. Most persons recover if the exposure is stopped. Calcium gluconate is usually given intravenously to relieve the colic. Salts are given to sweep material out of the bowel. The calcium must be maintained at a high level since this helps to drive the lead out of the blood stream into the bones. Sodium citrate is sometimes given in order to produce a soluble lead citrate which is rapidly excreted from the body. BAL, or British anti-lewisite, has not been found especially helpful in lead poisoning.

A special warning is needed against the danger of lead poisoning in children. Babies who chew on toys, cribs or window sills which have been painted with lead pigments may be poisoned. Fortunately, lead paint is now limited almost entirely to use on the exteriors of buildings.

Cases of lead poisoning have also occurred from inhaling the fumes of old battery casings when these are burned as a substitute for other fuel.

Mercury—Acute mercury poisoning usually happens when a child in a home gets hold of tablets of bichloride of mercury poison which may be used as an antiseptic or for other reasons. No one really needs to keep bichloride of mercury around the house. When it has been used for any purpose, it should be promptly destroyed after that use is ended. Mercury poisoning occurs in industry from inhalation of mercury vapors. This occurs particularly among gold and silver refiners, instrument makers and laboratory workers. The fur and felt hat industry used to uncover cases of mercury poisoning but the material is no longer used to any extent in that industry. During World War II, workers making mercury cadmium dry batteries were found to be suffering with mercury poisoning. The great danger from acute mercury poisoning is the damage to all of the organs that are involved in absorbing and getting rid of mercury from the body. The chief damage is to the kidneys, with evidence of renal failure and eventually death from uremia. In the bowel, mercury produces colitis and often a severe, bloody diarrhea. One form of mercury called "calomel" has been used as a cathartic for many years.

First aid in mercury poisoning involves giving egg white or milk, washing out the stomach with copious amounts of fluid and finally giving a saline cathartic to sweep the material out of the body. British anti-lewisite, or BAL, has been found to be a specific antidote against acute mercury poisoning.

Chronic mercury poisoning comes on insidiously, with a variety of symptoms. One of those first noticed may be increased amounts of saliva with a metallic taste in the mouth. Associated may be loss of appetite, indigestion, and diarrhea. Finally, such workers may develop tremors. Mental aberrations are seen, with excitability followed by periods of dullness. Ulcers occasionally occur on the skin. The one important measure is to withdraw the person immediately from exposure to the mercury and then to sustain him in every possible way with adequate diet and necessary stimulating drugs for the blood.

GENERAL TREATMENT OF POISONING

As will be noticed, the treatment of poisoning involves eliminating the bulk of the poison from the stomach as soon as possible by washing out the stomach, causing vomiting and giving cathartics. Second, the poison is inactivated by giving any specific substances which can combine with the poison and prevent its use by the body. Finally, the person must be sustained so that life will go on until the poison has been brought under control.

One must be careful that the poisoned person does not inhale the vomitus, since this may result in pneumonia. The stomach tube should not be used when strong mineral acids or caustics or ammonia have been swallowed, because the tissues will be damaged and the tube can actually puncture a hole in the tissues. The drugs that cause vomiting are not as effective as a thorough washing of the stomach. Among other things used to cause vomiting are a tablespoonful of mustard in a cup of warm water, also a strong warm salt solution. Doctors can inject substances which will produce vomiting by their effects on the nerve centers in the brain. Again, attention is called to various antidotes; alkaloid substances like morphine or digitalis can be controlled by small amounts of tannic acid in large amounts of water. Heavy metal poisoning involves the use of raw egg white or milk, and British anti-lewisite is effective against most of them.

When a specific antidote is not available, activated charcoal may be given in liberal doses. For irritative poisons, egg white, milk, flaxseed tea, starch water, barley or oatmeal gruel or gelatin solutions help to protect the walls of the stomach.

Poisons are eliminated by forcing fluids—preferably given by mouth, but if not, injected into the bowel or even under the skin. Most important is the use of substances to support the body, among which amphetamine or Benzedrine is helpful for sedative drugs against the depression of the nervous system. Caffeine and sodium benzoate may be used, and if depression is severe, other stimulants are considered of importance. Particularly to be mentioned is a knowledge of artificial respiration, which should be known by everyone. In severe cases patients should be taken immediately to hospitals, where inhalations of oxygen mixed with 5 per cent of carbon dioxide will not only supply oxygen to the tissues but also stimulate breathing.

CHAPTER XIX

EFFECTS OF PHYSICAL FORCES
ON THE BODY

HEAT

THE HUMAN BEING SUFFERS a variety of reactions when exposed to high temperatures. Usually there are three different forms of this reaction. They are called "heat cramps," "heat exhaustion" and "heat stroke." They may occur during exposure to the heat from the sun in climates where the sun is especially hot, and they occur particularly to people who have not been acclimated by exposure to the sun gradually over a long period of time. After a while the body accustoms itself to heat by a decline in the amount of sodium in the perspiration.

HEAT CRAMPS

Heat cramps occur in those who have sweated excessively and taken excessive amounts of water. The condition usually occurs in stokers and miners. Chief among the symptoms is pain which is due to a spasm of the muscles of the body. The taking of dilute salt solution instead of water for drinking purposes prevents heat cramp with certainty.

HEAT EXHAUSTION

Heat exhaustion comes usually during excessively hot weather and is accompanied by changes in the circulation of the blood. The chief symptom of heat exhaustion is weakness and faintness which may go

117

on to the coming of actual unconsciousness. The sweating is profuse, but the temperature of the body does not change.

It is easy to prevent heat exhaustion by reducing the amount of physical activity during excessively hot weather and by regulating the atmosphere by the use of electric fans or other similar devices. Whenever anyone is exposed to excessive sweating during the hot weather, dilute salt solutions should be taken instead of ordinary drinking water.

HEAT STROKE OR SUNSTROKE

The chief manifestations of heat stroke or sunstroke include rapidly mounting fever and a dry skin. Under such conditions the temperature of the body may go as high as 110 or even 112. With these high temperatures comes apathy and, finally, the person becomes unconscious. Apparently this disorder is more common in old people and in alcoholics. Heat stroke is also fairly frequent during the first few days of a heat wave when people keep right on working hard without regard to the height of the temperature. The condition occurs more often with a high humidity than when there is low humidity. The recommendation has been made that hospitals keep available tubs filled with water and ice, so that persons with heat stroke may be cooled off as rapidly as possible by being immersed in cold water and given massage to promote circulation of the blood at the same time. Just as soon as the high temperature is brought down to 100 degrees, the person is put in bed and the temperature is controlled by the use of wet sheets and an electric fan. The purpose of this is to stop as rapidly as possible the effects of the heat on the vital organs of the body. Under such circumstances everything possible is done to keep the heart and circulation of the patient in working condition.

COLD

FROSTBITE

Experts say that cold was the most important disabling condition encountered by military personnel in World War II. In the British army alone there were almost 85,000 cases of frostbite. In the fighting in Korea, exposure to wet and dry cold was the most serious condition confronting the doctors who had to keep patients or soldiers in condition to carry on their work. The human being can withstand extreme cold as low as 50 degrees below zero, with proper clothing and proper nutrition. The greatest danger comes from exposure to cold without adequate protection. When the body is exposed to cold, the first defense is for the blood vessels in the skin to become constricted so that there is a fall in the skin temperature without much change in the temperature inside the body. One does not experience discomfort from extreme cold in the fingers and toes until their temperature hits about 60 degrees Fahrenheit from a normal of 80 to 85 degrees Fahrenheit for this portion of the body. There is great discomfort when the temperature of the shoulders, back, or legs drops below 80 degrees Fahrenheit from a normal of 90 to 95. The body responds with intermittent shivering in an attempt to raise the temperature. Even the warmest clothing will not protect the wearer in temperatures below the freezing point unless there is exercise. Fingers and toes suffer from cold more than any other part of the body, first becoming painful, then numb and finally frostbitten. The disappearance of pain is a warning sign of great danger.

Not long ago an attempt was made to control certain difficult and uncontrollable diseases by causing the person to be kept in extreme cold. One patient with cancer survived a body temperature of 74° F. under these circumstances. On the other hand, flyers who fell into cold water in the Arctic, where the temperature of the water was between 41 and 50 degrees, have died in less than thirty minutes. When, however, the water temperature was 68 degrees, the flyers survived for several hours. In the German prison camps extensive chilling experiments were carried out on human beings. Consciousness was lost when the temperature in the interior of the body fell to 86 degrees. It took from seventy to ninety minutes' exposure to extremely low temperatures to reach a temperature inside the body of 86 degrees. The Germans report that death occurred when the temperature of the inside of the body was between 78 and 86 after exposures of one to two hours. The most effective treatment of freezing is rapid rewarming. Dr. Tinsley Harrison says that chilling drafts and sudden temperature changes are more important than cold itself, because they predispose to disease by lowering resistance to infection. Local chilling may produce nerve pains, muscle pains, sore throat, bronchitis, or pneumonia when resistance is lowered and the germs infect.

COMPRESSION

The chief effects of high altitude and changes in barometric pressure are dependent on the way in which this affects the use of oxygen by the body. The most common symptoms associated with compression, as in diving or descending suddenly from high altitudes, is pain in one or both ears, particularly when the tubes are obstructed. To this the name of *aero-otitis media* has been given. After or during the breathing of oxygen this condition may develop during sleep, because the Eustachian tubes, which go from the back of the throat to the middle ear, rarely open during sleep. The rate of compression is important in governing the degree to which an individual suffers from high altitude. If descent is made reasonably slowly, the difficulties do not arise. In commercial passenger aircraft the rate of descent from high altitude is limited to 300 feet per minute. Under these circumstances pain in the ears seldom occurs. Sometimes people who have been exposed to compression develop pains in the frontal sinuses because of blocking. The pain is due to the same conditions that result in pain in the ears.

A remarkable condition is the expansion of abdominal gas that occurs under some circumstances. When helium was used in diving, the mouthpiece produced flow of saliva and considerable amounts of gas were swallowed. When the men came to the surface rapidly, the gas in the stomach expanded and the pressure brought about so much pain as to induce collapse. Now it is generally known that swallowed air or gas, rather than food, is the source of most abdominal gas. Certain foods, however, tend to produce abdominal gas, including melons, beans, and carbonated beverages.

The big problem of high altitudes is little oxygen and this, of course, is being governed in aircraft by the use of oxygen chambers, so that oxygen is then released into the cabins and the pressure is kept at a proper level. Nowadays provision is made for a supply of oxygen on all flights above 10,000 feet and on all flights of more than four hours' duration between 8,000 and 10,000 feet.

When divers and compressed-air workers are subjected to rapid decompression, air bubbles form in the blood and they may produce such symptoms as pains which are called "the bends," asphyxiation which is called "the chokes," and paralysis. The most common manifestation is the dull, throbbing type of pain in the joints and in the muscles and bones which is known as "the bends." Normal breathing becomes shallow and rapid and then the worker seems short of breath. This condition is called "the chokes." If this is not relieved, the skin becomes cold and moist, the circulation impaired, and the person may actually have symptoms like those of shock. The treatment includes prolonged recompression and the use of oxygen and fluids, and then slow decompression so that the worker does not suffer from these difficult symptoms. The condition is a serious one and should always be recognized and treated promptly.

RADIATION

People are continually exposed to minute amounts of radiation that come not only from the various forces in the atmosphere surrounding the world but also from naturally radioactive materials that occur in soil and water and in other materials in our environment. Fortunately this radiation is so small in amount that it does not seem to have any significant effect on the body. Also a certain amount of radiation may come from X-ray tubes or from radium or from the taking of various radioactive isotopes. There is no way in which an untrained person can find out whether or not he is being subjected to radiation. For that reason, various means have been developed for determining the presence of radiation in our atmosphere. These include the exposure of photographic film and devices like the Geiger counter.

The physicists have classified the radiation into various types of waves and particles which vary greatly in their effects on the living tissue of the body. Some rays penetrate more than do others. The irradiation affects the protoplasm of the tissues and brings about certain chemical and physical effects. Some cells of the body are more sensitive to radiation than are others. When radiation is used against tumors, the physician knows the sensitivity of the cells to the radiation and the extent to which it can be counted on to stop cellular growth.

Radiation sickness results from absorption of the products of disintegration of the protein of the body. The chief symptom of radiation sickness is mild to severe nausea and, in some instances, there may be diarrhea due to the response of the intestinal tissues to the irritation.

Another type of radiation sickness results from irradiation of the entire body over a short period of time. This begins suddenly with severe illness that may go to the point of prostration. There may be thereafter a phase of relative well-being, followed by severe illness and ultimately by death.

The most sensitive cells of the body are the white blood cells of the blood. Radiation can damage the blood-forming organs so that the cells fall below normal with subsequent hemorrhage due to destruction of the thrombocytes in the blood and increased permeability of the capillaries from damage to the cells. Obviously, with loss of blood comes severe anemia. The effects of radiation can be such as to produce

121

sterility, but permanent sterility is not expected from irradiation because the dose necessary to sterilize the male sex gland is close to what is a fatal dose. In the woman also the radiation may produce transient sterility; permanent sterility is rare.

At present the best method of treatment for irradiation is the transfusion of whole blood, the use of antibiotic drugs to control infection, and forced nutrition to enable the body to overcome the damage that has occurred.

CHAPTER XX

THE INHALING OF DANGEROUS SUBSTANCES

SILICOSIS

PERHAPS THE MOST DANGEROUS and disabling of the diseases that come from inhaling foreign substances is the one called silicosis. This results from the presence of particles of silicon dioxide in the air. The condition was first discovered from an examination of the X-ray plates of workers in industries using silicon. First come the fibrous changes in the lung, and then small nodular infiltrations appear. Later there may be large masses in the lungs as a result of formation of fibrous tissue.

The occupations in which silicosis occurs most frequently are mining, sandblasting, foundry work, the prolonged use of polishing and cutting wheels composed of sandstone and, finally, stone cutting and polishing. Because the condition is one that affects the lung primarily, the changes that occur are related to the respiration, including some blueness, clubbing of the fingers, perhaps an increase in the total number of red blood cells. As soon as the condition is discovered, the patient, if a young person, should be immediately removed from the job. Men of advanced age who have taken many years, perhaps more than twenty, to develop the condition, may be permitted to continue at their work since the condition is not likely to become worse. The person with silicosis who subsequently develops tuberculosis has a difficult time.

ASBESTOSIS

Workers may inhale other substances than silicon and develop changes in the lungs. Asbestosis, which comes from the inhaling of

123

asbestos fiber, is one. These people, in addition to the lung changes, expectorate brownish formed material which contains the fibers and spicules associated with asbestos.

SIDEROSIS

Another condition called "siderosis" results from deposits of iron in the lung. This is seen in such occupations as those of the acetylene welder and workers with the electric arc.

BAGASSOSIS

"Bagassosis" is the name given to the results of inhaling bagasse dust. Bagasse is the name of pulverized and dried stalks of sugar cane. Bagasse is much used in manufacturing insulating board.

BERYLLIUM DISEASE

Beryllium disease of the lung is a new condition resulting from inhaling beryllium in the manufacture of fluorescent lamps. Most of the cases so far reported have occurred in women. The lungs in this condition observed with the X-ray are found to have what has been called a "sandpaper" appearance.

ALUMINUM DUST

The employees of smelters dealing with bauxite are found to suffer from the results of inhaling aluminum dust, which produces the formation of tissue in the lung. Another complication is a condition called "bissynosis" which is ascribed to the inhalation of cotton fibers. The condition is known to workers around cotton gins as "gin fever" and "Monday morning fever." The inhaling of almost any substance may have serious effects on the lungs, and among the latest noted is cadmium workers' disease which brings about lung changes. Finally, those who work with severe irritant substances like sulfur dioxide and other substances used in refrigeration may have damage to the lung, resulting finally in secondary chronic infections, from the inhaling of various irritating gases.

124

AIR POLLUTION

Polluted air is now recognized as a serious cause of inflammation of the lungs associated with bronchitis, bronchiectasis and even lung cancer. The air is polluted by smoke from industrial plants and by exhaust from motorcars. Some cities, notably London and Los Angeles, have recorded deaths from the pollution associated with fog in the atmospheric "smog."

CHAPTER XXI

FEVERS AND INFECTIONS

FEVER

BY FAR THE VAST MAJORITY of instances of fever result from infection. There are, however, cases in which fever occurs and in which the exact cause cannot be easily determined. Certain principles have been established by years of experience for the handling of fever.

Rest in bed is the number one step for any person with fever. Under such conditions the work of the heart, kidneys, and liver is reduced. The sense of fatigue is lessened. The blood flow to the kidneys and liver tends to be better in the lying-down than in the standing position. The disadvantages of bed rest include: less stimulation to breathing, a sluggish blood flow in the legs, and a noticeable diminution in muscular strength. Bed rest should always be used in association with a certain amount of activity suited to the condition of the person concerned. This may involve simply encouraging him to move, turn and sit up in bed, but might include controlled exercise or even moving of the patient's limbs by the attendant nurse or member of the family. In the nursing of those with fevers, special attention must be paid to giving plenty of fluids.

The fever patient usually loses appetite and needs to be encouraged to eat, and if necessary, must be fed by the nurse. Dryness of the mouth can be helped by the use of suitable mouth washes, or the nurse can cleanse the mouth by a piece of gauze wrapped around the finger. Profuse sweating may make necessary frequent changes of bedding and night clothes. The patient's skin must be protected against the formation of ulcers. If the sheets are kept dry and free from wrinkles, if alcohol rubs are used and if a suitable powder is applied, the skin is helped greatly. For dry skin, baby oil is preferable to any other system of softening. Movement of the joints by the nurse is helpful against stiffening.

People whose temperature gets above 102 degrees need at least three quarts of water a day. If there is vomiting and diarrhea, the amount must be increased by the amount of fluid lost in this way. If patients resist the taking of plain water, they can have fruit juice or vegetable juice, carbonated sweet beverages, milk, soups and similar fluid drinks.

The bowels become less active when there is fever and a person remains long in bed. The choice of a proper technic for getting rid of the waste material from the body is up to the doctor who understands the condition and the nature of the disturbance. He will have to prescribe the cathartic that is to be taken, whether something as strong as the salts or something like mineral oil or other lubricants or perhaps even a soapsuds or water-and-glycerine enema.

The doctor can always prescribe drugs which are known to be valuable in bringing down serious fevers. He can also prescribe sponges with alcohol or tepid water, which do a great deal toward controlling temperature through aiding irradiation of heat from the surface of the body. Cold compresses and ice bags are other types of cooling.

THE ATTACK ON INFECTION

Only a few decades have passed since physicians confronted with cases of many serious infections could only apply a sort of general treatment. This involved putting the patient to bed, stimulating the action of the bowel and kidneys, aiding the action of the heart and controlling the fever with drugs that have a tendency to reduce fevers. Medicine has had for only a few years powerful remedies called "chemotherapeutic" remedies or antibiotic drugs which definitely control the growth of germs or viruses or other organisms in the human body.

The use of drugs to suppress the growth of organisms that damage the human body is one of the greatest accomplishments of modern medicine. Naturally, the drugs must be able to stop the growth of the foreign invader without injuring the sick person. The new drugs attack germs in various ways. Quinine is a fine example of the way in which a drug can attack a single organism since it is a specific against the plasmodia which cause malaria. Some of the new antibiotic drugs can attack a great number of different germs of many different species. Some chemical substances damage certain cells of the human body and may interfere with their growth. Out of this fact may come, eventually, new and effective treatments for cancer.

The sulfonamide drugs and the antibiotics act by interfering with the ways in which the germs themselves live. In deciding which drug to use the doctor must know its effects on the patient. For instance, some patients do not react well to penicillin. In other instances the patient's germs have become accustomed to penicillin. Fortunately we now have streptomycin, chloromycetin, aureomycin, terramycin and other antibiotics, for each of which there is a long list of germs which it is capable of attacking successfully. Sometimes the medicine attaches itself to the tissues of the body and the germs cannot attack while the medicine is there. Sometimes the medicine relates itself to the way in which the germ feeds and grows.

The doctor chooses the remedy according to the dose he wants to give, the frequency with which the dose is to be given, whether or not the remedy can be taken by mouth or must be given by injection, whether it needs to be given by injection into the blood, into the muscles or under the skin, or for a number of other reasons.

SULFONAMIDES AND ANTIBIOTICS

At present the most significant antibacterial drugs are the sulfonamide drugs and the antibiotics. The sulfonamide drugs were known before the antibiotics; their chief period of use was between 1937 and 1945. Now thousands of different compounds of sulfonamides have been prepared and tested. The ones most widely known and used at present are gantrisin and gantanol; sulfadiazine and sulfamerazine; sulfathalidine; sulfasuxidine; and Kynex which is sulfamethoxy-pyridazine, together with combinations of other sulfonamides. The physician can determine the amount of sulfonamide in the body, and by that have a knowledge of its effectiveness. Usually the doctor prescribes a sufficiently large dosage to have an immediate effect; then he maintains the dosage by continuing a lesser amount at fairly frequent intervals.

Penicillin is still probably the most important and most widely used of the antibiotic drugs; it is much lower in cost and can attack successfully a wide range of germs. Few people are sensitive to the drug, perhaps as many as six out of one hundred, but we now have the antihistaminic drugs which are exceedingly useful in controlling effectively the reactions to other drugs. When people are sensitive, the penicillin can be stopped and by giving an antihistamine drug, a sedative, or a salicylate, the condition is controlled. Penicillin is now given by inhalation, in the form of a penicillin dust, by penicillin solutions, by tablets taken orally, by lozenges, by injections and, in fact, in ointments and in the treatment of the eyes.

Streptomycin has special effects against the germs of tuberculosis. Streptomycin is known in some people to have an affinity for certain changes in relationship to the nerves associated with hearing. Streptomycin has been used in bacillary dysentery and in a considerable variety of infections.

"Aureomycin" was given that name because it is gold in color and was derived from a mold. Aureomycin is not used by injection under the skin or into the muscles. It has been injected directly into the veins and can be given by mouth. People who get a little upset when they take aureomycin by mouth frequently avoid the reaction by taking the aureomycin with a glass of milk or some other food.

Chloromycetin, one of the most important of the new antibiotics that is obtained from a mold, was discovered in soil. It is the most effective of all of the antibiotics against the organism that causes typhoid.

Polymyxin is a new antibiotic obtained from a germ. Bacitracin is an older antibiotic, also obtained from a germ. Bacitracin is used more particularly in external treatment of ulcers, boils, carbuncles and wounds.

The antibiotic called terramycin was discovered in the earth, and has a wide range of action. It has been found particularly effective in controlling some of the infections by the larger viruses. Altogether about 141 antibiotics are now known by name, and the number being studied is almost infinite. Antibiotics have been found now in garlic, in radishes, in tomatoes, in hops, and in all sorts of specimens of soil, in molds, in fungi, and in germs. With this wide range of attack, the physician is now capable of controlling infections in a way never before possible.

Other antibiotics which have become widely known include Furacin, Ilotycin, Colymycin, Albamycin, Erythromycin, Staphcillin; Madribon; and hundreds of variations and combinations.

CHAPTER XXII

INFECTIONS AND IMMUNITY

WHEN LIVING ORGANISMS such as germs or viruses invade the human body, the tissues of the body undergo changes which help them to resist the poisons of the invader. By this reaction the tissues become immune to the poisons. Much depends on the virulence of the infections, the total number of germs invading, the place where they enter the body, the tissues or structures where they settle and grow. If you are susceptible to the infection, it will attack you; it may even overcome you. If you are resistant, the tissues of your body may develop antibodies which will overcome the germs or viruses or their poisons.

Certain environmental conditions may increase or lower your resistance to infection. Chilling of the body, excessive fatigue, absence of some essential nutritional substance, as proteins, or mineral salts or vitamins, or the presence of another disease at the same time may modify the resistance of the body to an invader.

The chemical composition of the invading organism may be significant in the way in which the body responds to it. An invading substance is known as an "antigen." Usually the response of the body to an invading germ is specific against that germ or against that type of germ. Bacteria may contain a number of antigenic substances, against each of which the body will rebuild resistance. An example of an antibody against infections is the immune globulin. This is a protein substance found in blood, in which we now know are accumulated substances that help to resist various infections such as those of measles or poliomyelitis. In man, most of the antibodies are found in the immune globulin of the blood. The amount of antibody that develops is also governed by such factors as the amount of infectious material that gets into the body. The doctors find that they can help you build resistance by repeatedly injecting small doses of an infecting substance. We know that a child gets resisting substances from its mother in her blood at the time of birth and in the first material that comes from the breast when the child begins to nurse. This is called "colostrum." The amount of antibodies may be unfavorably affected by starvation, exposure, reduced protein intake, alcoholism, or other poisoning.

TYPES OF INFECTION

For certain diseases there are certain specific types of causative germs, such as the viruses of measles, smallpox, infantile paralysis, or the germs that cause diphtheria, typhoid, gonorrhea or meningitis. The total number of germs, viruses, rickettsia, amebas, spirochetes, or other parasites that may infect the body reaches into thousands. Many germs have been described in groups according to their appearance under the microscope such as the streptococci that grow in chains, or the staphylococci that grow in clusters. The streptococci and the staphylococci may invade any portion of the human body and set up infection.

HEMOLYTIC STREPTOCOCCUS INFECTIONS

The streptococcus is one of the most widely distributed and variable organisms that attacks mankind. Such conditions as sore throat, sinus infections, scarlet fever, erysipelas, puerperal fever, or lymphangitis may be caused by streptococci. Other conditions associated with such streptococci include acute rheumatic fever and acute inflammations of the kidney.

Such infections are found in all races, in both sexes, at all ages, and they come on at any time of the year. Scarlet fever is said to be rare in the tropics. Very small babies, under three months of age, seldom have streptococcal infections, because they get some immunity from their mothers at the time of birth. Tonsillitis, pharyngitis, and scarlet fever are more frequent up to ten years of age. Streptococcal infections can result from contaminated food, milk, water but most frequently pass from one person to another with coughing, sneezing, spitting and what are known as "hand-to-mouth" infections.

Tonsillitis and pharyngitis are usually streptococcal infections which begin with sore throats. When there is a rash, the rash is said to represent sensitivity of the skin to the products of the streptococcus; this condition is scarlet fever. Infections of the sinuses usually follow infection

131

of the tonsils and throat. Ear infections occur in many cases and the streptococci are said to be responsible for 10 per cent of ear infections. Specific methods of inoculation against streptococci are difficult because of the many different varieties of the germ. The Dick test will indicate whether or not a child is susceptible to the streptococcus of scarlet fever and there are methods of building resistance against these streptococci by inoculating small doses of the toxin.

Regardless of the portion of the body that is attacked by the streptococci, the control of the condition is now possible through the proper use of the sulfonamide and antibiotic drugs that have been mentioned. Streptococci are especially susceptible to attack by the sulfonamide drugs. The complications of infected throats are more important than the sore throat itself. Penicillin is the antibiotic drug most frequently used in treating throats infected with streptococci. Penicillin is especially beneficial in laryngitis, pharyngitis, tonsillitis and scarlet fever. The complications of scarlet fever have in the past done more harm than the disease itself. In severe cases of scarlet fever convalescent serum may be used, and good results have been reported from use of the antitoxin.

Saline gargles and irrigations of the throat help to wash out the by-products of throat infection. One of the most significant advances is the use of sulfonamide drugs to prevent streptococcal infections. When there are outbreaks in large homes, in barracks, in asylums, or places where great numbers of people assemble, the sulfonamide drugs may be taken as a means of preventing infection with the streptococci. All sorts of attempts have been made to cut down respiratory diseases by the use of ultraviolet light in the air, by the spraying of medicated vapors or aerosols and by other technics for keeping the germs from floating in the air. These, in general, have not been successful.

THE COMMON COLD

Almost anyone can tell you right off when they have a cold, and yet there is no real agreement in the medical profession as to just what a common cold is. No single germ has yet been incriminated as the causative factor nor has any group of germs or viruses been established as responsible. At present the sequence of events seems to include a first period when the lining of the nose and throat seems to respond to some foreign invading substances by reddening and congestion and a profuse flow of mucus. With this may be frequent sneezing, stuffiness, difficulty in breathing, perhaps some fever, a feeling of lassitude, and some aching of the limbs.

132

Colds spread rapidly from one person to another, and the resistance established by having a cold lasts a very short time. Some people have many more colds than do others; the average for the country as a whole seems to be about four colds a year. Chilling, exposure to damp, sudden changes from a dry hot air to a cold damp atmosphere, sitting in a draft, getting the feet wet, and, particularly, working or playing in crowded rooms with others who have colds seem to be important factors in the spread of respiratory diseases.

The suggestions as to how to prevent frequent colds are numerous but some doubt prevails as to whether any of them really work. You may try to keep away from contact with others who have colds, but under the crowded conditions of our civilization this is well-nigh impossible. People have tried wearing face masks or gauze or paper during epidemics, but they permit contamination. Use of ultraviolet in the air has seemed to be useful but carefully controlled experiments with this technic and with spraying medicated vapors in the air have not yielded conclusive results. Mothers have tried to harden children by frequent cold baths, going without stockings, and hats and similar methods. These methods do not work, and the unnecessary hardship makes the children unhappy.

Most colds get well in from five to ten days. Complications are fortunately now controlled by the use of the sulfonamides and antibiotic drugs. Some claims hold that colds can be cured by taking an antihistaminic drug during the first twenty-four hours of invasion; most experts doubt that this is specifically helpful. The congestion in the nose is relievable by the use of decongestant preparations such as menthol, camphor, privine, amphetamine and other preparations which the doctor must prescribe. People feel more comfortable if they go to bed, take some aspirin or a small dose of an alcoholic drink. Frequently a hot bath and plenty of fluids, such as citrus drinks, secure relief. Secondary coughs are controllable with a variety of remedies. Particularly feared as a complication is secondary pneumonia. The doctor watches for signs of this in rising temperature, congestion and pain in the lungs, signs of congestion which he hears with his stethoscope, or can detect by percussion, or see certainly with the X-ray. Fortunately again, such secondary infections are now controllable with the new drugs.

INFLUENZA

Influenza is an acute infectious disease caused by several different viruses. It comes on suddenly with fever, muscular aches, chilliness, and

133

a cough. After an attack, serious weakness is common for some weeks. Although outbreaks of influenza have occurred for centuries only in recent years have the different forms of virus associated with epidemics been isolated. Many forms of viruses related to influenza have been isolated since 1933. Vaccines for inoculating against these forms have been developed but routine immunization is not advised because the uncomplicated disease is rarely fatal and because the type or nature of the virus varies from one epidemic to another.

The virus of influenza is transmitted from one person to another by droplets of fluid coughed out of the nose, throat, and lungs. An epidemic usually reaches its peak in two or three weeks and then subsides in from four to eight weeks. The worst period of the year is winter and early spring. The influenza virus seems to be constantly present among human beings and epidemics occur under the specially favorable circumstances that aid spread of the virus and lessen resistance.

Influenza comes on suddenly after an incubation period of a few days. The common complaints are headache, drowsiness, fatigue, and chilliness, but there may also be general illness with nausea and vomiting. The fever starts to rise and usually hangs around 102° F. but may get up to 104° F. A cough with dryness and irritation of the throat and tightness across the chest are common. A running nose is not nearly as frequent as with the common cold. The person with influenza feels really sick and is disinclined toward work or amusement or even reading. Pain in the eyes, with some redness, may occur. The disease itself is uncomfortable but not too serious, but secondary complications through invasion by other germs causing pneumonia, ear infection or even inflammation of the brain may make it dangerous to life.

The sulfonamides and antibiotic drugs can prevent secondary complications of influenza but do not act specifically against the viruses. Most doctors recommend rest in bed, plenty of fluids, aspirin or other salicylates, codeine to quiet the cough and, if necessary, drugs to help the patient sleep. The condition must be watched most carefully when it affects the very old or very young who are more likely to get secondary infections and to be less able to resist the wear and tear that influenza causes.

Vaccines against influenza have been developed based on various viruses that may be concerned in epidemics as of the Asian influenza type. These are recommended particularly for old people and pregnant women. Infection with one type of virus does not confer immunity against other types.

BRONCHITIS

Any of the germs that get into the nose and throat may secondarily invade the lung or the bronchial tubes and set up the inflammation called "acute bronchitis." This usually starts gradually with frequent coughing that is more severe at night. Slight fever may be present. If the amount of debris and infected material is profuse the coughing will raise a thick material that has to be expectorated. Young children do not spit, but swallow the material and then frequently vomit to get rid of it.

Bronchitis is not really a disease in itself, but far more often a complication of a common cold, influenza, measles, rhinitis, diphtheria, scarlet fever or rickets. Prompt attention to these conditions with special consideration for the inflammation that has extended into the lungs will help to prevent acute bronchitis and may do much to stop its becoming chronic. Bronchitis is chiefly dangerous to little children, and continuous inflammation with much coughing may make desirable removal to a warm climate to help the child get rid of the infection.

Since inflammation becomes worse when tissues are irritated, people with chronic inflammation of the bronchial tubes should avoid contact with irritating dusts, fumes, gases, or paints. Tobacco smoking must be stopped. The infected individual does better in a clean atmosphere where the air is neither too cold, too damp, too warm nor too dry.

All sorts of cough mixtures are known that will increase the flow of mucus and make the raising of the sputum easier. Inhaling steam seems to help many people. If there is sensitivity the use of antihistaminic drugs may be helpful and may aid also by a sedative effect.

MEASLES

Measles have been one of the most frequent of the childhood diseases. The condition is quite infectious, and is accompanied usually by a rash, with fever, cough, and inflamed eyes. Measles are caused by a specific virus which spreads easily from one person to another.

From ten to fourteen days after a child has been in contact with another who has had measles, symptoms like those of a severe cold develop. The child becomes drowsy and irritable. The eyes water and look red and the child avoids light. The appetite is poor. By the end of the third or fourth day the rash appears with individual spots that are at first pinhead size and pale red but then enlarge, become elevated and a darker red. The eruption is seen first usually on the face, scalp, and behind the ears, but then gradually covers the whole body. The fever increases as the rash breaks out. After the second or third day the rash begins to fade, the temperature falls and after seven days, usually, the patient is on the way to complete recovery.

During the first few months of life the child often has immunity from measles by antibodies derived from its mother. As the immunity wears off the child becomes susceptible, and most cases occur in children three or four years old. The child may be injected with globulin which provides immunity against measles. In 1962 a vaccine useful to prevent measles was developed by Dr. John Enders based on isolation of the measles virus.

Since the development of antibiotic drugs secondary complications of measles are more easily controlled. During the acute illness the child is kept at rest, given plenty of fluids, such as citrus drinks, a soft diet and good nursing. For itching of the skin a calamine lotion is used. The eyes are protected against irritation. For more severe cases convalescent serum or gamma globulin may be used. Measles are not a serious disease except for very small babies. Prevention and control of pneumonia at the earliest sign is most important.

GERMAN MEASLES OR RUBELLA

A virus like that of measles but distinct from it, as recognized by the different nature of the condition produced, causes German measles. This condition has assumed increasing importance recently, since it has been recognized that German measles infecting a prospective mother during the first three months of pregnancy can seriously damage the unborn child. German measles is a mild contagious disease with symptoms like those of a mild cold accompanied by a dark rash.

From ten to twenty days after exposure the condition begins with malaise, headache, a slight rise in temperature, and stiffness and soreness of the neck because of the enlargement of the glands at the back of the neck. The rash starts on the face and neck and spreads rapidly. The rash persists two or three days. The disease is more severe in adults and very young children. Usually one attack confers permanent immunity. Because of the dark red rash German measles is often confused with scarlet fever.

The disease is usually so mild that the only treatment is good nursing. Young married women need to be protected in times of epidemic. Often gamma globulin is given to help resistance. From 5 to 20 per cent of pregnant women who get German measles have babies damaged by the infection.

CHICKEN POX

Another common childhood disease caused by a virus is chicken pox. From ten to twenty days after exposure the symptoms begin with mild headache, loss of appetite and fever. Then after thirty-six hours the eruption appears. The rash usually is seen on the body and later on the face, neck, and extremities. Little red pinpoints enlarge to papules which change to blisters or vesicles. After a few days these break and are covered by dark brown crusts. The spots may become secondarily infected from scratching and pus infection will leave scars.

Chicken pox requires little treatment except to keep the areas free from secondary infection. The fingernails of children should be kept trimmed short. The itching is controllable by a calamine lotion containing 1 per cent of menthol or of phenol. If secondary infection occurs, antibiotic ointments will stop the spread. Chicken pox seems to be related to the nerve condition causing blisters known as *herpes zoster*. The common name for *herpes zoster* is "shingles."

WHOOPING COUGH OR PERTUSSIS

A germ called the *Hemophilus pertussis* is now recognized as the cause of whooping cough. The germ is spread from one person to another by direct contact or through coughing, sneezing, or talking.

The attack of whooping cough is usually divided into four parts, one stage running into another. About seven to fourteen days after exposure the condition begins with symptoms like those of a cold, such as sneezing, running nose, and hoarseness. The fever is mild. In the second stage a cough gradually becomes hard, dry, and annoying; it is more severe at night. The exudation makes this known as the catarrhal stage. During the third stage whooping develops with a wheezing inhalation of breath. The face becomes swollen and red, the tongue protrudes and the eyes water. After a whoop there may be a pause, followed by another spell of whooping and coughing. The difficulty may result in vomiting. During the fourth stage there is a gradual lessening of whooping and paroxysms of coughing. The total duration of the condition may be six to eight weeks or more.

Nowadays inoculation against whooping cough is possible with good vaccines. Children should be protected as they are protected against diphtheria.

In the treatment of whooping cough the new antibiotics have been found effective, and the disease is now much less feared. Streptomycin, aureomycin and terramycin are effective. The cough is controlled with suitable medication and sedatives. The nutrition of children must be watched carefully, as severe coughing with prolonged paroxysms may seriously interfere with taking and retaining food. Food can be given frequently and in small quantities.

DIPHTHERIA

Diphtheria is caused by a germ called the diphtheria bacillus and known scientifically as the *Corynebacterium diphtheria*. The disease is transmitted by droplets thrown into the air by coughing or sneezing. Children who have recovered from the disease may carry the germ. Indirectly the condition is transmitted on books, toys, clothing, and eating utensils.

Diphtheria develops usually from one to four days after exposure. The first signs are chilliness, slight fever, and loss of appetite, sometimes accompanied by vomiting and headache. Within twenty-four hours, sore throat occurs and a membrane or yellowish-white deposit is seen in the throat and over the tonsils. Membrane may also form in the nose or larynx. The symptoms become more severe, as the lymph glands in the neck enlarge. The fever may go to 102° F. or higher and is generally highest at the beginning of the disease. Often there is cough and, with severe infection, some prostration.

All children should be inoculated with antidiphtheria toxoid as soon as possible after reaching six months of age. The power of the toxoid is well established, and now there are many cities in the United States which haven't a single death from diphtheria in a year.

The treatment of diphtheria is of the greatest importance since the prompt giving of enough antitoxin will prevent spread to important nerves or other tissues of the body. Most dangerous is spread of the membrane into the larynx and serious interference with breathing. Recent research has shown the ability of penicillin to control the growth of the diphtheria germ and, conceivably, antibiotic treatment may eventually replace other forms of treatment.

RICKETTSIAL INFECTIONS

The Rickettsiae are minute infectious agents, smaller than most germs and larger than most viruses. Most classifications put them midway between the bacteria and the viruses. Rickettsia are too large to pass through a bacterial filter and are visible with an ordinary microscope. Like the viruses, they multiply only in the presence of living cells and many of them live inside living cells. They usually are transferred from animals to men by ticks, mites, fleas, or lice. Many of the rickettsial diseases of men have been identified as such only during the last fifty years. The word "Rickettsia" comes from the name of Howard Taylor Ricketts, a physician in Chicago who was one of the first to observe these organisms and determine their nature.

A form of typhus fever called "murine typhus" is an acute infectious disease caused by an organism of the rickettsia. The disease usually begins with a sudden fever that lasts two or three weeks; the rash is located mostly on the trunk. The disease was first described in the United States by James Paullin of Georgia in 1913. The chief mammalian carrier of murine typhus is the rat. The infection is transmitted from rat to rat by fleas. The rat louse will not feed on man but the flea will if given opportunity. The flea bite is not infectious but when the flea bites a man, the flea may deposit its excretions; then the human being scratches himself and thus may force these excretions of the flea into his skin.

About six to fourteen days after such infection has taken place, illness begins with a chill and muscular aching, headache, fever, loss of appetite, and cough; with this comes a feeling of severe illness. A skin eruption helps make the diagnosis. This eruption is present in 90 per cent of white patients, but of course is difficult to see on patients with a colored skin. The lesions of the skin are not hemorrhagic. In many patients the spleen is enlarged. Usually after eight to ten days the symptoms lessen and diminish—the condition clearing up in about three weeks.

Fortunately, two of the new antibiotic drugs—aureomycin and chloromycetin—have been established as valuable in controlling the symptoms of this virus infection. Most of those with murine typhus need lots of fluids while they are ill; if they cannot drink water, it is put into the body in other ways.

About one out of every one hundred people with the disease may be so severely sick as to die of it. The ones who die are usually the very old or sick people.

139

The extremely severe epidemic typhus that is seen in Russia is exceedingly rare in the United States. A form of typhus which occurred to our soldiers in the Far East is called "scrub typhus" and known to the Japanese as tsutsugamushi disease. In these conditions modern treatment involves the use of aureomycin, chloromycetin and sometimes para-amino benzoic acid which is effective in interfering with the nutrition of the virus in the body.

ROCKY MOUNTAIN SPOTTED FEVER

Rocky Mountain spotted fever is a severe infectious disease with chills, fever, prostration, and a hemorrhagic rash. It is caused by a Rickettsial organism and is transmitted by wood ticks. A disease called Brazilian typhus is identical, as are Mediterranean fever, South African tick-bite fever and Kenya fever.

Rocky Mountain spotted fever is largely a rural disease; it has been found in every state in the United States except Maine and Vermont. It occurs chiefly during the warm months of the year when the ticks are active. Indeed the only insects known to spread the disease are the ticks. These include the wood tick, the dog tick, the lone star tick, and the rabbit tick. The tick attaches itself to an infected animal and transfers the infection to man.

Two to fourteen days after being bitten, the illness comes on abruptly with chills, fever, severe frontal, or occipital headache, pains in the muscles and joints and sensitivity of the eyes to pressure and to light. Nausea, vomiting, constipation, nosebleed, a mild cough and similar symptoms appear, along with a fever which will rise rapidly from 103 to 105 degrees.

A rash is characteristic. It develops two to six days after the onset of the illness, usually first around the wrists and ankles and then spreading to involve the entire body surface. Several crops of the rash may appear, one after the other. Sometimes the rashes become hemorrhagic. The damage may be so great that gangrenous changes occur in the skin on the tips of the fingers, the toes, the earlobes and even on the soft palate. Secondary to these infections may be pneumonias, hemorrhages of the stomach and intestines and kidneys and serious inflammations of the eyes.

Vaccines have been prepared which are used to immunize people against Rocky Mountain spotted fever. Fortunately, chloromycetin, aureomycin, terramycin and para-amino benzoic acid have proved to be beneficial in Rocky Mountain spotted fever. The condition was formerly much more severe than since the new antibiotics have been developed. Once from 12 to 25 per cent of those infected died of the condition but it seems likely that with the new antibiotic drugs something less than 5 per cent of deaths will occur.

Q FEVER

Q fever is an acute illness often accompanied by pneumonia which results from infection with a form of Rickettsia. The first human cases of the disease were observed in Australia in 1933. Since they originated in Queensland, the infection was named "Q fever." Now a similar organism has been isolated from ticks captured in Montana and cases have been found in other areas of the United States.

Human beings are highly susceptible to Q fever; from 25 to 40 per cent of those exposed may be attacked by the disease. The condition was found much more often in Australia among people exposed to cattle. Before 1946 the disease was rare in the United States but has now been found particularly in epidemics in stockyards such as the one in Amarillo, Texas, in Chicago, and among dairymen in Los Angeles county. Workers in research institutes have frequently been infected.

From twelve to twenty-six days after exposure, the disease comes on with symptoms like those seen in other Rickettsial diseases. The two striking features that make Q fever different from other infections with Rickettsia is the absence of any characteristic rash and the almost invariable presence of pneumonia. However, pulmonary symptoms are often mild or absent. About one-half the patients have aches in the chest. X-ray of the chest shows that the lungs have been infected in at least 90 per cent of the cases.

Q fever may be confused with primary virus pneumonia, with tuberculosis, with psittacosis or infected bird fever, and must also be distinguished from ordinary influenza, sinusitis, undulant fever, dengue, and other Rickettsial infections.

Here again aureomycin, chloromycetin, and terramycin have been found useful in treatment. Relapses are rare. Most of the patients recover. Thus far only some eight or ten deaths have occurred among perhaps 1,000 cases that have been reported in medical writings.

GERM INFECTIONS—PNEUMONIA

Pneumonia was once one of the most feared of all human diseases. Its death rate was about a third of all those whom it attacked. The germ that caused it is one called a "pneumococcus" which lives ordinarily in the noses and throats of anywhere from 5 to 60 per cent of people. The condition comes on most often in the winter months and can affect people of all ages.

The pneumococcus gets down into the lungs and there sets up a severe infection which follows a typical course. For a few days the symptoms are like those of an ordinary respiratory disease. Then comes the sudden hard, shaking chill, rapid rise in temperature and pulse rate, with a severe pain on one side of the chest that the doctor recognizes as the beginning of pneumonia. The cough comes on painfully and with small amounts of pink or rust-colored sputum. Breathing is rapid, shallow and painful. There may be blueness because the blood is not getting enough oxygen.

The doctor, by the use of his stethoscope and by watching the motion of the chest, by thumping to discover areas of consolidation, recognizes that the lung is congested and unable to function. Usually after seven to ten days a crisis occurs. The body temperature falls to normal in from six to twelve hours, accompanied by profuse sweating, and the pneumonia as such is over.

The development of the new antibiotic drugs has changed the whole picture. Now, following the administration of penicillin, the pain in the pleura which lines the chest disappears in a few hours and the temperature, pulse, and respiration fall to normal in twelve to thirty-six hours. The spread of the inflammation can be stopped even before a single lobe is involved. This change in the nature of pneumonia is one of the most dramatic occurrences that has ever taken place in medicine and represents one of the greatest accomplishments of the present century.

For the treatment of pneumonia nowadays the chief reliance is on the drugs. The patient is kept in bed in a position in which he is most comfortable. He is given considerable rest but is permitted to sit up for examinations and for any other necessary procedure. He usually has little appetite and need not be urged to eat, but within a half a day after the specific treatment has been begun, he may be hungry and can take a soft diet. Formerly great efforts were made to keep the bowels moving; that too is no longer a serious problem for the doctor. If there is a real shortage of air and the person seems blue, oxygen can be given. It is customary to give oxygen now as soon as it is needed and not to wait until the patient seems actually to suffer from oxygen lack.

The pain in the chest can be controlled with suitable drugs. It is also possible to relieve severe pain by the injection of local anesthetic drugs or by strapping or wrapping the chest wall to prevent unnecessary motion.

142

The doctor is alert for complications. If penicillin is not as effective as seems to be desirable, aureomycin, the sulfonamides, such as sulfadiazine, and other methods may be tried. Particularly, however, the doctor must look out for complications such as secondary formation of pockets of infected material at the bottom of the lung.

The former fatality rate of 25 to 30 per cent has now dropped to less than 7 per cent. Pneumonia is still a particularly serious disease to those who have been long weakened by some other disease such as cancer or alcoholism or malnutrition, or some other serious complication involving the heart.

STAPHYLOCOCCUS INFECTIONS

Staphylococci used to be among the most feared of all the germs that attack mankind. In their various forms they could attack mucous membranes, the tissues of the heart, even the entire blood. Boils, carbuncles, and similar manifestations of staphylococcus infection were frequent. The germs would get into the centers of bones and cause the condition called osteomyelitis. Many a child was crippled for life by the inability of medicine to control this infection.

Occasionally staphylococci attack the bowel through entrance with food. Staphylococcus food poisoning results from the absorption of the toxin given off by the germ. The response is cramping pain, usually coming on two to four hours after the food is taken, with nausea, vomiting, and diarrhea. This lasts for a few hours, seldom more than a day. After twenty-four hours, the attack subsides, leaving the patient weak. The best treatment is to go right to bed and stop taking food for at least twenty-four hours. Paregoric is usually given to relieve the diarrhea and the cramping. Of course, a doctor has to make sure that the condition is not appendicitis or some similar disturbance.

Penicillin is the drug that is most frequently recommended for treating staphylococcal infections. When the germs are resistant to penicillin some of the other antibiotic drugs may be used, including the sulfonamides. Mixtures of several sulfonamides, such as streptomycin, aureomycin, or terramycin, are sometimes successfully used. The sulfonamides and the antibiotics are so effective in combating staphylococci that the only additional treatment usually required is good nursing. Surgery helps by opening accumulations of pus and draining away infected material, after which healing occurs promptly. A recent discovery is an antibiotic called staphcillin effective against staphylococci resistant to penicillin.

143

INFECTIOUS HEPATITIS

Infectious hepatitis is an infectious disease caused by a virus. Formerly the condition was simply called jaundice; now we know that catarrhal jaundice is produced by an inflammation of the liver resulting from an attack by the virus which is specific for that disease. Epidemiologists believe that the virus gets into the human being by two possible routes: 1) by inhaling a droplet from the throat coughed into the air by people who are infected, and 2) by consuming contaminated food or water.

A similar condition called homologous serum jaundice follows the injection of blood or serum from certain donors who harbor a virus that attacks the liver. This type of jaundice has a longer incubation period than infectious hepatitis—namely, from 50 to 140 days after the transfusion, compared to 25 or 46 days after receiving the virus by the routes previously mentioned.

Since the use of one syringe and a different needle for each person in a series of mass injections has been shown to be involved sometimes in causing homologous serum jaundice, doctors urge the only sure way to prevent this is to provide a heat-sterilized needle and a separate syringe for each person. Usually infectious jaundice causes gastrointestinal trouble, including nausea and loss of appetite, occasionally with fever, before the jaundice which is characteristic of this condition first appears. Symptoms include some upper abdominal pain on the right side and a loss of appetite associated with nausea. Vomiting and diarrhea occur in about one-fifth of the cases. Occasionally the liver is found to be enlarged and tender.

The jaundice and the symptoms gradually subside in from one to three weeks. When the jaundice has cleared completely and the patient is becoming convalescent, relapses may occur and the jaundice will reappear. Rest in bed is one of the most important treatments. Most of the patients get well and do not have any aftereffects; about 90 per cent recover without any damage. The number of people who die is exceedingly small, perhaps one in every 500 people who are infected with this virus. In 1 or 2 per cent of the infected chronic liver damage occurs, and these people can be troubled thereafter with hardening and scarring of the liver.

Certain factors seem to predispose people who have infectious hepatitis to having a serious case instead of a mild one. Probably the most important factor is a low state of nutrition. The high mortality observed in outbreaks among the native people in such areas as India where famine has been prevalent is not seen in healthy European countries, where mortality rates are much less. In undernourished communities, the mortality rate may be fifteen times that among well-nourished people. Severe injuries or burns associated with infectious hepatitis make the condition much worse, and pregnancy is reported to increase the risk of serious and permanent damage to the liver. Since malnutrition, injuries, burns and pregnancy all are related to disturbance of the protein metabolism, the massive damage to the liver that occurs when people have diets deficient in protein seems to bear a definite relationship to the severity of infectious hepatitis.

Although various methods of treatment have been tested, no specific chemical substance has been found which is effective against the virus of infectious hepatitis. Rest in bed for as long as the illness persists is one of the most important forms of treatment. When the bile had disappeared from the urine of the patient, he is allowed to leave his bed in order to attend to his toilet. Otherwise he must have complete rest in bed until the enlargement of the liver and the tenderness have disappeared. After infectious hepatitis, return to work must be gradual since the condition leaves patients seriously exhausted.

Protein is necessary to maintain the integrity and function of the liver. The diet in infectious hepatitis should be rich in protein and carbohydrate but poor in fat. The fats must not, however, be so severely restricted that the food will become unpalatable and the patient will lose his appetite and quit eating. The diets recommended are 150 grams of protein, 350 grams of carbohydrate and 50 grams of fat which provide about 2,500 calories. This is more than ample for a person confined to bed. Since the appetite is weak, the meals are to be small and given at frequent intervals. People who are severely undernourished and who sustain infectious hepatitis may have extra amounts of certain basic amino acids, methionine, cystine or choline, which deficiencies seem to enhance the virulence of the virus. British investigators suggest that water-soluble vitamins, particularly ascorbic acid, must be provided in adequate amounts to these patients, and also the vitamins of the B complex.

Therefore, in addition to rest and careful supervision of diet, the treatment of infectious hepatitis is applied to control of unpleasant symptoms like constipation, the use of sedatives to insure rest and sleep and other methods of treatment to control nausea and vomiting. If much water is lost by vomiting and diarrhea, the provision of extra fluid is important.

BRUCELLOSIS OR UNDULANT FEVER

The brucella germs are the cause of brucellosis or undulant fever.

Undulant fever has been known also as Malta fever. The condition is far more widespread now than formerly, although methods of prevention have been developed based on our knowledge of the fact that the disease is spread through drinking milk from infected cattle and through contact with the meat of infected animals.

Aureomycin has been found to produce prompt improvement in the symptoms of undulant fever with a lowering of the fever, a reduction in the size of the spleen and the other general symptoms of this disease which are so unpleasant. Streptomycin and sulfadiazine employed together are especially effective in controlling the organisms of undulant fever. Aureomycin seems to be preferred, however, to this combination of drugs because later reports show more satisfactory results and less of the toxic relations that accompany the use of the other antibiotics that have been mentioned. The results with terramycin appear to be about as good as those with aureomycin.

Before the antibiotic drugs were discovered and found to be so useful in brucellosis, patients were usually put to bed and given proper diet. Under these circumstances they seemed to recover gradually, although relapses were exceedingly frequent. Brucellosis is a rather chronic disease which may last for several months—even years—and be quite weakening. After the infection is over, people are weak, fatigued, nervous and often depressed. Loss of ambition is one of the most prominent symptoms of people who have had undulant fever.

Because the emotional reaction to the weakness may be so great, doctors are warranted in assuring patients that with proper treatment, complete recovery may occur and they can eventually regain their strength. In order to enable the person who has been weakened by a chronic disease to regain strength, rest, sunshine and a good diet with plenty of protein and vitamins is of the utmost importance.

POLIOMYELITIS OR INFANTILE PARALYSIS

For many years infantile paralysis has been the most feared of all the crippling diseases that affect mankind. The year 1955 marked the turning point toward elimination of infantile paralysis as a threat, just as typhoid fever and smallpox have been eliminated. This has resulted from the work of the National Foundation for Infantile Paralysis, which began raising funds for research on this disease in 1937. Up to that time the suspicion prevailed that this disease was caused by a virus, but the virus was not isolated. Today the viruses—there are several of them—have been isolated and grown in pure form outside the human

146

body. For this work Enders and his associates received the Nobel Prize. When the virus could be grown outside the human body on monkey kidneys in pure form, the preparation of a vaccine was attempted by Dr. Jonas Salk and early experimentation indicated that the inoculation of a mixture of killed viruses would produce in a child resistance against infection with this disease. After pilot experiments a vast experiment was undertaken under the auspices of the National Foundation for Infantile Paralysis in which great numbers of children were inoculated and compared with a similar number who did not receive the inoculation. Once this effective experiment was reported on April 12, 1955, at Ann Arbor, Michigan, the vaccine was made available by various manufacturers throughout the United States. Subsequently the research of Dr. Albert Sabin resulted in the development of a vaccine made of living attenuated viruses of infantile paralysis. Both the Salk and Sabin vaccines are now available for protection. The number of cases of poliomyelitis in the United States decreased from a high of over 57,879 cases in 1952 to less than fifty in 1972.

Since the virus of infantile paralysis seems to be spread by excretions from the bowel, the excretions of patients should be considered infectious and should be disposed of with precautions that they do not spread contamination. Little seems to be gained by adding antiseptic substances to the excretions but disposal of the material in a suitable toilet and thorough cleansing of vessels, such as bedpans, are important.

As soon as there is a question that the patient may have poliomyelitis, bed rest is important. The patient without paralysis must be confined to bed for at least three or four days after the temperature has returned to normal.

Most orthopedic specialists recommend the firm, hard bed from the beginning. The muscle tightness and paralysis can be helped by a suitable bed. The bed should be fitted with a footboard which is placed several inches beyond the mattress and allows room for pressure by the heels or toes of the patient when the patient lies on the back or on the stomach. This footboard also protects the legs from the pressure of bedclothing and gives opportunity to avoid muscle weakness by such use as can be made of the limbs. If the legs are weak, the knees are usually supported in a slightly relaxed position.

Since poliomyelitis is such a frightening disease, the doctor must do everything that he can to prevent fear and terror on the part of the infected child or of the parents. Early in the disease the whole family must be adjusted to the fact that there is a medical problem. Such attention given early in the condition is likely to avoid nervous and psychotic disturbances at a later date.

In the early stages, infantile paralysis is treated exactly as one would treat other infectious diseases, like measles, scarlet fever, or whooping cough. The treatment is usually rest in bed with a light diet but particularly with good nursing care.

During the early stages of inflammation, the patient must be provided with relief from pain. The use of moist heat is now considered most effective, including the application of hot baths for small children or for older ones, and the hot packs applied for thirty-minute periods every four to six hours. The extreme ritual developed by recent technics is not absolutely necessary. If patients revolt against hot packs, they should be discontinued.

EPIDEMIC ENCEPHALITIS

Epidemics of brain fever are not an excessively large cause of disability and death in the United States. There have, however, been outbreaks such as the one which occurred in St. Louis in 1933 in which there were more than 1,000 cases. In the St. Louis epidemic there were 100 cases for every 100,000 population and 20 per cent of those who were infected died. In various epidemics the number of cases varies from two cases for every 100,000 people to as many as twenty-two for every 100,000 people. A minor outbreak appeared in Florida in 1962.

Now it is established that the cause of epidemic encephalitis is a virus and that the outbreaks in human beings are closely related to certain similar conditions attacking animals, particularly an epidemic of a similar condition which concerns horses.

In several regions domestic birds such as chickens have been associated with the spread of the condition. In a California outbreak, the English sparrow and several species of blackbirds were involved. Research has also shown that various mosquitoes and mites as well as ticks may be associated with the spread of this virus.

In the prevention of encephalitis, control of the mosquitoes is of the utmost importance. Vaccines have been developed which may be used in outbreaks among horses. The condition is so serious that its appearance in any community should involve immediate investigation by competent health authorities.

CHAPTER XXIII

SOME COMMON SKIN DISEASES

ERUPTIONS ON THE SKIN result from a variety of causes. The rashes of measles, scarlet fever, German measles, Rocky Mountain spotted fever, and similar infectious conditions are typical. Most common of all skin eruptions, however, is that associated with the period of adolescence and called simply *acne vulgaris,* or referred to as pimples and blackheads.

ACNE VULGARIS

The eruption of acne is most frequent on the face, but spreads also to the neck, back, and trunk. Pinhead- or pea-size red swellings occur, many of them with little white spots of pus at the center. Blackheads are often followed by pimples. The skin around a blackhead or pimple is inflamed and red.

Germs are often found in pimples, but most physicians believe that the ordinary germs are secondary and are not the cause of the acne. The pimples come on after adolescence, and there is a tendency to relate their appearance to glandular changes associated with puberty. Constipation, overeating of sugars, oiliness of the skin, and anemias are also believed to be secondarily related to acne.

Perhaps the best advice for a boy or girl with acne is to make sure that his diet and nutrition are of the best. Scrupulous cleanliness is important. The face may be washed with applications of hot water, then the blackheads gently squeezed out, and after that an application may be made of a cream containing sulfur and resorcin which dries and disinfects the lesions. In some instances the use of the sex gland hormones seems to have been helpful. Large doses of vitamin A are now frequently prescribed. In the more severe cases doctors use X-ray and occasionally ultraviolet. For control of the pus-forming germs antibiotic ointments are tried; also Cortisone ointments as prescribed by the doctor.

PRICKLY HEAT

Frequently the skin becomes irritated due to excessive perspiration after exposure to heat. Wearing excessive clothing in hot weather is a contributing cause. The inflammation occurs most often in the folds of the skin about the neck, and under the breasts, but occasionally also on the chest and back and between the thighs.

The reddened skin develops little tiny, transparent blisters filled with a clear fluid. The itching and burning may be severe. Prevention of contact of the surfaces of the skin will give the inflamed area a chance to heal.

As recovery from the irritation occurs the dead skin may peel away. The greatest danger arises, however, from too much treatment, which increases the inflammation and gives opportunity for pus germs to invade.

The utmost cleanliness is important in all irritations of the skin, because damaged tissue gives opening to dangerous germs. The inflamed area may be washed with warm water and a bland soap, then dried carefully by patting without rubbing and powdered with a suitable powder. The physician will often prescribe a soothing lotion, like calamine lotion.

IMPETIGO

In impetigo, which is a rapidly spreading pus infection of the skin, the staphylococcus or streptococcus are most often involved. Once the infection has begun it may spread rapidly by the use of towels, or by squeezing or scratching with the fingernails. People find difficulty in letting themselves alone.

Impetigo begins as small blisters on the face, scalp, and hands. The blisters increase in size and spread, as new little blisters form at the borders. In infants, the blisters break and discharge a thin fluid, leaving a moist red spot. If secondary pus invaders come in, thick yellow matter forms. These areas may be covered by dirty brown crusts.

150

With proper treatment impetigo usually clears up rapidly. Nowadays the available remedies are so much more efficient than those previously known that most cases, when recognized, can be cleared in a few weeks. Formerly the blisters were opened, the area cleaned, and an ammoniated mercury ointment applied. Now antibiotic ointments are available which act specifically against the pus germs. Moreover, the doctor can inject adequate doses of the antibiotics into the body and attack the infection from inside. Washing the skin around the infection with alcohol helps to keep the infection from spreading.

Impetigo is most contagious, and a child with the disease should be kept away from other children. Epidemics are particularly likely to occur in the nurseries of large hospitals.

RINGWORM

Ringworm is the result of invasion of the skin by a fungus, and there are many different types. The scalp, skin between the toes, fingernails or toenails may be affected, as well as skin anywhere in the body. Occasionally the palms of the hands are attacked and the skin becomes softened and inflamed.

On the scalp, ringworm produces scaly gray spots from a fraction of an inch up to two inches wide. The hair falls out, and brittle stumps of broken hair may fill the area. On the body ringworm appears as small, pink, slightly raised spots, which gradually enlarge into ring-shaped areas. The centers of the spots are pale and white, while the edges are slightly raised and red. When ringworm attacks the feet the spaces between the toes are soft, scaling, tender, and occasionally blistered. Often there is a decaying odor to the peeling skin. Itching and burning are frequent symptoms of ringworm.

Once established in the scalp ringworm is difficult to control. The hair must be eliminated before remedies can attack the organisms in the roots. The hair may be pulled out or removed by X-ray, which may cause permanent loss of hair. The area may be shaved. Many cases are overtreated, and the resulting inflammation spreads the infestation.

Because ringworm is easily transmitted, those who are affected should wear a close-fitting skullcap and use only individual towels, combs, or hairbrushes. For years ringworm has been treated with Whitfield's ointment or other salicylic acid preparations. Applications include gentian violet, undecylenic acid and sodium proprionate. Newest is the use of an antibiotic called griseofulvin which, taken internally, acts to eliminate ringworm attacks.

The specialist in diseases of the skin will usually make some scrapings from the ringworm area and examine the material with the microscope. The nature of the ringworm may determine considerably the kind of treatment to be used.

PSORIASIS

The cause of psoriasis has not yet been determined. Many theories have been proposed relating the condition to the diet, to infection, to glandular disturbances, or constitutional disorders, but not one has yet been established. Psoriasis begins with flat, symmetrical reddish-brown spots or plaques on the skin, covered with silvery-white scales. Usually the condition is dry, without blisters or exudation. The spots are seen usually around the elbows, on the scalp, on the lower part of the back, and the upper chest. About 4 per cent of all the cases of skin diseases that come to doctors' offices are psoriasis.

Psoriasis is a chronic condition and once established tends to get better and worse and to disappear entirely for a while. For this reason innumerable technics have been announced as cures, only to be followed by subsequent disappointment when the condition recurred.

Many patients with psoriasis do well when put on a meatless diet. Some improve when treated with the appropriate sex gland extracts. Instances have been reported of psoriasis clearing up when treated by ultraviolet light, thiamin and other vitamins. Drugs taken internally, particularly derivatives of arsenic, have been reported helpful. Most recent in the treatment is the use of ACTH, the adrenal cortex tropic hormone, derived from the pituitary gland. This substance causes profound changes in the actions of various cells of the body and may act in that way to disturb the basic mechanism responsible for psoriasis.

URTICARIA OR HIVES

Hives are the response of the skin to sensitivity to some foreign protein substance. Hives are swellings, like long blisters, filled with a yellowish fluid which may come on any part of the body. Most frequently they appear on the legs, the back of the neck, the buttocks, and outer surface of the thighs. Like other forms of allergy the tendency to hives seems to run in families.

Among the foods most commonly associated with hives are shellfish, strawberries, and eggs. Light, heat, cold, the sun's rays, insect bites, contact with moths, nettles, and caterpillars and many similar contacts may result in the appearance of these itching eruptions in the skin. Following emotional upsets people with a tendency to hives may have attacks. The skin in such cases may be so sensitive that blisters or a white line may develop simply from stroking the skin, a condition called "dermographia."

The chief effort toward treatment of urticaria is directed toward finding the cause and removing the patient from contact with it. Obviously a saline laxative will wash the offending substance out of the bowel. The injection of adrenalin or epinephrine has been shown valuable. More recently the antihistaminic drugs like pyribenzamine, benadryl, neohetramine and others have been proved almost specific against urticaria and other forms of sensitization. The itching can be stopped by washing with baking soda solution, or by applying a calamine lotion with 1 per cent of menthol or phenol.

WARTS

There is no proof that warts are caused by a virus, but the vast majority of medical opinion now inclines to the view that a specific virus is responsible. Warts occur most frequently on the hands, the face, the soles of the feet, and the neck. Ordinary warts, called *verrucae vulgaris* are hard grayish-yellowish or brownish elevations on the skin of varying size. Juvenile warts are usually smaller. Unless the wart is in intimate contact with a nerve ending it is not likely to be painful. Warts may grow rapidly and spread, or they may remain isolated and stop growing or disappear, often without any special treatment.

Warts may be destroyed with acid, or with carbon-dioxide snow or with the X-ray. For ordinary juvenile warts a paste containing salicylic acid is sometimes effective. If warts are large or disfiguring, the best treatment may be simply removing them surgically.

A new method of treatment is simply action of cold water for a half hour.

HERPES

Herpes simplex is due to a virus which causes cold sores or fever blisters on the face (particularly the lips), occasionally also on the genitalia. Children between the ages of one and five frequently have herpes blisters in the cheeks and mouth and also on the genitalia. The cold sores are usually best treated by applying a cream or ointment that contains a small amount of Cortisone (0.2 per cent) which may be prescribed by the physician. This is applied twice daily. If sunlight seems to induce the blisters, sunlight should be avoided.

The more severe form of herpes is called herpes zoster or shingles. It is produced by the same virus that produces chicken pox. This virus may be latent in the body. It affects old people more often than younger ones. The blisters may be accompanied with pain, headache, sometimes fever. The condition is called shingles after the Latin word *cingulum* which means a belt, because the herpes go around the body.

Most people recover in about three weeks. Sometimes the burning and the pain require a pain-relieving drug. Physicians may also prescribe some of the Cortisone derivatives, either taken internally or applied as ointments.

CHAPTER XXIV

CANCER

CANCER IS A WILD, unrestrained growth of cells. Some disturbance occurs which disrupts the balance of cells of different kinds in the body. The cells seem to return to their primitive state or to the infantile or fetal type. The body of a baby before birth grows much faster than does a cancer, but the growth of the cells in the developing child is controlled or regulated by an internal mechanism.

Many substances have the ability to stimulate the growth of cells. Pure chemicals, glandular substances, or physical forces like heat or pressure may stimulate cell growth. The changes that initiate the sudden, rapid growth of cancer cells and the traveling of these cells into other parts of the body involve many different factors related to the chemistry of the body, its nutrition, damage to tissues by inflammation and infection, and modifications of growth brought about by glandular action.

A variety of chemical products, particularly those related to tar, are known to be able to stimulate the growth of cancer. In tropical areas white people who do not protect themselves against the sun develop cancer in amounts out of all proportion to that which occurs among the native people with darker skins. To a large extent farmers also, as well as sailors, suffer from cancers of the skin.

Irritation is still a basic factor in the production of cancer. Continuous rubbing, irritation by irregular or jagged teeth, and heat from a pipe carried always in one corner of the mouth are known to be types of irritation that can excite the growth of cancer.

SUSPICIOUS SYMPTOMS

Certain symptoms are suspicious and should be given serious consideration. Not long ago a state cancer organization asked 158 people with cancer why they had delayed so long in seeking medical attention with their problem. One half of them said that they had not taken it seriously. Two had hesitated because they were afraid of cancer and two because they were afraid of doctors. Ten per cent said that they just had not bothered about it, and another 10 per cent were afraid that it would cost them something to see the doctor. This information is enlightening, since we know that hundreds of thousands of lives could be saved today if people would just bring their symptoms soon enough to the attention of competent physicians and surgeons.

Whenever a lump appears underneath the surface of the body and does not go away the symptom must be considered suspicious. Whenever there is bleeding or a discharge, from any portion of the body, that is not easily explainable the symptom is a warning sign. Whenever a sore or rubbed area in the body does not heal promptly, investigation should be made immediately. Cancers that may be seen and felt easily are those on the skin, in the mouth, or in the breast. Women are much less likely to suffer cancers of the skin than are men, because women are much more careful about the appearance of the surface of the body. Men suffer more cancers of the mouth than do women. Cancers of the breast, however, are far more frequent in women than in men. The most frequent cancers which cannot be seen or felt but which warn of their presence by unusual symptoms such as bleeding and discharges are cancers of the urinary bladder, the kidney, or the organs concerned in childbirth.

Pain is a relatively late symptom in cancer. Pain is likely to cause people to seek medical attention promptly; but other symptoms usually come before pain. Cancers which cannot be seen and which do not give any external signs of their presence are those of the stomach, the bowels, or the lungs. Hoarseness that persists more than a short time, and particularly hoarseness that does not go away after the voice has been rested, may be considered a danger signal. Many a man with serious symptoms affecting his stomach satisfies himself with a dose of baking soda. This is like pouring water on a fire bell when the fire is burning in the house.

DIAGNOSIS OF CANCER

One of the most important single procedures used by the physician is the use of his hands in order to palpate or feel changes that have occurred underneath the surface of the body. As medicine is practiced in some parts of the world, patients seldom get time even to remove the necessary clothing to permit the doctor to look at the skin or to put his hands on various portions of the body in order to feel changes that have taken place.

When there is a suspicion of a new growth the doctor will look to see if there is any visible sign of a change on the surface of the body. He will then press with his fingers to determine whether or not lumps may be felt underneath the skin, or whether the outlines of various organs in the abdomen have been changed from what is usually felt.

New instruments have been developed that enable the doctor to project his powers of observation in a way that was not possible fifty years ago. There is now an electrically lighted instrument for every entrance and exit of the human body. The cystoscope, the bronchoscope, the esophagoscope, and the gastroscope are types of instruments which enable the doctor to look into the urinary bladder, the bronchial tubes, the stomach, and many other portions of the body.

With the X-ray the doctor can detect changes in the outlines of organs inside the body, and by combinations of the use of the X-ray with the use of certain drugs that can be taken internally he can get pictures of changes in outline and in functioning of various tissues of the body. He can even see tumors which project into the cavities inside the brain. In addition, there are devices such as the electroencephalograph which enable the doctor to determine changes in the function of the brain. There are also functional tests for the kidney, the stomach, the liver, the heart, and other vital organs.

Transillumination means that light is thrown through the tissues of the body; this is one of the tests that is used particularly in studying the breast for the presence of new growths.

New also in the study of cancer is the use of radioactive isotopes. We know today that certain chemical substances taken into the body will be carried by the blood to certain organs or tissues, where they are deposited. Thus, more than 90 per cent of iodine taken into the body goes directly to the thyroid gland. Calcium is deposited in bones and teeth. Some substances go directly to the liver. Radioactivity attached to these chemical substances goes with them, and they can then be detected in various portions of the body by use of the device called the Geiger counter, which shows the presence of the radioactive substances by a

157

clicking sound. All over the country research is now being made to determine how valuable radioactive isotopes can be in aiding not only in diagnosis but also in treatment of cancer.

New also in the study of cancerous changes are the studies that are now being made on the blood. Certain conditions such as excessively rapid growth of the red blood cells, called polycythemia, or excessively rapid growth of white blood cells, as in leukemia, can only be detected by examining specimens of the blood under the microscope. Since these conditions come on insidiously, a proper examination will always include the taking of a specimen of blood and an observation of this blood under the microscope. It will include also counting of the cells in the blood, because there are several different types of cells and the relative percentages of various types of cells in the blood may be of the greatest significance in relation to determining the existence of these conditions that are called cancer of the blood.

Some conditions that occur in the body, while not necessarily cancerous, may be considered precancerous, or early stages of changes in the tissues that might eventually lead to cancer. Thus, women should be examined after childbirth to determine the presence of injuries of the tissues, and the proper repair of damage may prevent subsequent irritations that lead to cancer. Erosions, which are rubbed spots on the surface of the organ, need to be given proper care. Ulcers of the stomach occasionally develop cancerous manifestations. Continued irritation of the gall bladder by gallstones may in some instances bring about the kind of irritation that results in excessive and wild growth of cells. Bear in mind that none of these conditions is the cause of cancer. They are contributing factors which have to be studied. In the absence of the stimulus that leads to cancer the contributing factors alone do not result in cancer, but the combination may be deadly.

Cancers of the lung, the intestines, or the stomach usually come on insidiously, and the person affected may not be aware for some time of the nature of his condition. Often people are reluctant to let the doctor know when the symptoms first appear; sometimes they fail to pay attention because of fear or ignorance. Doctors believe that many more cases could be saved if only people would come to the doctor sooner.

Great numbers of women disregarded irregular bleeding from the organs of childbirth. Some people have opposed campaigns of education about cancer because of the fear that they might create phobias and develop neurotics.

The Papanicolaou test involves removal of a scraping from the organ concerned—cervix of the uterus, stomach lining or bronchial tubes—and examining this under the microscope for cancer cells. Every woman past thirty years of age should have such an examination of the cervix of the uterus at least once annually. A new device, the Gravlee jet washer can put fluid into the inside of the uterus and then cause it to flow out by creation of a vacuum, bringing along loose cells from the lining for examination.

Cancer of the skin, breast cancer, and cancer of the uterus give indications of their presence early, and a high percentage of these patients can be cured if the condition is diagnosed early and properly treated.

Much has been printed lately about the definite increase in cases of cancer of the lung, which a few relate to smoking. The relationship is not definitely proved. Early diagnosis in such cancers depends chiefly on paying attention to symptoms affecting the lung and getting promptly a good X-ray study. The mass X-ray studies for presence of tuberculosis have helped to locate some cases of cancer.

TREATMENT OF CANCER

Modern medicine has four chief means for eliminating cancer from the body. These are surgical operation, radium, X-ray and new specific drugs. By surgical operations the entire cancerous structure is removed and usually with it the organ that contains the cancer, if that is not a vital organ. Some cases of tumor are especially susceptible to radioactivity. They are called "radiosensitive." Other types are resistant to the radioactive rays. The X-ray, particularly the modern type of high-voltage, deep-penetrating X-ray, can be used in areas in which radium cannot be implanted and to which radium cannot extend.

This does not mean that every case of cancer can be treated by just one method. Every cancer is different from every other cancer. The doctor must decide in each instance the forms of treatment that will be most helpful. In some instances not only surgery, X-ray, and radium are employed but also other technics. The female sex hormone or estrogens are used in the control of cancer of the prostate. All over the United States studies were made under the direction of the Therapeutic Trials Committee of the Council on Pharmacy and Chemistry of the American Medical Association to determine whether or not testosterone, the male sex hormone, is valuable in treating cancer of the breast. Apparently it is helpful in preventing spread from cancer of the breast to other portions of the body.

With cancer of the breast early attention is vital. If a cancer of the breast comes to proper medical attention within the first few months the woman can have practically her normal life expectancy. If she delays to the time when the cancer has extended to the glands under the arm her life expectancy may be greatly reduced. Studies made of thousands of cases of cancer of the breast prove with certainty that early attention prolongs life. Delay is likely to be fatal.

Not so many years ago a cancer of the lung was invariably fatal. In 1933 a surgeon for the first time removed an entire lung by operation, because of the presence of cancer. The patient was another doctor. That patient is still alive. Today there are hundreds of people throughout the United States who have had all or part of a lung removed and who have survived the operation successfully. Thus what was an invariably fatal condition now yields in a considerable percentage of cases to modern methods of treatment, and patients recover. Similarly, cancer of the stomach was formerly considered invariably fatal. The percentage of recoveries in cases that are diagnosed early and that submit to proper surgical treatment is considerable. Unfortunately, far too many wait too long. The prolongation of life includes years which are exceedingly valuable, because these conditions do not generally occur in extremely young people but usually in men and women at the top of their productive periods.

Drugs called nitrogen mustards and other drugs that stop cell growth are now available for use against cancer. All are powerful and can be used only as prescribed by the doctor. A drug called methatrexate is specific and saves lives in cases of choriocarcinoma, a cancer of tissues involved in childbirth. Sarcolycin and actinomycin D have been used against other forms of cancer.

The death rate for cancer is still high. Two hundred thousand Americans now die of cancer each year. The new knowledge that may come through research may even serve to prevent the appearance of cancer among great numbers of people whose fathers or mothers or ancestors may have had cancer and died of it and who therefore form something resembling a stock or type in which cancer is more likely to occur than among the population generally.

DIAGNOSTIC TESTS

Investigators are using several diagnostic tests for cancer, as the Wassermann test is used in syphilis. If it can be found that these changes in the serum of the blood come early in the disease and can be quickly detected, an intensive search can be made for the manifestations of cancer in the body.

RESEARCH

Certain substances of the nature of folic acid have been found capable of stimulating the growth of body cells. Cancer, too, is an excessively rapid overgrowth of body cells. Other substances have been found which act against folic acid in this activity. The scientists are determining the value of anti-folic compounds as a treatment of such conditions as acute leukemia in which there is excessive growth of the white cells of the blood.

Cell chemistry is fundamentally involved in the production of cancer. For instance, one investigator painted the skin of baby chicks with a chemical called methylcholanthrene, which acts as an irritant and which is known to be a carcinogenic agent. Chicks are particularly resistant to this substance. The skin did not respond except with the appearance of a few warts. Then the chicks were injected with considerable doses of the male sex hormone, testosterone, and cancers appeared, some of which were large. This shows the effects of hormones on cell growth.

Previously, Dr. Huggins and his associates at the University of Chicago had shown that estrogenic hormones, the female sex hormone, can be of help in controlling the prostate gland cancers of men, and other investigators have shown that testosterone definitely modifies activities of breast cancers in women.

Many different chemical substances have been tested for their effects on the human body, with particular relationship to their ability to prevent the excessive growth of cells. When it was found that the constituents of the war gases known as nitrogen mustards could lessen the production of white blood cells, a series of studies were made involving 100 different nitrogen mustard compounds. Four, which seemed to be best, were eventually tested against human leukemia and also against Hodgkin's disease, which is a form of cancer of the lymph glands. The effects were interesting but did not prove of sufficient value to be adopted as a common treatment. Out of such studies came also trial of the anti-folic acid compounds. These studies warranted the conclusion that the substances that antagonize folic acid have a definitely beneficial, although temporary, effect on cases of acute leukemia. This is not a specific cure for the disease, but is so definitely a specific action that it represents a real advance in the treatment of acute leukemia. Urethane is one of several chemical compounds that have seemed to offer some usefulness against leukemia.

In 1956 several new substances were being tested in the chemical attack on cancer. Domagk who discovered the sulfonamides has a drug called 10[7]—ethylene—imino—quinone which stops growth of cancer cells without injuring normal cells. An antibiotic called Sanamycin acts similarly.

In the fight against cancer one of our most potent weapons is education of the public. Since cancer comes on insidiously and since it is controllable in great numbers of cases in its earliest stages, people have to be told again and again about the early signs and symptoms of cancer.

How can you help yourself against cancer? First, resolve to have an annual physical examination, which is a fine insurance not only against cancer but various insidious degenerative diseases. Look out for the cancer danger signals which should send you for an immediate investigation: 1. Any sore that does not heal. 2. A lump or thickening in the breast or elsewhere. 3. Unusual bleeding or discharge. 4. Any sudden change in a wart or mole. 5. Persistent indigestion or difficulty in swallowing. 6. Persistent hoarseness or cough. 7. Any change in normal bowel habits.

VIRUSES

In chickens and in mice viruses have been found which cause leukemia in these animals but such viruses have not been found in human leukemia. Viruses have also been related to other tumors. The body may build antibodies against foreign substances and conceivably vaccines against cancer may be developed.

CHAPTER XXV

EYES

YOUR EYES ARE AMONG the most valuable of all your organs. For that reason, they ought to have fairly frequent examinations by competent persons to make certain that they are free from disease and capable of doing an efficient job.

A good examination of the eye must detect symptoms and signs of difficulties such as swollen and inflamed lids, pain with or without redness, and any change in vision, such as double vision or dimming of the eyesight. Among the common difficulties with eyes are irritations of the lid such as sties and crusting of the lids. Overwork of the eye may lead to such signs of fatigue as discomfort, dizziness, scowling, rubbing of the eye, frequent blinking, or inability to do close work.

Some people quite obviously use only one eye, and turn the head to make that eye more effective. Other people hold the head in an unusual position in order to see better. This is due to the fact that they do not see objects in the normal positions. When there are crossed eyes or eyes that do not focus together properly the difficulty is easily apparent.

The inability to see distant objects is another indication that changes have taken place. In fact, when people hold reading material or other fine work unusually near or unusually far from the eyes they should have an immediate examination, probably with the intent to secure glasses that will meet their needs.

People who do not see clearly incline to stumble over objects in their path or fail to appreciate the height of steps. They get their fingers caught in machines. They have auto accidents. They fall downstairs. Good eyesight prevents innumerable unnecessary accidents.

MECHANISM OF VISION

We do not see with the eye but with the brain and the nervous system. The chief factors involved in seeing are the optic nerve and the center in the brain for vision. Next comes the retina, a tissue back of the eye, which is a part of the nervous system and which conveys what is seen to the optic nerve. The lens is actually a lens, and serves to focus objects on the retina. The muscles control the size and shape of the lens in its focusing. There are also accessory muscles which move the eyeball. The iris makes up the pupil. By dilating and contracting, the iris controls the amount of light which enters the eye.

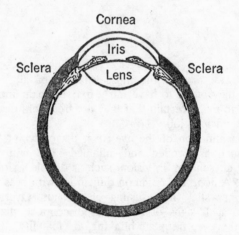

CROSS-SECTION OF EYE

The eye can adapt itself to various conditions of light, but even this mechanism of adaptation may be exhausted by overuse. It is better to provide suitable lighting than to strain the eye by insufficient light. The eye may also be strained by too much badly distributed light or glare. The effects of glare and of eyestrain result in the fatigue of the eye, with increased danger of accident.

Devices for measuring the amount of light in use at any point in the office, the shop, or the home are now available. Shades are made to distribute light suitably and thus prevent glare. Walls are painted and ceilings enameled to reflect a maximum amount of good light where it is most needed. Attention to these factors may mean many more years of good vision for those who otherwise would soon be incapacitated.

An eye which is fatigued and unable to work satisfactorily becomes easily irritated. Moreover, it is more likely to be invaded by foreign bodies like cinders and dust, simply because the tissues do not react to get rid of such foreign material. People with bad eyesight frequently have red rims on the eyes, swollen eyelids, and constant watering. The eyelids will be crusted together in the morning.

EYESTRAIN

Eyestrain is one of the common conditions that everyone talks about. Unsuspected eyestrain may be associated with twitching of the eyelids and face. It may be responsible for nausea and vomiting, for headache, bad nutrition, loss of appetite, and many other similar conditions. Yet the only way to determine whether or not eyestrain actually exists is to make a suitable examination of the ability of the eyes to see, and then to overcome the condition by rest and the provision of eyeglasses.

Motion pictures have been incriminated as a cause of eyestrain and tiredness. Under normal conditions moving pictures do not cause serious fatigue of the eye. However, the wrong type of lighting in a motion-picture house, films that are jerky or spotted or badly lighted, and long periods of projection without change in the light will produce serious fatigue of the eye. Televison used in moderation does not hurt the eye but flickering, glare, bad light may be harmful.

Suitable eyeglasses are prescribed nowadays for vision that is deficient or for the correction of the curves in the eyeball that result in astigmatism.

When eyeglasses first became popular they were frequently prescribed when they were not necessary. Everybody who had his eyes examined felt that he simply had to have glasses in order to justify the examination. Today the reaction against this results in the development of fakirs who try to get people to throw away their glasses.

There are three chief reasons for wearing glasses: to protect the eyes, to see well, and to see without fatigue. An eyeglass is a crutch to aid a deficient or weakened eye, exactly as an ordinary crutch aids a weakened limb. A crutch lends support until the limb is capable of working for itself. A permanently deformed limb or an eye of which the structure is anatomically wrong demands permanent use of a crutch or eyeglass. Proper glasses can relieve eyestrain; improper glasses may make the condition more severe. Contact lenses must be prescribed and fitted by experts and the users trained in how to take care of them.

Not only is your eye the window of your soul, but it is a barometer for measuring the health of your body. By looking into your eyes, visualizing their interior through the use of the ophthalmoscope, and by measuring certain of their reactions the physician can tell a great deal about your body generally.

Not only does the body reflect to some extent bad conditions of the eye, but the eye can reflect troubles elsewhere in the human body. When the doctor notes that your eyes are clear and bright, he diagnoses at once a fairly good state of health. A condition such as jaundice shows itself in yellowness of the eyeball. Frequently trouble in the brain or in the nervous system may be found by looking into the back of the eye with the ophthalmoscope. Certain conditions, such as alcoholism, rheumatism, gout, diabetes, and poisoning of the body by various metallic substances, reveal themselves in changes back of the eye.

DEVELOPMENT OF THE EYES

We depend so much on our eyes that we ought to give ourselves every benefit that we can in relation to their education, their hygiene, and their control. Here are some interesting facts about the development of the eye from birth.

The eye of the newborn child is about 70 per cent of the size of the eye of the person fully grown. It is a shorter eye than the eye of an adult; the lens of the eye of the newborn child is a sphere or circular globe. During the first few years of life the eye grows rapidly, and it reaches adult size at about the age of eight or nine years. The lens of the eye continues to grow throughout life.

The pupil of the eye is small at birth and remains small until about the end of the first year. During childhood and up to the age of youth the pupil of the eye develops its maximum size. Then it gradually becomes smaller, so that in older people the pupil depends to a large extent on the adaptation of the retina of the eye to light.

The retina is the nerve tissue at the back of the eye by which we are able to see. If a great deal of light suddenly pours into the eye the pupil will become smaller by contracting. Gradually the retina will adapt itself to the increased illumination. Then the pupil will again enlarge to approximately its normal size. There are, however, many different factors which may modify the size of the pupil from time to time.

The iris of the eye is the colored portion. People of dark races have

166

a darker color in the iris than those of the blond races. Most children are born with a blue iris, the color being due to the appearance of the color layer at the back of the iris. The color changes during the first years of life as the material becomes thicker. Then the eye may gradually become brown or even darker. If there is a lack of pigment the eye has a strange pinkish color such as is seen in albinos.

As the child grows the eye becomes longer. The retina is farther back, and the lens becomes flatter. This occurs mostly between the ages of six and sixteen.

If the rays of light which enter the eye focus short of the retina the child is nearsighted. If, for example, the eye of the child focuses normally at the time of birth, it is sure to become nearsighted as the eye becomes longer.

The lens in children is quite flexible, but as people grow older this flexibility tends to decrease. It is apparent, therefore, that parents should have the eyes of children tested regularly, to make certain that they are getting the best vision possible with the type of eyes they have at the time they are born.

Children must also be taught to use their eyes correctly. This involves co-ordination of nerves and muscles and of the brain, which can be improved with proper training. As the child grows older it develops what the specialists call "binocular vision"—that is to say, it uses both eyes in seeing. Sooner or later one eye becomes more important than the other and we tend to rely more on one eye than on the other. As Dr. W. S. Knighton has said, "One of the two assumes the role of the master eye."

SPOTS BEFORE THE EYES

One of the most common symptoms complained of by many people is a sense of spots floating before the eyes. Scientifically, these are called *muscae volitantes*. The specialist in diseases of the eye attaches little significance to these spots, unless such spots can be seen on special examination of the eye with the ophthalmoscope, the instrument with which the specialist looks into the eyes. These floating spots have been attributed to irritations of the eye, to congestion of the tissues, to eyestrain, and various constitutional diseases. Generally speaking, they are not important. If the person concerned has the right kind of glasses and keeps himself in good physical condition the spots will disappear.

SPARKS AND FLASHES

Many persons complain also of sparks or flashes of light. These are sometimes due to disturbances of the circulation of the blood of the eye. In cases in which one of the lining membranes of the eye may be inflamed the sensation of dazzling flashes of light of various colors may be very pronounced.

Some people complain particularly of constant showers of golden dust or of large numbers of black specks floating in front of the eyes or of stationary spots of large sizes. In many instances these are due to difficulties of color vision or of vision generally. Sometimes the wearing of blue-colored glasses, which cut off the red rays, will relieve the person concerned of his symptoms.

No doubt the best advice that can possibly be given to people generally is to tell them to see a competent specialist in diseases of the eyes at least once each year, and not to take lightly any disturbance of vision. The eye, once damaged, does not recover with ease; neither does any other highly specialized organ of the body. Disturbances seen early are treated to better advantage than if there is considerable delay.

INJURIES OF THE EYE

Eyes may be injured by the entrance of cinders, dust, pieces of glass or metal, which get imbedded in the tissues of the eye. The eye may be cut or wounded, may be bruised or burned, or damaged by chemicals.

The commonest difficulty with the eye is the entry of a particle of dust or a small cinder that gets caught under the eyelid. This causes pain, a flow of tears, difficulty with vision. A particle under the upper lid is worse than one under the lower lid. People who have been properly trained can evert or roll back the eyelid, detect the foreign substance, and remove it with a sterile, moist cotton applicator. If you have not been trained, do not try this procedure. You may do more damage than good. The simplest step in first aid to the eye is to cover it with a sterile bandage or a recently washed-and-ironed clean handkerchief and then to get the person to someone who understands the nature of the problem and who can do what needs to be done.

If an eye is burned by a chemical such as an acid, an alkali, lime, or an irritating gas the eye should be washed immediately with plenty of fluid. A simple way to do this is to put the whole head under water and then to open the eye under water. The doctor will irrigate or wash or flush the eye with a suitable solution, depending on the nature of the substance that has entered the eye. Boric-acid or sodium-bicarbonate solutions are the ones most frequently used. One of the most important aids to immediate care for injured eyes is the application of local anesthetics. These are now available in the form of ointments or solutions. They stop the pain of an injury and, above all, allay the fright and nervousness of the person who has a foreign body in the eye or who has suffered a burn or injury.

Remember: if you are not familiar with first aid to injured eyes let the eye alone. Simply cover the eye with a sterile bandage and get help from someone properly trained.

COLOR BLINDNESS

A Quaker bought himself some scarlet stockings when he thought he was purchasing dark brown. His name was John Dalton, and he is the first scientifically recorded instance of color blindness. Dalton was an eminent English physicist. It is said that he was walking down the street wearing his cap and gown and the red stockings at Oxford, where a degree had just been conferred upon him, and that one of his brother Quakers promptly took him to task for wearing such colors in public.

Color blindness is more common in boys than in girls. It is exceedingly important today, because the signals on the railroads and on street corners are most frequently red, green, and yellow, but occasionally also blue, and these are the colors most frequently concerned in color blindness. Certainly no one who happens to be handicapped with this condition should attempt to drive a motorcar in modern traffic. The difficulty of distinguishing between red and green is the most common form of color blindness. The blue-yellow difficulty is much rarer. People who have color blindness see objects as lighter or darker but are unable to distinguish the shades. Sometimes they distinguish between the red and the green lights on roadways by their difference in brightness.

There is no specific cure for color blindness, since the defect is one of structure of the eye. However, as has already been mentioned, there are various ways in which the color vision may be developed or substitutions found. In testing for color blindness the most common test involves the sorting of a number of colored worsteds. The person who is being tested is given certain pieces and asked to match them with others. There are other tests in which colored strips of paper are sometimes employed.

One color-blind woman, who was an excellent seamstress, was able to do sewing provided her family would tell her the colors of the thread. She was able to remember them by having each color in a different place in the workbox.

So significant is color blindness today in relationship to accident that every person who attempts to drive a motorcar or to indulge in any other occupation in which color detection is significant should have a test as soon as possible.

The Navy and the Air Force do not admit men who are color-blind. A few have gained admission by learning the tests. There is no cure for color blindness. If a boy is smart enough to learn the tests so that he can pass them, the Army can probably find a place for him.

CONJUNCTIVITIS

The tissue which lines the eyelids and runs out over the eyeball is called the conjunctiva. An inflammation of this tissue is known as conjunctivitis. When the conjunctiva becomes inflamed there is burning and smarting of the eyelid, formation of pus, and reddened eyelids. Usually the eye when inflamed becomes exceedingly sensitive to light, and tears flood it constantly. In the morning the eyelids will be found crusted together. Doctors treat this condition according to the character of the germ that causes the inflammation and according to the severity of the infection.

Pinkeye is a common type of conjunctivitis. Shortly after this special type of germ gets into the eyes they become reddened, the lids are swollen and puffy and usually glued together in the morning. Pinkeye is usually spread by the use of common towel, and sometimes by soiled hands.

In some instances the eyes become inflamed by germs which get in from contaminated swimming pools. Physicians are able to prescribe new preparations of sulfonamides and antibiotics which quickly bring infections under control.

It is easy to transfer germs from one person to another. The safe step is for people with infected eyes to use individual towels and to make certain that the hands are always thoroughly washed with soap and water whenever any contact is made with the eye.

TRACHOMA

One of the most widespread diseases of the world is an inflammation of the eyes called trachoma, now believed to be due to a specific virus. The condition is so common in Egypt, Palestine, and India—except among the upper classes—that it is almost a universal disease.

The infection is carried by the transfer of the secretions from the eyes through the use of the hands, towels, handkerchiefs, pillows, or even by sneezing. It has been thought, indeed, that in some areas the infection is carried by flies.

In this condition the eye becomes inflamed and red; then blisters and crusts form. The scarring and injury may change the shape of the eyelids. If the infection of the cornea of the eye becomes sufficiently severe the eyesight may be destroyed.

This infection should be avoided with every possible effort. People who are in an area where trachoma is common should be exceedingly careful about the use of common towels and about rubbing the eyes with the hands.

The modern treatment of trachoma using the sulfonamide drugs has been exceedingly helpful in stopping the progress of the disease.

In treating the symptoms of trachoma, including the inflammation and the secretion, attempts are made to check and remove the granules and to overcome the enlargement of the tissues of the conjunctiva. This is accomplished by the application of caustic substances such as sulfate of copper or nitrate of silver and by mechanical and surgical methods, such as the scraping or cutting away of the excess material. This demands the utmost judgment and care on the part of the physician, since overirritation demands soothing treatment. Consequently there is no routine treatment—each patient must be treated according to the condition that exists at the time he is examined. It becomes necessary to keep the eyes clean for some time by the frequent use of solutions of salt or alkaline washes, or other preparations which the physician may prescribe.

TUBERCULOSIS OF THE EYE

Among the most difficult of conditions that confronted physicians in years past was the infection of the eye by tuberculosis. Tuberculosis and syphilis are two diseases that can affect any portion of the human body.

Almost everyone knows by this time that streptomycin has a special quality in attacking the germ of tuberculosis, but few people have realized that certain preparations of sulfonamide drugs, such as promizole, promin, and diasone, are also known to have capabilities in stopping this germ. Incidentally, one phase of the most recent studies relates to certain observations made with other diseases. Undulant fever was one of the most difficult conditions to control by various methods, and eventually physicians found that a combination of an antibiotic and sulfonamide was more effective in controlling the conditions than either antibiotic or sulfonamide drugs alone. Now, careful studies made at Johns Hopkins University Medical School have proved that a combination of streptomycin and promizole is the most efficient method yet known for controlling tuberculosis of the eye. Before the method of treatment was tried on people with such infections, each of the drugs was tried separately and then a combination was tried on tuberculosis of the eye of rabbits. The eyes of all rabbits with such tuberculosis were found to be free of any evidence of tuberculous infection after four weeks of treatment with a combination of these drugs.

Thirteen out of fourteen people with tuberculous infections of the eye and with evidence of tuberculous infection elsewhere in the body were given the combination of streptomycin and promizole, and with results far superior to those which physicians had seen previously in treating such cases. The inflammatory symptoms disappeared, a change for the better began anywhere from nine days to three weeks after the treatment was begun, and the only disadvantage was the appearance of occasional toxic reactions to the drugs. Of course neither these drugs nor any others can replace dead tissues. They cannot remove the scars resulting from damaged tissues, nor can they overcome cataracts or any other irreversible changes. Inflammatory changes, however, which had not resulted in complete destruction of the tissues were completely controlled. Unquestionably this investigation with these favorable results means that a condition of the eye, which has been formerly responsible for a great deal of blindness, is now amenable to treatment.

IRITIS

The iris is the colored portion of the eye. It can become infected and inflamed, due to various causes. When it is infected it becomes swollen, dull, and discolored. The pupil gets small, gray, and sluggish. There is pain, radiating to the forehead and to the temple, which is worse at night, and there is much disturbance of vision. In most infections of the eye the person who has an inflammation of the iris cannot stand to look at the light, and there is constant watering of the eye.

The iris may become infected by various germs and may be involved in rheumatic conditions. It is of the utmost importance to take care of this condition immediately, because the inflammation and infection may result in scarring which will either block the pupil entirely or bind the iris down in such a manner as to prevent its motion. Obviously, this will cause a permanent disturbance of vision.

When a doctor takes care of this condition he applies drugs which relieve the congestion and put the part at rest. Dilatation of the pupil will prevent the scarring and tend to break up the smal scars that have already formed. Various preparations of atropine are useful for this purpose. There are other drugs which are anesthetic in character and which prevent pain. The doctor may prescribe also moist, hot compresses for several hours, which will tend to diminish the pain and the inflammation.

Of particular importance, however, is the treatment of this, as of other conditions, through the body as a whole. Syphilis affecting the eye means syphilis elsewhere in the body, and demands the kind of consistent and persistent treatment that is necessary for this condition. The rheumatic condition with which iritis is associated must be treated for the general rheumatic disturbance, with the detection, if possible, of the focus of infection in the body, and with the elimination of that focus when it is found. Other types of septic infection must also be controlled. When there is diabetes the treatment of the condition by diet and insulin, so as to control the diabetes throughout the body generally, is even more important than the treatment of the condition as it affects the eyes. Once the condition is healed, surgical operations of various kinds, including plastic operations, may be necessary to bring about normal restoration of the iris and thus to aid vision.

GLAUCOMA

When the pressure within the eye becomes increased, usually because of more fluid forming than is usually there, the condition is called glaucoma. The fluid in the eye circulates. When this circulation is blocked so that the fluid does not drain, glaucoma appears. Inflammation or hemorrhage into the interior of the eye may also cause increased pressure. With glaucoma, vision is lessened. Physicians use a device called a tonometer to measure the pressure. If a person frequently sees colored rings around a lighted center, called a halo, glaucoma may be suspected. The ophthalomologist may prescribe drugs which lower the tension. Several operative procedures are used which control glaucoma. The tension may also be lessened by prescribing drugs which increase elimination of fluid from the body. Occasionally people with glaucoma have mild headaches and pain in the eye.

RETINA DETACHMENT

Among the most serious of the conditions which may affect the human eye is detachment of the retina. The retina is a tissue at the back of the eyeball, which apparently receives the images focused upon it by the lens of the eye and passes them to the optic nerve, so that they will be suitably recorded by the brain. Under certain circumstances this tissue may become detached, which results promptly in loss of vision.

Operations are performed for the cure of detachment of the retina. This condition usually afflicts men slightly more often than women. Usually it affects older rather than younger people. Cases of detachment of the retina also are recorded in persons as old as seventy-five. In a considerable number of cases detachment of the retina seems to follow an injury of some sort.

Most of the operative procedures now used involve application of chemical cauterizing substances or else application of heat for purposes of cauterization. The subsequent scarring causes the retina again to become attached to the field in which it should lie. The laser can throw a light beam, pin-pointed to the area of detachment, and thus bring about reattachment.

ASTIGMATISM

The human eye can be farsighted or nearsighted, in the latter case the rays of light are focused in front of the retina—the seeing tissue of the eye—in the former, behind it. When the eye is at rest and parallel rays are focused exactly on the retina the eye is said to be normal. When parallel rays of light coming into the eye are focused at different meridians or angles the eye has astigmatism.

Astigmatism is usually due to a change in the curvature of the cornea or outside membrane of the eye, with or without some shortening or lengthening of the diameter of the whole eyeball. Occasionally astigmatism is also caused by defects in the curvature of the lens of the eye. The exact causes of these anatomical differences are not known, beyond the fact that the shape of the eyeball differs in various people, so that there is a tendency for astigmatism to appear in members of the same family. The shape of the eyeball itself is inherited.

There are, however, cases in which injury, inflammation, or operative procedure on the cornea of the eye will change the curves and thus produce astigmatism. There are also instances in which, apparently, pressure on the eyelids may distort the eyeball and thus may produce astigmatism.

Probably every eye has some astigmatism. However, many people do not have enough disturbance of this type to make any attention necessary. In other cases, however, the blurring of vision brought about by the astigmatism makes it necessary to wear corrective eyeglasses for focusing the rays of light properly on the retina. Whenever there is a considerable degree of astigmatism the acuteness of vision diminishes both for distant and near objects.

The specialist who examines the eyes is likely to suspect there is some astigmatism when the eye cannot be brought by the use of spherical lenses to see the line of letters numbered twenty at twenty feet distance. One of the simple tests is to use what is called the astigmatic dial, which is a clock with lines radiating to each of the hours. If the person is unable to see all of the rays with equal clearness, astigmatism is responsible. The lines that are seen more distinctly and the lines seen less distinctly indicate the principal meridians. By the amount of blurring or the place of the blurring the expert who examines the eyes is enabled to determine the areas in which the curvature of the lens needs correction.

CROSS-EYES

For a long time any attempt to control cross-eyes in children was prevented because people superstitiously thought that cross-eyes were due to fright, shock, or prenatal impressions on the mother. A squint or walleye may develop from excessive strains placed on the external muscle of the eye by the extra effort in seeing which is required when there is an extreme degree of nearsightedness. Any straining of the eye or imbalance of the muscles may result in cross-eyes or squint.

Many people believe that children outgrow cross-eyes. This may happen, but in other instances the sight of a crossed eye may never develop, and in many instances the squint or crossed eye becomes worse as time goes on. Early diagnosis and treatment are essential for the best results in this condition. As soon as you notice that a child is cross-eyed a specialist in diseases of the eye should be consulted. He will make a sufficiently thorough examination to evaluate the factors in the case and decide on the proper treatment.

In at least half the cases of cross-eyes there seems to be some hereditary anatomical weakness in the eye; there will usually be a record of other cases somewhere in the family. Most people have some minor muscle out of balance in their eyes. One muscle will pull harder than the other, and the strong one will overcome the weak one. When both eyes are open the stimulus coming from the brain can supply enough extra effort through the weak muscle to keep the eyes lined up. With both eyes open and seeing, we will see double if one eye turns out of line with the other. In the case of cross-eyes the person affected may avoid seeing double by using only one eye at a time. This happens also in people who have one eye farsighted and the other nearsighted, if they are not balanced suitably with proper eyeglasses they will use only one eye at a time for seeing. If this is not corrected the good eye will be used and the weak one will turn. Sometimes good results are secured merely by prescribing eyeglasses which will tend to hold the two eyes in position. Children have been found quite able to tolerate eyeglasses at the age of fifteen months. The earlier the glasses are used, the more valuable will be their effect.

It has also been suggested that the weak eye be exercised by various training devices to overcome the habit of suppressing the image of one eye. In certain types of cases, when the deficiency is very slight, this so-called "orthoptic" training is successful. Many types of apparatus have been developed by specialists in diseases of the eye for giving training of this character. The most favorable age for training is between three and six years of age. After the age of seven years the results are rarely satisfactory.

The surgical procedure for overcoming cross-eyes is most certain. Proper placement of the eye muscles will tend to bring the eye back into proper relationship to the other eye and will permit binocular vision. The operation will not improve the vision of the eye but will prevent the vision from being lost from failure to use the eye successfully. Moreover, the correction of cross-eyes is very important for establishing a proper mental attitude in the child. Children with cross-eyes may become so shy and so sensitive to laughter that they will become "shut-in" personalities and their lives be thereby ruined.

EYE EXERCISES

For a good many years now, attempts have been made to get people to train their eyes by exercises to improve the strength of the eyes in various ways, thus permitting these people to avoid glasses. The original slogan was "Throw away your glasses and have perfect sight."

Unfortunately, the majority of experiences of eye specialists during the past twenty years has inclined definitely to limit the extent of usefulness of eye exercises as a means of improving vision. The modern ophthalmologist, or specialist in conditions affecting the eyes, knows the limitations and insists that such methods cannot be applied indiscriminately to all sorts of defects of the eyes. There are certain disturbances which are not affected in any way whatever by exercises; these include cataracts, destruction of the optic nerve, opaque scars of the cornea, and serious changes in the retina. A cataract is a cloudiness of the lens of the eye. The nerve must be alive and normal to permit vision. An opaque scar of the cornea is like a window blind drawn over a window; such scars render vision impossible. The retina is the tissue back of the eye which is responsible for vision, and permanent change to the retina obviously means permanent damage to vision. Exercises can do nothing to help such vision.

The psychologic treatment associated with education of the eyes helps to reconcile people to difficulties with vision, even though it does not cure them.

In certain instances skillfully chosen exercises can improve the ability to see. Studies made with patients who are color-blind show that it is possible by education to improve the ability to discriminate between colors but that it is impossible to cure color blindness, since the condition is due to permanent changes in the tissues concerned. People who are extremely nearsighted can be taught how to make better use of their vision, but it is not possible to reduce the nearsightedness by any kind of exercise. People who have severe scars of the cornea may be helped to some extent by exercises and education, because they can be taught to make the most of the amount of vision they have.

CATARACTS

One of the most serious manifestations of increased age is a gradual loss of transparency in the lens of the eye, a condition commonly called cataract. The word cataract came from a Greek word meaning waterfall. Experts in language say that the term was applied to the

177

formation of a cataract in the eye because the gradual loss of vision was related to something dropping in front of the eye. The condition was known in the third century B.C., and the operation for removal of the lens, so that people with cataracts could see, was first done in 1745. However, in 300 B.C. a procedure was known for depressing the lens, so that the vision would improve.

The degree of loss of vision depends on the location and extent of the cataract in the lens. In some instances vision is gradually reduced until only the ability to see light remains. Nearsightedness often develops. Cataract is not difficult to diagnose, particularly with the many instruments now available to specialists in conditions affecting the eye. Thus, a device known as the slit lamp will tell the physician exactly the character, nature, and extent of the opacity in the lens. While the cataract is developing, vision may be helped by appropriate eyeglasses. Once the vision is seriously impaired, surgical operation is necessary and desirable. A new technic involves the use of an enzyme, chymotrypsin, to loosen the attachments of the lens and make removal easy. New anesthetics and new antibiotic drugs have made the operation much easier and insured a high proportion of successful results. Specialists in such surgical procedures are now available in most of the medical centers in the United States and, in fact, in many smaller communities.

EYES OF THE AGED

The aging process is continuous from the time of birth to the time of death. Some human beings age more slowly than do others. Many of the changes in the vision of older people are associated with changes in the circulation, including hardening of the arteries. The eyelids of old people develop wrinkles.

Old people seem to cry easily, and sometimes suffer from an overflow of tears. This is often due to relaxation of the tissues of the eye, which do not hold the material as do the elastic tissues of the young. Surgeons have developed technics for maintaining the normal relationships between the tissues, overcoming this overflow of tears when it becomes a nuisance. Elderly people often complain of heaviness of the eyelids and inability to raise them, especially in the morning. The weakness may be due to a gradual disappearance of the elastic tissue from the eyelids.

In the old person the pupil of the eye becomes smaller and less movable, and the color of the eye becomes lighter. The lens of the eye grows and increases in weight throughout life. Sometimes a ring seems to form around the colored center of the eye. This is called an *arcus senilis* and is characteristic of aging. Cataract is typical of the aged, and the exact cause is not known. The decision as to whether or not a cataract is to be removed by surgical operation depends on many factors having to do with the patient's physical and mental condition, as well as the actual condition of the eye.

Old people need much higher intensities of light than do young persons. In fact, improvement of the light often decreases the need for stronger eyeglasses.

EYESIGHT AND TELEVISION

When motion pictures were first introduced much was published about the danger of glare, flickering, and long-continued intense looking at movies. When radio came in similar discussions began to be published about the effects of noise, strain of the sense of hearing, and other possible complications. People soon learned that the human mind could do a great deal in shutting out the unwarranted sounds.

Now comes television with a combination of strain on both hearing and seeing. Already great numbers of investigators have been trying to develop devices that can help the human eye and ear to make the most out of television without strain on the essential sense organs of the body. Recently several experts in conditions affecting the eye were consulted by the *Journal of the American Medical Association* to find out what they thought about the effects of television on eyestrain. Here are six considerations to which they agreed:

1. In general a large screen is considered better than a small one, because it allows a clearer vision at a greater distance and gives a large visual angle.

2. A distance of ten feet or more away from the screen would in general be better than a shorter distance, provided that the size of the screen and of the room would permit.

3. The nearer to the perpendicular the screen is viewed, the better. Too much of an angle produces distortion and makes co-ordination of the two images received by the eyes difficult. (It might be added here that since most of our visual work is done at the level of or below our eyes it would seem better, especially for children, to have the screen at eye level.)

4. Although there is not a definite time limit for watching television, some discretion should be used, and it should not be persisted in beyond the point of fatigue.

179

5. Daylight screens in general are considered better than the ordinary ones, because they are compatible with more light in the room, thus reducing the contrast between screen and surrounding objects.

6. Although television in itself does not produce eyestrain, viewing it requires all the important components of vision. Since we know that there is a very large personal factor and that people vary in their capacity to carry on various visual tasks, there will be more enjoyment if the rules given above are followed. People with defects in convergence, accommodation, fusion, and refraction suffer ocular discomfort sooner than others.

To these the editors of *New York Medicine* have added four more suggestions.

7. Distance glasses, if needed for driving, movies, and the blackboard, should be worn when viewing television.

8. The reproduction should be actually focused and no attempt made to view an indistinct picture. The viewer should sit directly in front of the instrument with the screen at eye level.

9. Because of pupillary and retinal fatigue from contrast and flicker, a dim light should be constantly used in the television room.

10. Colored or tinted lenses should not be worn while viewing television, whether they do or do not contain the person's correction.

Of course the people who do best are those who utilize judgment in the amount of strain that they put on their bodies.

CHAPTER XXVI

NOSE, THROAT, AND EAR

MIDWAY IN THE FACE between the eyes is an organ which gives the human being more concern for its size and prominence than any other in the human body. In more ways than one it is the center of interest. Compared with the eye or the liver, there is not really much to a nose: some small bones, cartilage, and soft tissues, which surround the two cavities called nostrils. The nose is lined with a membrane called mucous membrane, which is mostly responsible for the troubles that affect the nose. On each side of the nose and in back of and above it are the nasal sinuses. These are cavities in the bones of the head; all of them connect with the inside of the nose by small openings. In addition to the tissues mentioned, there are the usual blood vessels and nerves, which are responsible for bringing in blood and taking it out and for giving us the sensations of odor and also of pain, itching, and other disturbances.

SENSITIVE MEMBRANE

The mucous membrane of the nose is one of the most sensitive tissues in the body. When it is bruised or hurt in any way it responds promptly with swelling and inflammation. It can also become sensitive to various protein substances; in reacting it will swell and pour out a lot of fluid. Occasionally a small ulcer or infection in the nose will erode a blood vessel; then a crust forms and there is oozing of blood.

Inside the nose are hair follicles and hairs, which filter out dust or infectious materials. However, they also form occasional opportunities for the entrance of infection. The pus-forming germs such as the staphylococcus and the streptococcus are widespread, and will usually get into the human being whenever they come in contact with tissues that have been damaged in any manner. Then there is an infection which may eventually spread throughout the rest of the body.

A nose is best let well alone. The pernicious habits of picking the nose, pulling hairs, and trying to squeeze pimples or other infections may set up forms of inflammation that are most serious. When an infection in the form of a pimple, a boil, or an abscess occurs in the nose it is best to have prompt competent medical attention, to prevent the spread of these infections into a general poisoning of the body.

An infection in the lining of the nose manifests itself by redness, swelling, discomfort, and a pain which increases steadily. If the swelling is sufficiently great the outer aspect of the nose becomes swollen, and the swelling may extend even up to the eyelids. Whenever there is a swelling in the nose a physician should inspect the area to determine the presence or absence of infection and to provide for a release of infected material so as to obviate the danger of a generalized infection.

HYGIENE OF THE NOSE

The right way to take care of the nose is to remove carefully, by proper use of the handkerchief, such material as can be reached easily. Those which cannot be reached may be washed out by the use of a mild spray without pressure. There are now generally available all sorts of sprays, and materials which can be sprayed into the nose safely. Under no circumstances should materials be put in the nose under high pressure. This applies particularly to oils of various kinds, since it has been found that such oils may get into the lungs and, on occasion, pneumonia has resulted from such procedures.

FOREIGN BODIES IN THE NOSE

Children, particularly infants, are likely to put into their mouths almost anything they happen to pick up. Occasionally also they push things into the nose. A substance of fairly small size taken into the mouth is not likely to be harmful, providing it is clean, even after it is swallowed. The digestive passages are big enough in most instances to let it pass through. Usually after eighteen to twenty-four hours the foreign materials will have disappeared from the body.

The breathing passages are much smaller than the digestive tube.

Moreover, the breathing passages are curved and their walls are rigid. A substance forced into the nose is likely to remain there and serve as an obstacle which blocks the passage of air. Even more serious, however, is the fact that it will block the outflow of secretions.

Buttons, beans, pieces of chalk or erasers that have from time to time been pushed into the nose get lodged there. Occasionally they are inhaled and get into the windpipe. Then an exceedingly serious condition develops. The continuous presence of a foreign substance in the nose results eventually in the damming back of secretions and in the development of secondary infection. Soon there is a bad odor, a secondary swelling, and danger to life itself. A doctor can utilize some of the special instruments that he has available and get a foreign substance out of the nose without very much trouble. The great danger of trying to get out a hard object like a button or piece of chalk is the damage to the tissues that results from manipulation. In many cases it is necessary to give the child an anesthetic to prevent jerking and moving of the head or interference by the hands and arms.

When a foreign substance is inhaled into the tube that leads to the lungs or into the lung itself it is an immediate menace to life. Under such circumstances there must be no delay. An X-ray picture is taken as soon as possible, which aids the doctor in localizing the foreign substance. Special instruments have been developed, which permit the placing of a tube down into the lung, and forceps and similar devices have been developed, by which a foreign substance can be grasped and removed from the body.

THROAT

General inflammations of the throat, associated with redness, swelling, and excessive discharge of mucus, may have many different causes. Most common, of course, is exposure to cold, or an extension of inflammation from the tonsils, the adenoids, or the nose. Excessive use of tobacco, excessive exposure to dust, smoke, and irritating fumes, and sudden changes in temperature, excessive dryness and other atmospheric irritations may all cause irritation of the throat. People who are sensitive to certain food substances sometimes react with blisters on the tissues of the throat, which become secondarily infected and produce irritations and inflammation.

There may be severe pain associated with swelling and inflammation of the throat, including pain in the ears because of blocking of the

183

tubes which lead from the nose to the ears; there may also be a sense of fullness or obstruction, with much hawking and spitting.

The first thing to know about any inflammation of the throat is its cause. If the condition happens to be due to diphtheria, prompt action is necessary, including the giving of diphtheria antitoxin. If, however, it is due to some other type of germ, other methods of treatment are employed. The pain of an inflamed throat is best relieved by use of an ice bag filled with cracked ice. Most doctors are now convinced that gargles seldom go deep enough in the throat in sufficient quantity or strength to permit them to have much effect in killing germs or in curing disease. To have a definite effect from any antiseptic in the throat, it is necessary to apply it directly to the infected or inflamed part. This is best done by spreading with a cotton swab or by using an atomizer properly. In order to get the antiseptic into the back of the throat it may be necessary to hold the tongue or to use a tongue depressor.

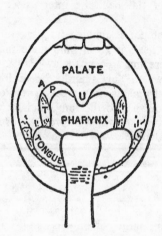

DIAGRAM SHOWING PALATE, UVULA, TONSILS, PHARYNX, AND TONGUE

The primary purpose of a mouthwash or throat wash is to clean and soothe. Many modern mouthwashes contain drugs capable of killing germs on contact. A good cleansing mouthwash is salt solution, made by adding a fourth of a teaspoon of salt to a half glass of warm water. If there is much mucus, the addition of a quarter of a teaspoon of bicarbonate of soda or ordinary baking soda may be beneficial.

ACUTE TONSILLITIS

The infection of throat and tonsils often first manifests itself with a chill, pain in the head and body, loss of appetite, and fever. The temperature may go up to 103° or 104° F. The tongue is usually coated, and the lymph glands at the back and side of the neck will be swollen. Swallowing is painful and even talking may be difficult. When you look at the throat it will appear red, swollen, and often covered with whitish-yellow spots. The symptoms in the throat last three or four days.

Many people seem to have throats that are easily infected, with trouble every time they are exposed to cold, fatigue, or sudden changes in climate. The streptococci are usually the infecting agent, and, since they are practically always present in the nose and throat of people, the explanation seems to be that they grow and multiply every time the resistance is lowered. In epidemics, streptococci from infected food or milk or from the hands of food-handlers are spread about, and attack those who cannot resist. If children have repeated sore throats with infected tonsils, the tonsils may be removed during an intervening period when inflammation is absent.

An abscess in the tissues around the tonsils is called quinsy. The doctor relieves the pain and swelling by puncturing the abscess and getting the accumulated pus out.

All streptococcal infections of the throat should be taken seriously because of the great danger of secondary rheumatic fever, arthritis, middle ear infection, or other complications. The sulfonamide drugs and penicillin, also aureomycin and terramycin, act powerfully against streptococci, and already the total number of severe and complicated cases has been greatly reduced.

LARYNX

The larynx, commonly called the voice box, consists of cartilage held together by muscles and ligaments so as to make a tubular structure holding the vocal cords. At its upper end is a structure called the epiglottis, which serves to keep food from going down the larynx and windpipe and causes it to pass instead from the pharynx into the esophagus and stomach.

The chief purpose of the larynx is to aid speech. However, it also is capable of helping with expectoration. When a moving column of air strikes the vocal bands, the column is set in vibration. Speech includes, however, not only the vibration of this column of air but the molding of the column with the help of the tongue, the teeth, the palate, and the lips. If any of these structures does not function properly, the voice can be greatly changed. The adult male possesses a deep voice because of the action of the long vocal cord during its relaxed state. A low-pitched voice is produced by a slow-moving cord, and a high-pitched voice is produced by a vocal cord that vibrates with an increased frequency.

The doctor looks at the larynx by means of several different technics. For the usual examination he wears a head mirror which casts light into the mouth. The person who is going to be examined puts out his tongue, which is held out with a piece of sterile gauze. While the tongue is held gently, the patient breathes through the mouth with short gasps of breath. Then the doctor puts a mirror, which has been slightly warmed to prevent condensation of air on its surface, into the back of the throat and requests the patient to say "Ah." This raises the palate, and the mirror may be passed a little farther into the throat. By regulating the angle of the mirror the doctor can see the vocal cords. As the patient makes various sounds, the doctor can determine whether or not the vocal cords vibrate properly. He can also see whether or not they have been modified by inflammation or swelling or growth of nodes. For some people who are sensitive the use of a local anesthetic may be necessary to permit passing the mirror into the back of the throat. Techniques have also been developed which permit the doctor to look directly at the vocal cords, with instruments designed for the purpose.

One of the first signs of inflammation of the larynx and of the vocal cords is hoarseness, so that hoarseness and laryngitis have become almost synonymous. There are, however, many causes of inflammation.

LARYNGITIS

Inflammation of the vocal cords may follow overuse of the voice, irritation by chemical substances, or infection. Men, who are more frequently subjected to exposure to irritant substances in their occupations and who indulge more than women in deleterious habits, suffer more from laryngitis than do women. Contributing causes to inflammation of the larynx include the swallowing of hot or spicy foods, the abuse of alcohol and tobacco and similar irritants. Occasionally the larynx becomes inflamed because there is an infection in the throat or the lungs. In fact, any condition that blocks breathing through the nose helps to cause laryngitis, because large amounts of air then pass directly to the larynx without having been modified, as is usual, in passing through the nasal tract.

In serious cases of laryngitis it is customary to go to bed and keep quiet. Nothing helps the vocal cords under such circumstances as much as continuous rest, speaking only in a whisper. The application of an ice bag or ice collar or moist compresses to the throat is soothing. Some people prefer warmth, which seems to be equally effective in its soothing action. A measure which comes down from ancient history is the inhaling of steam to which various aromatic oils can be added. Apparently the chief benefit is derived, however, not from the aromatic oils but from the moisture and the warmth. Nowadays many special devices have been developed that use electrical heat in order to produce such steam for inhaling. These devices are usually much safer than the old-fashioned dish or kettle of hot water. Many instances have been known of severe burns from accidents with open kettles of exceedingly hot water used in this way.

For serious laryngitis, particularly that complicated by inflammation or infection, the physician may prescribe many drugs that are helpful in securing rest and in soothing the area concerned.

TRACHEA

The scientific name for the windpipe is the trachea. It is often involved in infections of the throat and the bronchial tubes. Any virus or germ that can produce inflammation of the respiratory tract can also cause the lining of the trachea to become infected. It is possible for the experts to see the lining of the trachea by the use of the bronchoscope.

When the lining of the trachea becomes inflamed the most typical symptom is the cough. These coughs are non-productive, hacking, and metallic. They tend to be worse after the person goes to bed and during the night. An acute inflammation of the trachea is accompanied by rawness, tightness, and discomfort, sometimes even pain, in the lower part of the neck and behind the upper part of the breastbone, or sternum. As the inflammation goes on, there is mucus, and finally a good deal of sputum and mucus may be expectorated. If the infection is purulent, as with the staphylococcus or streptococcus, the material coughed up will be a mixture of mucus and pus.

These conditions can be helped by the usual treatment that is given to other inflammations of the respiratory tract. That means going to bed for a few days, applying warmth, and producing rest by the use of

187

appropriate remedies which the doctor prescribes. Often inhalations of warm vapor treated with medicated oils help to bring relief.

In some instances the acute inflammation of the trachea becomes chronic. In such cases the cough is irritating and frequent. When these symptoms are present it becomes necessary for the doctor to make certain that the patient does not have tuberculosis or any other condition affecting the lungs. In such cases it is customary to prohibit smoking. Often, residence in a warm, dry climate is advisable. The use of anti-infectious remedies such as the sulfonamides and penicillin are important in eliminating infection.

THE EAR

There is much more to the ear than appears on the outside of the head. That part, easily visible, if unusually prominent gives a lot of concern. In addition to the external ear, the apparatus for hearing includes the middle ear and the internal ear.

The external ear includes the portion that is on the outside and the small canal which runs down as far as the eardrum. It is a collection of skin and other tissue such as cartilage and muscle. In most human beings the muscles are merely remnants of the large muscles possessed by animals, so that few people are able to move their ears with any degree of celerity or satisfaction.

PLASTIC SURGERY FOR LOP EARS

There are really few conditions affecting the external ear that are disturbing. Sometimes large portions of the ear may be absent at birth. Occasionally the ears project in an extremely unsightly manner. All these extraordinary appearances are controlled nowadays by the use of plastic surgery. An expert is able to fasten the ear back if it projects exceedingly, to rebuild an ear out of other tissue if portions are missing, and to modify the shape of the ear if it is of extraordinary shape.

Many mothers feel that the ear became a lop ear because the child lay on his ear with the ear crumpled when he was small or because he wore his hat pressed down on the ears. There is no evidence that these factors are really of any importance. The fault is one of anatomical development. Manipulation of and bandaging the ears to hold them against the head will not correct the condition.

Occasionally, small tumors will develop on the outer ear; these may be removed if they show the slightest tendency to growth or irritation.

The ear may be infected by pimples or boils or by an infection of the type of erysipelas, in which it swells to a tremendous size. Such conditions should have the best available surgical treatment, in order to prevent destruction and damage that would require plastic surgery for repair.

"TIN EARS"

One of the most common forms of injury to the external ear is the development of what the pugilist calls a "tin ear." Repeated pounding on the ear results in the pouring out of blood into the tissues of the ear and surrounding areas. At first such swellings are bluish-red; they feel to the touch like dough. In the worst cases surgeons open the tissue and remove the clot of blood to prevent permanent thickening and swelling. They also apply special bandages to mold the ear and hold it in shape while repair is taking place.

INSECTS IN EARS

Cases are on record in which living insects have entered the ear. They died and their bodies remained, gradually becoming surrounded by hardened wax, so that eventually the external canal was blocked and hearing lost entirely. Outside of the loss of hearing, no damage is likely to result. More damage comes from attempts to remove material from the ear than from the entrance of the material itself. It is not advisable for anyone to try to remove a foreign body from the outer ear if it cannot be washed out, unless he has had special training in this type of work. (The technique of syringing the ear is explained fully under "Hygiene of the Ear" later in this chapter.)

REMOVING FOREIGN OBJECTS

Several instruments have been developed for removing foreign objects. A bean or piece of chalk has been removed by the use of a probe with some adhesive material on the end. This becomes adherent to the bean or piece of chalk, which is then gradually withdrawn. Such performances are, however, best left to the experts.

A pimple or boil or any other infection in the tissue lining the external ear canal will cause intense pain, inflammation, swelling, and some fever, and should have prompt medical attention.

INFECTIONS ARE MORE EASILY
PREVENTED THAN CURED

Without special instruments and devices with electric light it is not possible for the average person to see the eardrum or to recognize trouble in the middle ear. The physician has devices, an otoscope and also an ear speculum, which permit him to see the lining of the canal and to throw light directly on the eardrum. When the eardrum is observed, it is possible to determine whether or not everything is normal, whether there is any obstruction in the external ear canal, and whether or not there is any infection.

It is also necessary in an examination of the ears to determine whether or not the Eustachian tubes are infected in any way, because infection or inflammation of these tubes will interfere seriously with hearing. The Eustachian tubes pass from the back of the nasal cavity to the middle ear. Frequently infection spreads from the tonsils and adenoids by way of the Eustachian tube to the ear canal.

HOW TO AVOID EAR INJURIES

Far better than the attempt to treat such conditions when they develop is the application of simple laws of hygiene that tend to prevent infections in the ear. Increased bathing and swimming have multiplied the number of cases of infection in the ear arising from that source. Children should not be permitted to swim more than fifteen or twenty minutes at a time. If they tend to have trouble with the ears they should not be permitted to dive. The child who complains of difficulties in hearing or of fullness in the head after swimming should give up the sport. This is nature's way of warning against trouble.

Unhealthy tonsils and adenoids may be the source of infections which extend into the ear. The vast majority of infections of the ear are secondary to colds in the head and influenza. About 10 per cent of children with scarlet fever and measles develop infections of the ear. About 5 per cent of those with diphtheria develop infections of the ear. Other cases develop after mumps, typhoid fever, whooping cough, and similar infections.

Prompt care of children with various infectious diseases will determine the presence of infection early, and immediate application of proper treatment can prevent extension of the infection into the mastoid or inner ear.

Before the age of twelve, children acquire infections of the ear more easily than do adults. Infections with virulent streptococci are more likely than others to cause infections of the ear. Removal of the tonsils and adenoids, when repeatedly infected, is important in preventing infections of the ear.

HYGIENE OF THE EAR

An Irish doctor said that there are two kinds of deafness—one due to wax in the ear, which can be cured by washing it out, and the other not due to wax. Most people nowadays know enough about personal hygiene to keep their ears clean. Boils and pimples still occur, and there are still cases in which the removal of hardened wax is necessary. The cerumen, or wax in the ear, when it becomes hardened is most easily removed by the use of the ear syringe filled with slightly warm water. Harm can be done by needless or too frequent syringing. The syringe should be sterilized by boiling before using, and water should be previously boiled and used warm but not hot.

The person whose ear is to be syringed should sit in a good light, a towel should be put around the neck and tucked inside the clothing so as to prevent soiling it, a pan should be held at the edge of the ear so that the fluid which runs in will run into the basin and not down the patient's neck. The ear is pulled slightly upward and backward to straighten out the passage. With the ear held in this position, the nozzle of the syringe, which has been filled and has all the air expelled, is placed just inside the outer opening of the ear. The water is then permitted to flow along the back wall slowly and without too great pressure, so as to permit return of the excess flow of water as the water goes in.

Special instruments are usually needed for removing foreign objects. A probe with adhesive at the end may attach itself to a foreign object which can then be pulled out. Usually experts have the instruments and can do this performance easily.

A pimple or a boil or any other infection in the tissues lining the external ear canal will cause intense pain, inflammation, swelling, and some fever. Prompt medical attention is required. With modern antibiotic drugs such infections are usually controlled.

OTITIS MEDIA, OR MIDDLE EAR INFECTION

Infection of the interior of the ear after a sore throat is not nearly so frequent as such infections used to be. The specific action against staphylococci, pneumococci, streptococci, and other germs that infect noses and throats wrought by the antibiotic drugs and sulfonamides has enormously reduced such complications. However, neglect of a sore throat or a virulent infection may occasionally be followed by spread of the germs to the middle ear. One or both ears may be infected. The condition usually begins with a pain in the ear and a high fever. The pain is continuous, but may be irregular, and is usually worse at night. When the doctor looks at the eardrum it is seen to be bulging. If the drum is not opened the pressure may cause it to burst. Then a thin watery discharge will come out, often changing to thick creamy pus. When the eardrum is cut or bursts the pain stops immediately and usually the temperature falls. The discharge may persist for a long time.

BLOW THE NOSE PROPERLY

Often the middle ear is infected because a child has not learned how to blow the nose properly. The worse technic is to hold both nostrils tightly when blowing, since this forces the infected material from back of the nose into the middle ear. The proper technic requires that only one nostril be held and that blowing be gentle. Preferably, the handkerchief or disposable tissue should be held quite loosely over the opening of the nostrils.

Middle ear infection may lead to some degree of deafness and, rarely, to permanent loss of hearing. Following an infection the child should be taken to a specialist—an otorhinolaryngologist—who will test the loss of hearing and do everything possible to stop the progress of infection and restore action to the damaged tissues of the ear.

Mastoiditis used to be frequent after infection of the ear, but now the total number of cases of mastoiditis has been greatly reduced by the antibiotic drugs. Pain and tenderness in the region behind the ear are the first symptoms of inflammation of the mastoid. The skin may be swollen so that the external ear seems to be pushed away from the head. Early treatment of infected ears will usually prevent this complication. Surgical treatment of mastoiditis involves an operation in which the infected area is opened and the infected material cleaned out. Unless controlled, a secondary inflammation of the coverings of the brain —meningitis—is possible.

CHAPTER XXVII

THE VENEREAL DISEASES

WHEN I WAS A MEDICAL STUDENT, between 1908 and 1912, clinics for the care of venereal disease were packed with sufferers from all ranks of society; whispers circulated in the dormitories of the colleges about students whose entire careers had been ruined by attacks of venereal disease. The end results of gonorrhea were horribly depicted, as were those of syphilis, in fake clinics conducted by venereal disease quacks. The museums of horrors were conspicuous in the districts devoted to honky-tonks and night clubs in every great city. The armies of the world were overwhelmed with the costs of caring for venereal disease; great numbers of men had constantly to be hospitalized and taken away from military service because of these infections. Moreover, at that time one hardly dared to speak either the word "gonorrhea" or "syphilis." No newspaper, at least in the United States, would dare to print the words.

The steady progress of medical science has now enabled us to determine the exact cause of each of the venereal diseases; to establish positive methods of diagnosis; to develop capable technics of prevention; and, best of all, to find methods of treatment which can cure gonorrhea within twenty-four to forty-eight hours and bring syphilis under control within a week.

Serious is the spread of venereal diseases associated with the rise of juvenile delinquency. The infected adolescent fears to consult medical advice. With the decrease in venereal disease doctors do not take seriously enough the necessity for detecting and following up contacts.

With the elimination of gonorrhea has gone the host of complications, including infected tubes and prostate glands and infected sex organs, with accompanying sterility. Surgical operations necessitated by gonorrheal infections are no longer frequent. Gonorrheal arthritis, a terrible disabling and crippling disease, is so infrequent that it is hardly suspected in making a diagnosis.

In New York City an appropriation of several hundreds of thousands of dollars usually made each year for the operation of venereal disease clinics was eliminated from the budget. Venereal disease is and always has been a problem among troops.

GONORRHEA

Gonorrhea is caused by a germ known as the "gonococcus." The finding of the germ in the secretions that come from the infected tissues is a means by which the presence of the disease is determined with certainty. The bacteriologists have established rather simple technics for detecting the presence of the gonococcus. When this germ invades the sex organs pus appears, and the presence of the infection is accompanied by burning and frequency of urination, which begins two to fourteen days after the exposure. When the condition infects women the symptoms are not easily detectable; the infection may proceed for a long time before the woman seeks medical attention. With men treatment is begun just as soon as the obvious symptoms appear and is not delayed while the necessary laboratory studies to confirm the diagnosis are being made. When the germs have invaded other tissues of the body, such as the eyes or the joints, the treatment is best conducted in a hospital.

The number of gonorrhea cases began to increase again in the United States in 1965, increasing steadily each year. By 1972 the frequency of gonorrhea in the United States was greater than that of any other communicable disease that requires treatment. For a time penicillin appeared to control the disease quickly. Now physicians realize that treatment alone will not eradicate gonorrhea. The ease of modern treatment led to the belief that gonorrhea is an inconsequential disease. However, women were not always adequately treated. Their fallopian tubes became infected and they became sterile. Even though men could be quickly cured of pain and the appearance of pus, the urinary tube was frequently damaged and a stricture resulted. Moreover, in many instances the prostate became infected, leading to disturbances later in life. Many different antibiotic drugs are now used in treating gonorrhea. In addition to penicillin, several other drugs are available. The germs may become resistant to penicillin so that change to another antibiotic may be necessary. In former years, massaging the prostate gland was used as a means of getting out the inflammatory residue; also the seminal vesicles were stripped in order to bring out any latent germs. This is no longer considered necessary. Because gonorrhea sometimes hides a simultaneous infection with syphilis, anyone found with gonorrhea should be instructed to have a blood test for syphilis after the gonorrhea has been cured. Occasionally tests may be made later to make sure that syphilis infection has not been hidden.

SYPHILIS

First in importance in the history of the control of syphilis by scientific medicine is the discovery of the organism that causes the disease, known as the *Treponema pallidum,* or the *Spirochaeta pallida,* which means the pale, corkscrew-like organism. Next is the discovery of positive blood tests for syphilis, of which there are now several generally accepted.

The discovery by Paul Ehrlich of the drug that was known as "606," or salvarsan, later named arsphenamine, marked the beginning of the chemical attacks on the disease, which included the use of drugs of the arsenic and bismuth type. However, the discovery of the antibiotic drugs has completely revolutionized the treatment of syphilis.

From ten to sixty days, but usually about three weeks, after sexual exposure the first sign of syphilis appears, as a sore on the genital organs. This sore is called a chancre. Every person with a sore of any kind on the genital organs should be suspected of having syphilis. Examinations of the material from the sore must be made with the special microscope that permits what is called "dark-field examination." Moreover, blood tests determine positively the nature of the disease. A single positive test is not usually accepted as being certain; it is customary to repeat the tests once a week for a month, and perhaps once a month for six months, to make certain that the condition is not present.

If the initial infection with syphilis is not controlled, the secondary forms may appear within a few weeks. Sometimes these are confused with other skin eruptions. All sorts of skin eruptions are associated with this condition. The blood test is necessary to confirm the diagnosis. Sometimes symptoms may appear as headache, fever, pains in the joints, and, in fact, a general illness affecting the whole body. Syphilis is an infection which may attack any or all parts of the human body.

To eliminate syphilis our armed forces give six injections into the muscles of 600,000 units each of procaine penicillin G; these are given at forty-eight- or seventy-two-hour intervals over a period of eleven to seventeen days. Some doctors prefer to give eight injections into the muscles, once each day for eight days.

The serious character of this infection is recognized in the recommendations that repeated blood tests be made and also, to make certain that the condition has not invaded the central nervous system, that tests be made of the spinal fluid.

If patients fail to respond to penicillin, the doctor's armament against the disease now permits the use of arsenical preparations like mapharsen; this is given by injections into the veins over a long period. Also, bismuth subsalicylate is injected into the muscles once a week for five weeks, followed by subsequent periods of treatment with both mapharsen and bismuth. Sometimes patients show sensitivity to penicillin, with eruptions including itching and wheals. In these cases the use of the antihistaminic drugs, such as benadryl or pyribenzamine, can control the condition in most instances.

Syphilis is such a dangerous disease that the mere disappearance of the symptoms or of the infectious character of the condition should not permit any person to cease watchfulness. There must be repeated examinations for a long time, including examinations of the blood and the spinal fluid, to be certain that the organisms have been eliminated from the body.

Occasionally a mother may be infected with syphilis, and the infection is discovered during pregnancy. The proper treatment of syphilis in pregnancy will prevent infection of the child in practically every case. Penicillin is the drug that is used, and it is given as soon as the infection is discovered.

When the child is born, repeated examinations are made to be certain that the child has not been infected. If infection is found, again the use of penicillin has been found sufficient in most instances to bring about cure of the disease.

CHANCROID

Chancroid is a localized venereal disease caused by a germ known as the Ducrey bacillus. This germ attacks the sex organs and produces ulcers and infections of the lymph glands in the groin. The condition is found chiefly among people who live under dirty and unhygienic conditions.

In the United States this condition is seen relatively infrequently, but it is rather frequent in tropical and semitropical countries. The condition is usually spread from one person to another during sexual contacts.

The ulcer is usually shallow, with ragged and undermined edges, and covered with a grayish flow of pus. The glands in the groin are enlarged in at least half the cases; they may eventually develop abscesses. If they are not treated they become soft and rupture to the surface. In every case a careful examination of the material from the ulcer needs to be made to make certain that the condition is not syphilis. Moreover, the necessary blood tests must be made to rule out a syphilitic condition.

Fortunately, sulfadiazine has been found most effective in controlling this condition. Sulfadiazine is given four times a day for from eight to twelve days, and with it some baking soda to prevent any secondary complications. Streptomycin has also been found effective, as are also chloromycetin and aureomycin. However, the antibiotics should not be given until repeated tests have shown with certainty that the condition is not syphilis.

LYMPHOGRANULOMA VENEREUM

Another venereal condition is called *lymphogranuloma venereum.* This condition is due to a virus which is usually acquired by sexual contact. Associated with this infection are large glands in the inguinal region and also systemic symptoms.

Lymphogranuloma venereum is seen in all parts of the world, but mostly in tropical and semitropical climates. A positive skin test determines with certainty the diagnosis of this condition; it is called the Frei test.

Usually from one to four weeks after exposure, the condition begins with an ulcer or an erosion at the place where the organism attacks the body. Frequently this little spot will be considered insignificant, and nothing done about it. Gradually the lymph glands in the groin will begin to swell and form a large mass, which may later break down. The infection may spread to the lower opening of the bowel, causing inflammation with bleeding and a purulent discharge and serious scarring.

Here sulfadiazine is the drug most commonly recommended for treatment. The drug is given four times a day for twelve to fifteen days, and this usually clears up the condition. The antibiotic aureomycin has also been found effective.

GRANULOMA INGUINALE

Another chronic ulcerative venereal disease of the skin and mucous membranes, caused by a germ known technically as the *Donovania granulomatis,* is called granuloma inguinale. This condition is spread

197

all over the world but is seen most widely in tropical and semitropical countries. Although the condition is generally believed to be transmitted by sexual contact, the condition is not especially infectious and is not seen nearly as frequently as are other venereal diseases.

The condition is suspected when the characteristic symptoms occur but, of course, has again to be differentiated from other similar venereal diseases, and particularly from syphilis.

Fortunately, granuloma inguinale heals rapidly when the patient is treated with streptomycin, chloromycetin, aureomycin, or terramycin. The drug is given in adequate dosage by injection over a period of seven to ten days, with a good result.

The patient is studied carefully again and again to make certain that he has not any other venereal disease. If there are secondary infections with pus germs, these are treated with penicillin.

PREVENTION OF VENEREAL INFECTION

Early treatment of people with venereal disease is absolutely necessary to secure maximum benefits and to prevent the spread of infectious venereal diseases. Our soldiers are routinely educated as to the nature of venereal infection and as to what can be done about it.

As soon as a soldier reports with a venereal disease attempts are made to secure the names of all persons with whom he may have had sexual contact, from whom he may have acquired his infection, and to whom he may have given an infection. The information is kept confidential, but it is absolutely necessary that such information be secured, in order to control the spread of venereal disease.

While the person is under treatment he must abstain from all sex contact and he must, of course, be informed of the great danger to himself and to others of any sex contact while he is infected.

There are nowadays many excellent methods of preventing venereal infection, including, principally, cleanliness. Thorough washing with soap and water is of utmost importance in getting rid of infection of all kinds. The taking of a tablet of penicillin in a dosage of 250,000 units is said to be effective in preventing gonorrhea, and usually does not mask an infection with syphilis. In the armed forces of many nations the use of such tablets is considered routine.

CHAPTER XXVIII

THE CARE OF THE FEET

PEOPLE WHO LIVE under primitive conditions need shoes only to keep the feet warm and to protect them against the roughness of the ground when walking. Soft leather moccasins were therefore worn by Indians and Eskimos. In modern cities people walk on cement, wood, and brick surfaces, against which the feet must be protected. Because of changes in weather and other environmental conditions, feet must also be protected against heat, cold, moisture, and infection. Modern conditions of work demand that some people stand for long hours, whereas others may sit three or four hours at a time.

The shoes of babies and growing children and the shoes of women are constructed quite differently from those of grown men, because the needs and desires are different. Children run and jump in their shoes. As the feet grow, the muscles and the ligaments need room to move. Little babies really do not need any foot coverings, but custom demands little stockings and bootees. Later, the infant has to have a shoe with a stiff sole, but with plenty of freedom above so that the foot can be moved without any difficulty.

Experts recommend that the shoe for a growing child have a straight inner margin, with plenty of space for the toes. The heel should be low. The sole should be of thick leather, flexible, and with a toe above it thick and hard enough to prevent damage from bumping the toe. If the foot of the child is distorted out of the normal position, so that it turns too much to one side or the other, or if the child walks too much on the toe or walks flat-footed the mother will do well to have the foot studied by an orthopedic specialist, who can often modify the shoes so as to overcome the condition. The foot of the small child seems often to the mother to be distorted even when it may still be quite normal. Disorders of walking in any child over five years of age should certainly have study by a competent specialist.

BLISTERS, CORNS, AND CALLUSES

Blisters, corns, and calluses on the feet come to remind us that perhaps the shoes do not fit, the stockings wrinkle, or we walk in such a manner as to put most of the burden of the weight of the body on some single spot on the foot. A burning pain on the inner side of the ball of the foot, itching between the toes, or pain anywhere in the feet may indicate that something is wrong. The feet become hardened to work by more use, but hastening of the hardening can be helped by alcohol rubs. Massaging the feet at night is conducive to restful sleep. The foot powders are helpful because they help to reduce the friction between the feet and the stockings and shoes. Most foot powders are chiefly boric acid and talcum. A little salicylic acid or menthol may be added to relieve itching. Physical therapists have found that alternate bathing of the feet in hot and cold water, about two to five minutes in each kind, is helpful to the circulation of blood in the feet.

Blisters are painful. The pain comes from pressure. If a blister is punctured with a germfree needle, one that has been passed through a flame, the fluid will be released and the pain will stop. Preferably, the area where the blister is to be punctured should be wiped with alcohol before the puncture is made.

A corn is an inflammatory response to irritation. A callus is a similar hardening of the tissue, usually occurring on the sole of the foot, wherever the bones press particularly against the shoe. A corn or a callus may be a symptom of some underlying difficulty with the mechanics of the foot, which may be due either to the shoe or stocking, to some anatomical difficulty, or to a wrong way of walking.

Few people have both feet of the same size, yet shoes are usually made with the right and left shoe similar except for the curve. People with great differences between the feet need to have their shoes made especially for them.

Recently, attempts have been made to fit shoes more accurately by X-raying the feet in the shoe store. Actually this is a technic which is not of much benefit to the people who buy the shoes. Probably you can tell better by the way a shoe feels whether or not it fits you right than an untrained clerk can tell from looking at a poor X-ray.

A "soft corn" is an area between the toes which has become rubbed and, usually, secondarily infected with ringworm. If the area around a corn becomes infected the tissues become red, swollen, and painful. Under such circumstances the foot may be kept elevated and treatment applied, such as wet packs soaked with boric acid or some similar mild antiseptic, until the condition improves.

A hard corn can be removed by cutting it away, but such surgery is not for amateurs. People have died from secondary infections resulting from careless and even unsanitary cutting of corns. Unless the persistent pressure and rubbing on the foot are controlled, the corn will return promptly after treatment. The pressure can be modified by wearing suitably prepared pads in the shoes, and otherwise protecting the area.

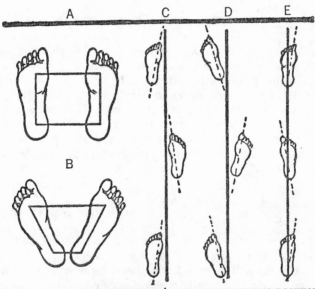

RIGHT AND WRONG FOOT POSTURES. A—CORRECT STANDING POSITION. B—MILITARY STANDING POSITION (WRONG). C—CORRECT WALKING POSITION. D—MILITARY WALKING POSITION (WRONG). E—INDIAN POSITION, WALKING

Most so-called corn cures contain salicylic acid, which softens the hardened material so that it can be scraped away. Corns can also be removed by use of the X-ray or radium, but such treatments are safe only when applied by experienced specialists.

Soft corns will not disappear unless the area is carefully and thoroughly cleaned. The ringworm must be eliminated by suitable treatment. Pads are worn between the toes to get rid of the pressure and the rubbing. If there is a projection from the bone inside the toe the rubbing may be most difficult to prevent. Such deformities may be removed by the orthopedic surgeon.

Calluses on the bottom of the feet are seen often on golf players who pivot on the sole of the foot and on women who wear shoes that are high-heeled and too short. The calluses get thick and hard and are therefore painful. They may be pared away with a sharp knife or razor blade, but they return unless the conditions that produced them are controlled.

WARTS ON THE SOLE OF THE FOOT

Among the most painful of all warts are those that occur on the sole of the foot, commonly called plantar warts. These are probably caused by infection of the rubbed skin with a specific virus. A part on the sole of the foot becomes so painful as to interfere with walking.

Plantar warts are treated in a variety of ways. The hard skin on the bottom of the foot must be softened, and the wart removed. The damaged tissue is protected by proper bandages and antiseptics during the process of healing. Such warts may be removed by surgery, by electrocoagulation, sometimes by radium or X-ray.

INGROWN TOENAILS

When stockings are too long or too short pressures occur on the sides of the toenails, with overgrowth of the tissue around the corners of the nail. Eventually the nail grows into the tissue, forming an ingrown toenail. The nail on the large toe is the one usually involved. Usually the person who suffers with ingrown toenail tries all sorts of poultices, antiseptics, and ointments on his toe, in addition to a little home surgery, before he limps into the doctor's office. The doctor finds the toe red and swollen and, often, with pus oozing from under the nail onto the stocking or the cotton the patient is using for protection. People seldom sterilize the scissors or even the razor blades they use at home for first aid to afflicted feet.

One surgeon has suggested the following procedure for the cure of ingrown toenails: It is necessary to cause the middle of the nail to catch up with the corners. One therefore cuts a small V or U in the center of the nail. This slows the growth at the side of the nail and takes the pressure off the corners. If the foot is kept scrupulously clean, if stockings are worn thick enough to afford protection, if the shoes are loose enough to prevent pressure but not so loose as to cause rubbing, and if the toenail is kept properly trimmed during the process of healing, the nail will gradually become normal. Proper foot hygiene will keep the nail in normal condition.

FOOT STRAIN

Long hours of work under conditions of stress put an extra burden on the feet. The ligaments that connect the muscles with the bones become overstretched, tender, and swollen. When your feet get painful you concentrate on them instead of the work.

Work at a bench or a machine usually involves standing in such a way that the weight is carried not by the heel but by the front of the foot. A bar attached to the shoes will shift the weight, or an inclined platform may be built on which the worker stands.

When feet become strained and painful they should be studied by an orthopedic surgeon. The examination may include X-ray study to rule out inflammation or infection of the bone. Then the feet are put at rest. When the inflammation and pain have disappeared, routine alternate hot and cold bathing, massage and manipulation of the feet will help to restore the tissues to normal. In some instances it becomes necessary to put the feet in plaster casts, so as to eliminate the disturbance for a period long enough to permit complete recovery.

Sometimes flatfoot, hammertoes, and corns are primarily responsible for painful feet. Hammertoes may require a surgical operation. Control of flat feet may involve a wide variety of procedures, including the necessary muscle training to build the strength of the relaxed tissues.

CHAPTER XXIX

INSECT PESTS

ALL SORTS OF INSECTS attack and prey upon human beings. Most common of those that attack the body directly are the lice and the itch mites. Less frequent are bedbugs and spiders. In the woods and in tropical areas chiggers and mosquitoes, ticks and the biting flies annoy mankind.

CHIGGERS

Chiggers are known scientifically as *Trombicula irritans*. They hook themselves on to the skin. The skin becomes irritated, and an intolerable itching begins. Red blotches appear, and blisters form. The chiggers do not burrow into the skin, but they inject a substance which dissolves and softens the tissue, and this causes the itching.

Infestation with chiggers can be prevented by putting flour of sulphur or sulphur powder into the stockings or underclothing when going into tall grass or weeds. Protection can be had by wearing leggings and by closing off the bottom of the trousers.

If you have been seriously bitten by chiggers, wash the skin thoroughly with soap and water and allow the lather to remain on the skin ten minutes before removing. Then any of the anti-itch preparations can be applied to keep the itching under control until healing has occurred.

Insect repellents such as freon with pyrethrum, and similar preparations can be used to remove chiggers from infested areas, as well as mosquitoes, moths, and other insects.

LICE

The louse is an annoying inhabitant on the human body. Head lice are such a frequent annoyance among children in schools that health departments usually give special instructions for their control. Several specialized mixtures have been developed for getting rid of head lice, body lice, and pubic lice.

To kill head lice, ordinary crude petroleum or kerosene mixed with sweet oil or olive oil, half and half, is rubbed well into the scalp. Then cover the hair with a piece of muslin for at least two hours or, better, overnight. Petroleum is poisonous and inflammable. Never let the hair get close to any open flame, such as a gas jet or a lighted match. When the muslin is removed wash the hair and scalp with soap and hot water and rinse well with clear water. Repeat this process as long as live vermin are found in the hair. Nits may be removed by wetting the hair thoroughly with hot vinegar, then combing with a fine-toothed comb. Dry the hair completely after such treatments before going out.

For body lice, the body, all clothing, and all bedding may be thoroughly dusted with a suitable repellent powder.

Pubic lice are commonly called "crabs." Specialized ointments including the old-fashioned "blue ointment" and "Gammexane" ointment, are used, rubbed thoroughly into the infested areas. If such lice get into the eyelashes, they should be picked off, with their nits, by a forceps.

Itching from the bites of lice or other insects in controllable by ointments or lotions containing small amounts of phenol or menthol or camphor, such as 1 per cent phenol or menthol in calamine lotion or phenolated camphor in mineral oil.

SPIDER BITES

The only venomous spider in the Western Hemisphere is the black widow. When a person is bitten by a spider the first step is to stop the absorption of the poison into the circulation. The wound can be disinfected with tincture of iodine or any other good antiseptic. If any considerable amount of poison has been taken into the body, the area of the bite can be put under suction.

Following the bite of the black widow spider, one feels a sharp pain. Then comes swelling and redness at the bitten spot, and the whole body reacts with dizziness and weakness, tremor of the legs, and even abdominal cramps. Small children may have difficulty in breathing and even stupor or convulsions. A serum or antitoxin has been developed, but has to be secured in most cases from the health department or directly from the manufacturer.

FLIES

Flies are not as frequent an annoyance as they used to be. Cleaning up of surroundings, the use of flypaper and fly swatters and the various insect repellents are serving to eliminate them. Such flies as the common housefly, stable flies, greenbottle flies, bluebottle flies, blowflies, fruit flies, and others feed on contaminated garbage and may spread viruses and germs. Such filth-feeding flies have been incriminated in the spread of epidemics of typhoid, dysentery, diarrhea, cholera, infectious hepatitis, and other diseases.

A female housefly can lay as many as 2,000 eggs during a lifetime— i.e., the fly's lifetime. In warm weather these eggs hatch in from eight to ten hours and the new flies go right on breeding. Here are some simple recommendations for getting rid of filth-feeding flies:

Clean up yards, vacant lots, and all surroundings.
Get rid of accumulations of decaying material.
Keep all garbage cans covered, and wash them frequently.
Don't spill garbage around the can or permit it on the sides of the can.
Fill in all low spots where water is accumulated after rain.
Screen all doors and windows in the home and keep the screens in repair.
Cover the baby carriage with mosquito netting when the baby is sleeping outdoors.
Keep flies out of any sick room.
Be sure that all food is kept covered, and do not buy food where it is constantly exposed to flies.
Swat the fly, and be sure the fly swatter is scrubbed once in a while.
Always wash your hands with soap and water after handling a fly.
Outdoor privies should be soundly constructed and screened. Application of quick lime or crude oil or any other permitted insecticide should be made frequently to the contents of the pit.
Remember, if there is no exposed debris or filth there will probably be few flies.

BEDBUGS AND FLEAS

A bedbug bite usually appears as a raised blister with a red spot in the center. It itches and sometimes has a burning sensation. Bedbugs do not live on the human body but they do infest beds, bedding, upholstered furniture, walls, woodwork, and draperies. They usually come out at night, drawn by the odor of the human body. When crushed, the bedbug gives off a foul odor.

Because the bedbug bite itches, the bitten area may be masked by the results of scratching and secondary infection. The spots most commonly bitten are the parts not covered by the night clothing. People who wear pajamas, if bitten, are usually affected in the areas around the ankles, the wrists, and the neck. Sometimes the spots are found in a line, as the bedbug feeds along its way. The only treatment usually required for a bedbug bite is application of a lotion of calamine, with menthol or phenol or camphor to relieve the itching. Ordinary rubbing alcohol or wet dressings of boric acid may be applied.

The bite of the flea resembles that of the bedbug, but the flea injects an irritating fluid when it bites. The spot is usually surrounded by an area of redness, and groups of bites may be close together. The flea bites are usually on exposed portions of the body, but the fleas may get under the clothing and bite anywhere. Any of the lotions usually used for itching may be applied to flea bites.

Fleas that infest rodents can carry diseases such as plague. Fleas are found everywhere. They may pass to human beings from dogs, rats, or pigs. When human beings are bitten by fleas the source of infestation should be found and eliminated. Flea powders are easily available at any drug store.

SCABIES

Scabies, also called seven-year itch, Cuban itch, prison itch, and similar names, is caused by the itch mite. It spreads amidst poverty, overcrowding, and uncleanliness. Usually scabies is transmitted by body contact.

The itch mite does not have the same habits as the body louse. The body louse lives in the clothing and feeds on the body, but the itch mite lives in the body under the skin. Any infestation of clothing or bedding by the itch mite is accidental. Only about 3 per cent of all cases are infested from clothing or bedding.

The itch mite tunnels under the skin. If the skin is cleaned and is free from crusting and secondary infection the little spots of invasion can be seen. The female mite burrows into the skin through the hair follicles and travels along a tunnel, which she creates. At the inner end of the

207

tunnel she lays her eggs. After three to five days the eggs hatch, and the larvae burrow along new tunnels or come out of the old one.

Most common areas of infestation are between the fingers, on the backs of the hands, elbows, under the arms, in the groin, under the breasts, around the navel, sex organs, the shoulder blades, and the back.

During World War II several new treatments were developed for scabies. Emulsion of benzyl benzoate, 23 per cent, is most frequently used. Several proprietary preparations like Kwell and Eurax embody this principle. After the body has been thoroughly scrubbed with hot water, the emulsion is applied with a brush or with an insecticide gun and the whole body is covered from the neck down. The emulsion is allowed to dry, and then after ten or fifteen minutes a second application is painted on. The patient then puts on his clothing and refrains from bathing for twenty-four hours. Then he is given another painting with the benzyl benzoate emulsion. After a second twenty-four-hour period he is instructed to bathe and put on all clean clothing. If these instructions are carried out carefully 95 per cent of patients are cured. The failures are given another course of treatment. The ointment called Gammexane, which is hexachlorocyclohexane, is also used effectively against scabies. The new treatments tend to replace the older use of sulphur ointment, pyrethrum ointment, and rotenone ointment.

MOSQUITO BITES

The mosquito is proof of Kipling's famous statement that "the female of the species is more deadly than the male." The male mosquito does not bite. The female mosquito is out for blood. The mosquito does not really bite, but saws through the skin.

Investigators have found that mosquitoes prefer to bite some people rather than others. They have found, moreover, that some people react severely to mosquito bites, whereas others do not react at all. The attractiveness of an individual for mosquitoes varies from time to time. Mosquitoes that bite prefer places with lots of people, rather than those with just a few people or places that are empty. Mosquitoes are more attracted by numerous or unwashed sleepers than by a few people who are sleeping and who are well washed. Thorough cleansing with soap and water decreases the attractiveness of any individual for mosquitoes. Mosquitoes are attracted by warm objects, by lights at night and by dark objects during the day. Dark clothing is more attractive than light clothing for mosquitoes, and rough clothing is more attractive than smooth clothing. Mosquitoes prefer damp weather to dry weather, but in the cold seasons they prefer dry weather to damp weather. Mosquitoes prefer adults to children and men to women.

If you watch a mosquito as it alights on the skin you will find that it begins to move back and forth, causing the saw to penetrate the skin. If it feeds rapidly it swells up, and if you smack the mosquito a spot of blood will appear on the skin, indicating the amount of blood that has been taken. When the mosquito first inserts the proboscis into your skin it injects some saliva which keeps the blood from clotting.

Mosquitoes carry malaria, yellow fever, and a number of other diseases. The mosquito can be eliminated by getting rid of pools of stagnant water in the surroundings, by spraying surfaces of water with oil, by the widespread use of DDT, and by other well-established health-engineering technics. The itching of the mosquito bite can be controlled by the use of 1 per cent menthol or phenol in calamine lotion or by the application of the ointments of antihistamines such as neohetramine, neoantergan, thephorin, pyribenzamine, benadryl, diatrin, and others.

CHAPTER XXX

MENTAL HEALTH

HEALTH IS GENERALLY CONSIDERED to be freedom from disease. However, health also involves the state of the mind. If you are satisfied with life, if your mind functions accurately, and if you possess enough force, driving power, and impetus to give you confidence in yourself and the ability to accomplish your work, you have good mental health.

Happiness has been described as a balanced flow of energy and the satisfaction of desires. You are happy if you get what you want. Many people do not know what they want. People differ in the things they want. Everyone who is ordinarily healthful is interested in getting enough to eat and enough rest, and in satisfying the ordinary desire for reproduction. There are different levels in fundamental desires. Some people get hungry without really needing food; others require far more rest than do average people. The nature of any desire is conditioned by experience and knowledge, and a person who has never eaten strawberries is not likely to crave strawberries.

An unsatisfied wish is a driving stimulus until it is satisfied. Good mental hygiene requires rationalization. Rationalization is a term used to describe the ability of a human being to satisfy himself with what he gets rather than constantly to be wanting something that he cannot have.

Because it is possible to find happiness with less than a maximum of the desires we have, mental hygienists suggest that everyone develop as a major interest not only a job but perhaps some hobby or game in which he may achieve the success that it is not possible to reach in another field. The basic rule for a happy and contented mind is to cultivate certain standards of living against unexpected changes and then, so as not to be incurably depressed when you fail to achieve something you want, maintain a flexible attitude of mind.

WORRY

Worry is a protracted or recurrent act of the mind, which always fails to result in a constructive solution of the question and usually ends in confusion, fatigue, and emotional instability. You can concern yourself about an important problem, if this means merely a careful consideration in an orderly manner, leading eventually to an acceptable conclusion. Even when the conclusion happens to be contrary to your wishes, it may be accepted as a conclusion and thus worry can be avoided. Such an effort is constructive, whereas worry is always destructive.

The ordinary dictionaries describe worry as feeling or expressing a great deal of care and anxiety, manifesting unrest or pain, fretting, chafing, being anxious or fearful. Since all of these reactions are undesirable from the point of view of their effects on the body, worry is a most undesirable characteristic.

Many people insist that they never worry. These are the people who have learned to reason themselves out of anxiety over situations in which they find themselves. The process is known as "rationalizing." Other people develop mental tranquillity or peace of mind by accepting a belief which eliminates from consideration anything displeasing to them. Such a process is not rationalizing, but may achieve the same effect if the person can shut out completely any problem that disturbs him.

Most people find peace of mind necessary if they are to accomplish their responsibilities in the business world or in the home. Without such peace of mind there is a constant feeling of insecurity, a constant fear of a threat to life itself or to the life situation of the person concerned. As a result, energy is squandered and the reserve of the nervous system is exhausted, so that the person becomes tired, worn, distressed and may have what is commonly called a nervous breakdown.

When worry appears to this extent, the effects manifest themselves on different portions of the body. If the worry is related to the heart the person feels palpitations, extra and light beats of the heart, and similar manifestations; such a person may focus attention unduly on the pulse or the blood pressure or some other factor related to the circulation. If the nervous condition brings the focus of attention on the stomach and bowels there may be constipation, diarrhea, or other manifestations even more serious.

Many a person endeavors to escape from worry by fleeing into an addiction to drink, to drugs, to sedatives, to gambling, or to other practices that are known to be against his best interests. The escape is only temporary, and the trouble returns just as soon as the liquor or the drugs have worn off. A restful night's sleep, a vacation, indulgence in outdoor sports, or even the theater or the movies may be utilized to better advantage as means of escape from the reality of worry.

EMOTIONAL HEALTH

Emotional health is necessary for physical health. Human beings often become mentally and emotionally disturbed because of self-condemnation related to problems of sex which they do not understand. Social and cultural considerations which regulate human sex behavior are more rigid than the biological considerations. These considerations define what is moral much more definitely than do biologic and medical science.

In various portions of the United States the attitudes of people vary a great deal as to the ordinary relationships between the sexes. In some portions of the country people would consider it a gross violation of domestic relations for a married man to have lunch with a married woman other than his wife. In other branches of American society, and this refers of course particularly to our larger cities, such ordinary meetings are within the pattern of everyday social existence.

When a young man moves in the United States from one community to another he may require several months to find out the restrictions on conduct which are considered suitable to the new community. Up to 1915 people paid little attention to inhibitions, and did not fret much about these matters. Since that time public education on psychological subjects has created fear among people of being considered "inhibited."

Professor John C. Whitehorn of Johns Hopkins University has classified maturity of human beings on a five-point scale. People who are infantile in their emotional attitudes are likely to be dependent on their parents or substitutes for the parent—a governess or nurse—and to expect infinite amounts of service and tolerance from the parents. Sometimes men and women of advanced years retain this infantile attitude until the death of the parent or some forced separation, which may be quite tragic in their lives. Thus, a woman thirty-eight years old, who was subject to repeated moody spells, had that kind of dependence, and had to have someone strong on whom to lean in all her difficult situations. The child who has been "teacher's pet" will have to be the "boss's favorite" when he gets a job.

The second level is the childish level. The child develops some sense of personal responsibility but can always get rid of it by an excuse. The child still has to have complete trust in some other person. People who grow up and maintain their childish level are those who always find excuses for the failures, alibis for their weakness and who "pass the buck" whenever confronted with difficult situations.

The child during the period of puberty with its development of secondary sexual characteristics really goes through two periods, which may be called early adolescence and late adolescence. The child in early adolescence begins to have a drive for self-assertion and begins to resent parental domination. Just as the male animal shows his best characteristics for the attraction of the female, so also the boy in early adolescence begins to show off and indulge in contests in which he can demonstrate superiority. The boy's room begins to be filled with trophies won at the track or in the swimming pool or at other sports. The girl's room begins to be decorated with programs of dances, souvenirs of parties, and knickknacks accumulated on dates.

As late adolescence develops "dating" becomes the most important aspect of life. If this passes on to what boys and girls call "going steady," difficult mental situations may develop. Parents frequently try to dominate the situation, because of economic, religious, or purely emotional factors. These situations may lead to emotional disturbances in the young that may mark the life of the growing youth for many years thereafter.

Finally, adults are supposed to have a balanced perspective and to adjust themselves to various social roles, but adults still need affection, security, and well-established relationships toward other people. If the adult has failed to mature and depends heavily on the affection of others, if he requires definite signs of favoritism he is unlikely to be able to develop a satisfactory marriage, and may react emotionally to situations which he himself cannot solve. Professor Whitehorn is convinced that the chances for good marriage adjustment among people who reach mature years without overcoming infantile dependence on affection are slight. It seems to be an American trait to strive toward perfection in marriage relationship, and most psychologists believe that a little less perfectionism would lead to much greater satisfaction in many disturbed marriages.

EMOTIONAL DISTURBANCES

Most people have minor emotional disturbances that are not recognized but, because of their effects on the general health, have medical significance. Many people in industry, in labor, and in public life get along, although they suffer at all times with difficulties of adjustment to their environment. An analysis of the people who come to doctors' offices revealed that from 30 to 60 per cent come as patients primarily because of complaints due to emotional disorders, which are reflected as physical disorders. Therefore, frustrations, anxiety, and fear may appear as headaches, ulcers of the stomach, asthma, or similar conditions. Indeed, emotional factors may be present in the great majority of physical illnesses. Treatment is not fully satisfactory unless it takes care of the mental as well as the physical factors.

Our population has become an aging population. People live much longer than was common fifty years ago. As people get older they tend to develop more emotional experiences, and this has greatly multiplied the need of psychiatric help. According to the available figures, one out of every twenty people will need advice or guidance from an expert for severe emotional illness at some time during his lifetime. This is indicated by the fact that more than one half of all the veterans in veterans' hospitals are psychiatric patients. Thirty-seven per cent of releases from the army for medical reasons were for psychiatric disorders. A total of 51 per cent of all medical separations from the military service were due to personality disturbances. In addition, people who are mentally disturbed constitute about one-half of all of the patients in hospitals in the United States.

While modern medicine has much knowledge of psychiatric conditions, far more still remains unknown than is actually known. Methods of treatment developed in recent years include the successful use of the tranquilizing drugs (see below), psychic energizers, electric shock, psychoanalysis, the use of occupational and recreational therapy. Since the number of competent experts capable of treating such patients is insufficient, study is now being made of the treatment of mentally ill patients in groups. This is called group psychotherapy.

THE TRANQUILIZING DRUGS

When Sir William Osler made his valedictory address to the University of Pennsylvania in 1889, he chose the subject "Aequanimitas." He said, "In the physician or surgeon no quality takes rank with imperturbability." Then he defined the word: "Imperturbability means coolness and presence of mind under all circumstances, calmness amid storm, clearness of judgment in moments of grave peril, immobility, impassiveness, or, to use an old and expressive word, *phlegm*." He was doubtful that it could be acquired except by inheritance, and he thought that some of his students, "owing to congenital defects," might never be able to acquire it. He counseled, nevertheless, that education with practice and experience might help to attain imperturbability in fair measure. The doctor, Osler felt, should develop an "inscrutable face by education of his nerve centers." In concluding this discussion of imperturbability he said:

"Cultivate, then, gentlemen, such a judicious measure of obtuseness as will enable you to meet the exigencies of practice with firmness and courage without, at the same time, hardening the human heart by which we live."

The mental equivalent to imperturbability, which Osler called "a bodily endowment," is a calm equanimity. He considered that one of the first essentials in securing a good equanimity is "not to expect too much of the people amongst whom you dwell." Osler recognized that prosperity is an aid to equanimity and enables us to bear with composure the misfortunes of our neighbors.

One wonders what Sir William Osler might have said had he had available in 1889 such aids to imperturbability and equanimity as have come with the new tranquilizing drugs. Statistics of institutions for the mentally disturbed and for the alcoholic already indicate the results of an administration of these new remedies.

At a regular meeting of the Society of Biologic Psychiatry, the president, Dr. Harold E. Himwich, said, "A few short years ago it would have been impossible to read a paper on the new tranquilizing drugs but now we know that Chlorpromazine and Reserpine are valuable in the treatment of disturbed psychotic patients." Since that paper was read, many other drugs and combinations have been added to the list. These are the drugs that affect the brain. Both Reserpine and Chlorpromazine depress the hypothalamic mechanisms, particularly that part concerned with the patterns for emergency, for fight, and flight. Chlorpromazine depresses not only these mechanisms but also the sympathetic and parasympathetic nervous systems. Other research has indicated that Chlorpromazine prevents the awakening, alerting, or arousal reaction producing what is in effect a pharmacologic lobotomy.

The mechanism by which these drugs have their effect is not clearly established. However, some evidence indicates that a neurohormone is involved. When it is insufficient in amount to produce its normal effects, abnormal behavior may be observed. In concluding his address Dr. Himwich wrote, "These new drugs are not a flash in the pan but their therapeutic values have been widely corroborated. However, they are not a complete answer to our therapeutic problem because no one drug is able to ameliorate the condition of all of the patients and none of them is as efficacious for melancholia as is electric shock."

In addition to the drugs already mentioned consideration must be

215

given to the pharmacological properties of tranquilizers. All these drugs must be prescribed by the physician for the individual patient. The doctor prescribes the dosage, the frequency of use, and the possible side-effects are told to the patient. They are used to quiet patients and to relax them. These drugs have brought about a great change in the care of psychotic and disturbed people. Other tranquilizers include Ultran, Trepidone, Trilafon, Taractan, Mellaril, Librium, Atarax, Dartal, and many others.

DEPRESSION

People who are depressed have in the past been treated frequently with benzedrine, or amphetamine, which stimulates but which has the undesirable effect of raising the blood pressure. New drugs have been developed called psychic energizers which are used to overcome depression. If the central nervous system is underactive, these drugs seem to restore it to a more normal level of activity. Obviously drugs of this type are not given to people who are overexcited. The drugs have been useful in the condition called narcolepsy, in which there is a sudden irresistible desire to sleep. This condition has also been treated with amphetamine. In cases of fatigue, drowsiness, or what is called a low-down feeling they may be prescribed by the physician. Other psychomotor stimulants include Ritalin, Marsalid, Meratran, Ambar, Nardil, Deaner, Elavil, and Tofranil.

MENTAL HYGIENE IN BUSINESS

Suitable adjustment of workers to their surroundings is important in establishing a smooth-running condition in any business or industry. Ask the average businessman if he needs a psychiatrist in his business, and he will think you are mentally disturbed. Psychiatrists, most people believe, spend practically all of their time finding people who need to be confined in institutions because they are wholly irresponsible.

Most large industries have employment interviewers, who have knowledge of the positions to be filled, of the persons in the department, and, therefore, of the kind of employee who will fit best and serve most satisfactorily under the circumstances. Most employment interviewers can recognize easily a prospective employee who is so far "off the beaten path" from a mental point of view as to be unsatisfactory for any job. No one suggests that employment interviewers should be replaced by psychiatrists or psychologists. What a business-man wants is a worker who can respond to the particular problems and procedures of the job for which he is employed. The boss seldom wants to be troubled about the general personality of an employee or the question of how he gets along with his wife. Nevertheless, that very situation may be important in relation to the quality or amount of work. Problems may arise which are due to a neurosis or psychosis in some employee whose mental condition has not been recognized.

Mental hygienists are convinced that training ought to be made available to employment managers or to the workers in the personnel divisions of industries. Workers are frequently transferred into personnel departments because they appear to be able to get along well with other people—but sometimes because they are hard and skeptical. Generally they work out their own techniques, whether for the handling of personal problems or for the selection of new employees.

Already there are plenty of reports of instances in which employees who failed to respond acceptably to their executives were given scientific study and thus saved for the organization. We have learned how to modify the attitudes of parents and to improve their relationships with their children. Similar tactics are needed for executive businessmen to improve their relationships with their employees.

MENTAL DEFECT

Among the great unsolved problems of modern medicine are many of those associated with mental disease. People still fear the sudden appearance of the "loss of the mind," or the birth of a child apparently without normal mental ability. Over 4,000,000 children are born in this country every year. Actually from 150,000 to 200,000 of those born will eventually be committed to hospitals for mental disease or defect.

Much can be done to prevent or overcome many of the conditions that disturb the mind. With modern methods of treatment, improvement can even be secured in certain forms of complete mental breakdown. Problems of mental defect and of mental diseases are not only approached by putting the patients in institutions but also by applying some of these new forms of treatment.

Parents, teachers, and those organizations concerned with the supervision of children must realize the importance of recognizing strange behavior at the earliest possible moment. Children who are mentally retarded or who are slow in their mental development should be submitted to expert advice as soon as possible. These children will be brought into social and economic competition, and the contrast with normal children, coupled with pressure from forces behind them at home and even from their association with competitors, may result in a reaction and in the formation of attitudes which lead to permanent disturbances.

There are many causes of mental breakdown and many classifications of mental disturbance. Research has been intensified on dementia praecox, in which the so-called insulin shock, metrazol shock, and electric shock treatments are being tried. Modern medicine also offers new forms of study, including analysis of the mental processes, leading to recognition of the underlying factors in mental disturbances.

The wise man need not fear such a catastrophe. He should know that scientific methods of diagnosis and treatment are now available.

CHAPTER XXXI

FAMILY MEDICINE CHEST

AMONG THE STRANGE ITEMS found in a half-dozen family medicine chests that I looked over were old cloths to be used as bandages, cracked atomizer bulbs, horehound candy, shoehorns, curling irons, dried sponges, packages of seeds, hair grease, mange cure, face bleach, shoe polish, empty tooth paste and shaving cream tubes, fifty different remedies for colds, combs for permanent waves, bobby pins, the remaining partners of divorced cuff links, nail polish, bath salts, and discarded sets of teeth.

The number of antiseptics found, and their efficiency, varied tremendously. One or two antiseptics were found in some cases, and as many as six different antiseptics in others, individual members of the family having their own likes and dislikes in these matters.

A household remedy should be one with a certain definite action. If the thing is worth keeping in the medicine chest it should be something which is used fairly frequently.

Dangerous poisons have no place in the family medicine chest. A dangerous poison is one which is likely to produce serious symptoms or death if taken in even moderate amounts.

Prescriptions ordered by the family doctor for a certain illness should never be kept for the future. If any of the material remains in the bottle it should be poured promptly into a safe place of disposal. Since useful bottles are rare around most homes, the bottle may be thoroughly washed with hot water, dried, and stored away. Few people realize that most drugs deteriorate with age and that a prescription for a certain illness is not likely to be useful for the future.

The wise person will go over the family medicine chest at least once every three months and discard all materials not constantly in use. It is also well to have the family doctor take a look at the materials, offer his advice on those worth keeping, and make suggestions as to what is needed.

SUITABLE ITEMS FOR MEDICINE CHESTS

Items that should be in any first-class family medicine chest may include a laxative or cathartic. Under certain circumstances any laxative or cathartic may be exceedingly dangerous, most conspicuously in appendicitis. Appendicitis is at first just an infected spot on a little organ which extends from the large bowel and which, apparently, has no serious function in the human body. If this infection develops, as a boil develops from a pimple, it is in danger of bursting and spreading throughout the body. Therefore, no laxative or cathartic should ever be taken when the abdomen is exceedingly painful.

The most common laxatives used include liquid petrolatum, or mineral oil, which is a mechanical lubricant without possibility of serious harm. Other common preparations much used include, of course, the old-fashioned castor oil, Seidlitz powders, psyllium seed, sodium phosphate, aromatic cascara, mineral oil mixed with agar, methyl cellulose, and phenolphthalein.

The next most commonly used preparations in a family medicine chest, aside from the cosmetics, are pain relievers. Most of these are used for headaches, although sometimes they are used for what are called "neuritis" and "neuralgia," for other pains of unknown origin, and for toothache, as well as to produce sleep. Most headache powders bought under patent trade-marks contain phenacetin or acetanilid. Aspirin is the safest pain reliever.

Other drugs much used to produce sleep are derivatives of barbituric acid, of which some of the best examples are veronal, trional, and combinations of barbituric acids with other drugs.

The family medicine chest is better off without preparations of this character, as the possibilities for harm are sufficiently great to suggest that these preparations be not used except with medical advice.

The widely publicized milk of magnesia and sodium bicarbonate, or baking soda, are two preparations which can safely be kept in the family medicine chest and which are frequently advised by physicians for alkaline purposes.

Some families keep paregoric as a useful preparation in case of cramps that affect women at periodic intervals.

Most modern women prefer to keep their cosmetics in their own boudoirs, but the man of the house is likely to put his into the family medicine cabinet. They should include, in most instances, a razor, which should be kept in its box and not permitted to lie around loose, also some shaving soap or cream, some face lotion, which may be either witch hazel or a special lotion which he prefers.

The most commonly used general pain reliever is acetylsalicylic acid, commonly called aspirin. So far as is known, aspirin is relatively harmless, except for a few people who are especially sensitive to it. Such people cannot take even small doses. One aspirin is as good as another, provided it is up to the standard of the United States Pharmacopoeia.

Among the strongest of medicinal preparations are the narcotics and anesthetics. Narcotics should never be used by anyone without a physician's prescription and, indeed, no drug that has to be administered with a hypodermic syringe should find a place in the average family medicine chest.

There are some people with diabetes who have been taught by their doctors to inject themselves with insulin. Even these people should keep their syringe outfit separate from the materials in the family medicine chest.

There are all sorts of antiseptics available for use on the skin, in first aid, and also for gargling and for washing various portions of the body. The most widely known skin antiseptic is tincture of iodine. Antiseptic mouthwashes and gargles are available for the destruction of germs in the mouth and throat. If the antiseptic is applied directly on a swab, so that the material is held in direct contact with the localized infection, it is more likely to be effective.

ANTISEPTICS

Among the antiseptics approved by the Council on Drugs are preparations of hexylresorcinol and preparations of metaphen, also merthiolate, zephiran, cepryl, and neutral solutions of chlorinated soda and hydrogen peroxide. The Council has not approved antiseptics commonly represented as being useful in the relief of all sorts of infections of the throat and also for the prevention of various types of infectious diseases, including colds.

FIRST AID

In these days when everybody takes the chance of needing emergency first-aid treatment, because of the use of the automobile and wide indulgence in sports and gardening, first-aid supplies may be kept in the family medicine chest. Among the materials needed are adhesive tape of various widths, sterile cotton, sterile gauze bandages, sterile gauze pads, and a scissors which should be kept in the medicine chest exclusively for such purposes. You should also have the ready-made combination of a piece of adhesive tape with a tiny piece of sterilized bandage, that can be used to cover small wounds after they have been treated with iodine or mercurochrome.

Most people should know that the proper way to stop bleeding of small wounds is simply to press upon them with a sterile piece of gauze.

In cases of very serious wounds affecting arteries, and thereby difficult to control, it may be necessary to put a tourniquet around the limb. The tourniquet should be fastened just tight enough to stop the bleeding. An ordinary piece of rubber tubing or a narrow towel tied and twisted with a stick will serve most purposes satisfactorily.

The family medicine chest may also contain aromatic spirits of ammonia, which is sometimes given when a prompt stimulant is needed, following fainting. Half a teaspoonful in water, for a sudden fainting spell, is a fairly safe thing to give in most cases of this emergency.

It is not advisable to use a styptic in the form of a stick of alum to stop slight bleeding after shaving. Much better are any of the astringent surgical powders, of which a small amount may be taken from the box on each occasion and applied directly to the bleeding point.

Finally, any good talcum powder may be used after shaving and after bathing, according to the individual preferences of the users.

It is taken for granted that every modern household has a good clinical thermometer, a hot water bottle, and an ice bag. These are three exceedingly useful devices in any home, and when they are available in an emergency the comfort they give is tremendous.

In addition to the materials used for first aid, most families will have bedpans for use in cases of illness, glass drinking-tubes, syringes for giving enemas, atomizers, and sometimes special devices for creating steam to be medicated with small amounts of tincture of benzoin for relief in various forms of hoarseness or other conditions affecting the larynx and the lungs.

TAKING MEDICINE

Medicines rightly used can be of immense aid and comfort to the afflicted; wrongly used, they may cause serious damage to the human body. When a doctor prescribes medicines for a patient, they are for that particular patient and not for anybody else in the family.

When you measure out the medicine think of what you are doing and pay no attention to anything else. Medicines are usually prescribed in dosages of drops, teaspoons, fractions of teaspoons, and spoons of larger sizes. Because spoons are nowadays in many fanciful shapes and sizes, each family should have a medicine glass with measures of various spoons recorded. When a doctor prescribes a certain number of drops they should be measured with a medicine dropper and not by guesswork.

If liquid medicine is being prescribed the bottle should be thoroughly shaken each time before the medicine is measured. Most medicine should be mixed with a little water when taken, but sometimes the medicine may be put in the mouth and washed down with a swallow of water. Pills and capsules should either be handed to the patient from the original package, so that he may help himself, put the pill or capsule on the back of the tongue, and wash it down with a drink of water, or else be brought to the patient on a spoon, so that he may take the pill or capsule from the spoon. The person waiting on the patient should not carry the capsules or pills in the palm of the hand, where they may be softened or disintegrated by moisture or contaminated from the hands.

There are several ways in which medicines of unpleasant taste may be made more palatable. If very cold water is taken it will serve to cover up the taste. It is not advisable to give medicine to children in foods, particularly in milk, as this may create a distaste for the food or milk which lasts for a long time afterward.

There are lots of ways to disguise castor oil. One of the simplest is the so-called "castor-oil sandwich," in which the castor oil is poured on a layer of orange juice and covered up with another layer of the same substance. Water will not mix with castor oil and will not disguise the taste. Nowadays there are available tasteless castor oils and flavored castor oils, which serve the purpose without the disagreeable taste.

HELPFUL RULES FOR THE FAMILY MEDICINE CHEST

1. Don't save poisonous preparations of any kind.
2. Never keep in the family medicine chest bichloride of mercury, pills containing strychnine, or solutions containing wood alcohol.
3. Never keep samples of patent medicines of unknown composition.

4. Never permit any preparation of opium or morphine to be loose in the family medicine chest.

5. Never save any prepared preparation after the specific need for which it was ordered by the physician has ended.

Keep It Orderly

6. Go over the family medicine chest at least once every three months and discard all useless or spoiled materials.

7. When measuring out a medicine think of what you are doing and pay no attention to anything else.

8. Have a measuring glass for measuring doses of medicines and several spoons of various sizes available for administering liquid medicines.

9. Always measure drops with a medicine dropper and not by guesswork.

10. Always shake a bottle containing liquid medicine each time before pouring out the medicine for use.

11. After removing the cork from a bottle, put the cork top-down on a table, washstand, or tray. Put it back in the bottle immediately after the medicine has been poured out.

12. Never take a cathartic for abdominal pain unless the cause of the pain is known. It may be appendicitis.

13. Never take pyramidon or tablets which contain pyramidon without a doctor's prescription.

14. Never drop any medicine in the eye unless a doctor has recommended it.

Don't Crowd It with Cosmetics

15. Women's cosmetics should be kept in their own place, preferably where they are used by the woman concerned.

16. Never take sleeping powders, pills, tablets, or solutions unless in the amounts recommended and at the times recommended by your doctor.

17. Persistent pain is a warning signal of danger of disease or damage to your body. Do not disregard it. Do not mask it with pain-relieving remedies.

18. Do not treat the baby for pains, spasms, skin rashes, or disorders of digestion which you would not try to treat if they affected you. Call your doctor. Give the baby the same chance you would want for yourself under similar conditions.

CHAPTER XXXII

EXERCISE

THE ROAD TO HEALTH does not involve the cultivation of enormous muscles. Innumerable systems of exercise have been exalted as leading to healthfulness. All sorts of extraordinary springs, bicycles, walking machines, dumbbells, and similar apparatus are alleged to lead the user directly into vim, vigor, and vitality, the three objectives of the physical culturist.

Exercise is a means of stimulating the action of the muscles, improving the co-ordination of nerve and muscle, and improving the circulation of the blood. The chief value of exercise is to stimulate the general chemistry and physiology of the body through its effect on the circulation and on elimination. That's why a healthy person feels better after exercise.

Everyone should have sufficient strength of muscle to carry on the ordinary activities of life, and to permit some exceptional use in time of emergency. For young people exercise has the value of stimulating body growth. Competitive sports of a vigorous kind, such as running, tennis, handball, football, and baseball, are useful, but should never be tried by those not physically fit to undertake them. Among muscular activities suitable to people of all ages are swimming, walking, golf, horseback riding, fishing, and gardening. These sports cultivate endurance and grace. They may not make the heart beat faster, but neither will they make it hesitate or stop. Before undertaking any kind of strenuous physical activity let your doctor determine the capacity of your heart.

Here are the proper amounts of muscular activity for people of various ages: four hours of muscular activity at the age of five years, five hours daily from the age of seven to nine, six hours from nine to eleven, five hours from eleven to thirteen, four hours from thirteen to sixteen, three hours from sixteen to eighteen, and two hours from eighteen to twenty. One authority has said that one hour should be given daily to activities involving the use of the large muscles of the body after twenty years of age, and that anything less will result in physical deterioration.

EFFECTS OF EXERCISE

Just why do we exercise? People who do not exercise do not have positive health. They do not seem to have the vigor, vim, and vitality of those who take a reasonable amount of exercise. The muscles of our chests and hearts and of our bodies generally need a certain amount of activity in order to give them a factor that is called "tone." Tone includes the ability of a muscle to respond when called on.

The chief purpose of exercise is to obtain a normal development of tissues, so that they will be capable of performing their ordinary functions. The muscles of the trunk and of the back must be well-developed to maintain good posture. The muscles of the back, legs, and feet are needed to make walking, running, and jumping easy and graceful.

Exercise increases the circulation of the blood, and thus aids nourishment of the individual cells of the body. Improved circulation also helps to remove waste material from the body. The proper circulation of the blood is related to the regulation of the heat of the body.

Exercise also increases the depth and rate of breathing, thus giving the red blood cells more oxygen to carry, and helps to eliminate the waste carbon dioxide from the body.

Following a reasonable amount of exercise in the open air, the body feels refreshed and not exhausted. With such refreshment comes the relaxation that is exceedingly important for rest and good mental hygiene.

Finally, there is a sense of satisfaction associated with being able to swing a golf club, a tennis racket, or an ax as well as the next man, or in being able to row a boat or to swim when such an activity may be required.

There is apparently no absolute evidence that physical training produces a condition which helps to protect the body against disease. There is general belief that the hardy mountaineer, who has to keep climbing and who is constantly in a state of physical activity, is more healthful than the lazy inhabitant of the tropics, who sleeps through large portions of the twenty-four hours, but there is no proof that the mountaineer has better health than the lazybones who sleeps in the sun.

The chief value of exercise is that it increases the competence of the body to do physical work, lessens fatigue, increases endurance, and produces perfection of movement.

THE MUSCLES

The main virtue of exercise does not lie in any increase of muscular strength but in its maintenance of the normal activities of the tissues. When a muscle contracts it uses up a substance called glycogen, which is present in muscles in large amounts. A waste product, lactic acid, accumulates. The blood takes up carbon dioxide, which develops from waste material, and carries it to the lungs, where it is eliminated from the body.

If carbonic acid and lactic acid accumulate in them, the muscles become acid in their reaction. If lactic acid accumulates in considerable amounts the movement of the muscles will stop. Oxygen is required to aid continuous movement of the muscles. When oxygen comes in, the lactic acid disappears, the glycogen accumulates again, and the muscles become alkaline instead of acid. Large amounts of oxygen are necessary for continuous work by the muscles.

A person who is doing hard muscular work requires ten times more oxygen than he needs when he is resting. The extra oxygen, which is provided by speeding up the circulation, increases the rate of breathing and sometimes raises the pressure of the blood in the blood vessels.

During exercise the pulse rate becomes more rapid, the blood pressure rises, and more blood goes through the tissues. The amount of increase depends on the rapidity and continuity with which, and the length of time during which, the muscles are being used.

In addition to the value of exercise for improving the general health, there is its value in improving the condition of tissues that have been weakened by disease. Therefore, restricted exercise is prescribed for people who have such conditions as heart disease or high blood pressure. These exercises must be controlled by trained attendants, so that the sick person never becomes fatigued, exhausted, or subjected to overexercise.

The balance between beneficial effects and bad effects is so delicate that it is impossible for anyone to regulate the exercise in relation to disease for himself. Even doctors who have such conditions cannot regulate for themselves the amount of effort they may put forth.

Serious harm, at times even death, has resulted from having a doctor tell such patients casually that they need exercise, without specifically prescribing the character and the amount. The tragedies of the handball and tennis courts and the golf course bear eloquent testimony to this fact.

In determining physical fitness the doctor studies the pulse, the blood pressure, the breathing, and the condition of the blood.

THE PULSE

Everyone should know how to measure the rate of the pulse. The rate is much faster in children than in adults. It varies from just over 100 beats a minute for a three-year-old to eighty-one for a boy of twelve; sixty-eight or seventy for a youth of eighteen, and sixty-eight for a man of sixty. The rate for women is five to nine beats higher in each age group.

Here is how the pulse gauge works in relation to exercise. Count your pulse beat after you have been sitting for a while and have not had any exercise. Then stand up and simulate running for a few minutes. Running of this type for five minutes will speed the heart and pulse more than the same exercise for three minutes. The longer the exercise, the longer time required for the rate to return to normal.

Among a group of boys who ran the 100-yard dash there was an average increase of forty-five beats per minute in the pulse at the end of the race. The pulse of a sprinter who had run 400 yards was still sixteen beats above normal after he had rested one hour and twenty minutes.

BLOOD PRESSURE

The blood pressure averages from 110 to 120 above the age of twenty years and up to the age of forty. From ten years to twenty years it averages about 100.

Exercises of strength, such as weight-lifting, will raise the blood pressure. Exercises of speed, such as tennis or speed swimming, will cause the blood pressure to rise somewhat less rapidly and to return to normal more slowly.

When the blood pressure of a woman who had run up three flights of stairs in forty-five seconds was measured, it was found to have risen forty points. In exercises of endurance, such as thirty-six holes of golf, a long hike across the country, or a slow bicycle tour, the blood pressure will not rise as high as it does in speed exercise. At the end of the trip it may actually be lower than ordinary.

BREATHING

Breathing also varies according to the nature of the exercise. Training in breathing makes the difference between winning and losing an athletic event. In the short dashes the racer breathes normally through the time when the starter says, "On your mark." At the order "Get set" the sprinter will take a breath and hold it until the gun indicates the start. He will retain this breath until he is under way. Better sprinters hold their breath longer than those who are untrained.

Swimmers mostly shorten the time when the breath is taken in and given out and increase the rate of breathing with the rate of the stroke.

Expert golf players take a deep breath before the drive and hold it during the swing of the club. This serves to stiffen the chest muscles and aids in control of the arms. After the drive the golfer lets out the air and breathes normally. During the putting, the breathing should be quiet and shallow.

The average person breathes from seventeen to twenty times per minute. Women breathe a bit more rapidly than do men. All of us breathe more rapidly when standing than sitting. The amount of air taken in with a single breath averages three quarts for a grown man, two quarts for a grown woman.

SUPERSTITIONS ABOUT EXERCISE

Big muscles are not necessarily a sign of strength or a guarantee of long life. Overdeveloped muscles may be a liability rather than an asset.

The length of life depends on the general physical condition of the body as a whole, and a great deal on the nature of the body that one has inherited from one's ancestors. People who live long tend to have children who live long.

Many peculiar devices have been developed for producing expansion or development of various portions of the body. Some contend that breathing exercises, which will greatly increase the expansion of the chest, are beneficial to health and long life. Actually the evidence shows that most such exercises are more harmful than beneficial.

Most of the important functions of the body related to health are automatic, including the work of the heart, the lungs, and the kidneys. This natural automaticity regulates the rate and depth of breathing in relation to the functions of the body of the person concerned.

Increased work brings increased need for oxygen and more and deeper breathing. Young people who participate regularly in a certain amount of wholesome physical activity, including ordinary games and competition, swimming, tennis, walking, rowing and bicycle riding, will not worry about their rate of breathing.

Large lungs and vital capacity developed beyond the usual needs of the body mean that much of the tissue concerned will not be called on enough of the time to be helpful. Unused tissue tends to become infiltrated with fat and to become weak. This happens to the man who develops tremendous muscles and an enlarged heart by exercising during youth, and then gives up all exercise suddenly as he gets older.

Young people need more exercise than do older ones, because their bodies are growing. They, therefore, take in more oxygen and give out more waste matter than does the ordinary adult.

Training improves an athlete and the quality of his performance. Training helps to co-ordinate the muscles, so that they give a better performance without using up as much energy as might otherwise be required. The danger of exertion may be overcome if boys and girls will be careful to warm up slowly before any activity, exactly as athletes do before football games or track meets. The warming-up process enables the body to reach its maximum requirement and prevents the short breath and discomfort which usually precede what athletes call the coming of the "second wind."

Training increases the vital capacity—that is, the amount of air that can be handled by the lungs. The average athlete has a capacity of four to five quarts of air, in contrast to three quarts for the non-athlete.

The increase in endurance resulting from good physical training is shown by the fact that the onset of fatigue is delayed. Most important in training is practice in using the correct form. Dancing is exercise, but not a graceful one until you learn the steps.

HERE ARE ELEVEN SIMPLE EXERCISES DESIGNED BY
HEALTH TEACHERS AT THE UNIVERSITY OF ILLINOIS

The exercises were designed for adults. Used daily, they will increase your vigor, muscular strength, body suppleness, motor reaction, and body posture.

Learn to do the exercises correctly, vigorously, and in good posture.

In the beginning, repeat each exercise the minimum number of times; then gradually increase the dosage.

Perform the exercises with enthusiasm. Count out loud; hum a march.

Go through the entire series without stopping. The investment of ten or twelve minutes of your time in this way cannot help but pay big dividends.

I. THE STRETCHER (Min. 4; Max. 10)

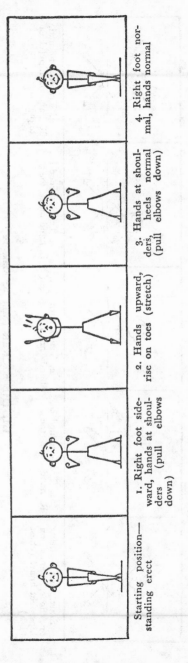

Starting position— standing erect

1. Right foot side- ward, hands at shoul- ders (pull elbows down)

2. Hands upward, rise on toes (stretch)

3. Hands at shoul- ders, heels normal (pull elbows down)

4. Right foot nor- mal, hands normal

II. THE TWISTER (Min. 6; Max. 15)

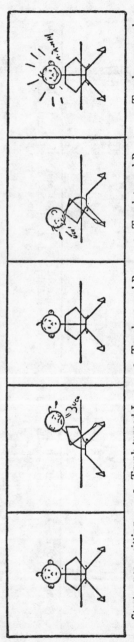

Start. pos.—sitting on floor, hands on hips, feet apart (chest high)

1. Trunk turned L., R. hand on L. toe

2. Trunk normal R. hand on hip (chest up)

3. Trunk turned R., L. hand on R. toe

4. Trunk normal, R. hand on hip (chest high)

III. THE KICKER (Min. 6; Max. 12)

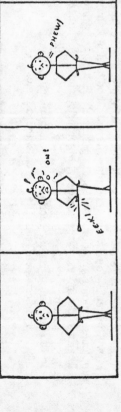

Start. pos.—standing erect, hands on hips

1. R. foot raised sideward (kick high)

2. R. foot normal

3. R. foot raised forward (kick high)

4. R. foot normal

IV. THE SIDE BENDER (Min. 6; Max. 15)

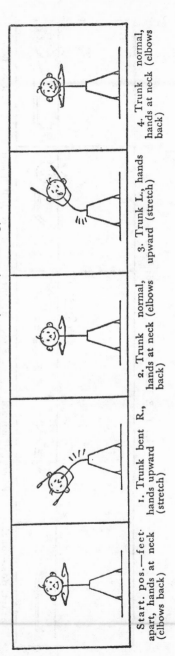

Start. pos.—feet apart, hands at neck (elbows back)

1. Trunk bent R., hands upward (stretch)

2. Trunk normal, hands at neck (elbows back)

3. Trunk L., hands upward (stretch)

4. Trunk normal, hands at neck (elbows back)

V. THE NECK PRESSER (Min. 6; Max. 15)

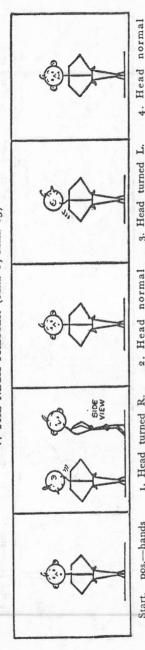

SIDE VIEW

Start. pos.—hands on hips

1. Head turned R. and drawn backward

2. Head normal (don't let head sag)

3. Head turned L. and drawn backward

4. Head normal (don't slump)

VI. THE SQUATTER (Min. 6; Max. 15)

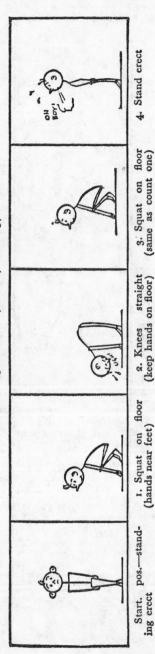

Start. pos.—stand-ing erect

1. Squat on floor (hands near feet)

2. Knees straight (keep hands on floor)

3. Squat on floor (same as count one)

4. Stand erect

VII. THE LEG LIFTER (Min. 6; Max. 15)

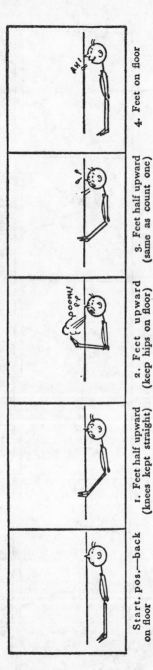

Start. pos.—back on floor

1. Feet half upward (knees kept straight)

2. Feet upward (keep hips on floor)

3. Feet half upward (same as count one)

4. Feet on floor

VIII. THE COMPRESSER (Min. 6; Max. 15)

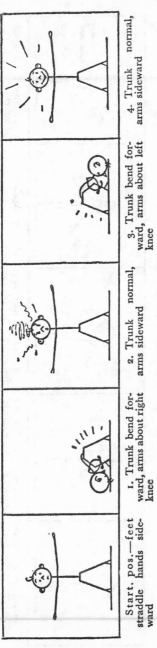

Start. pos.—feet straddle hands sideward

1. Trunk bend forward, arms about right knee

2. Trunk normal, arms sideward

3. Trunk bend forward, arms about left knee

4. Trunk normal, arms sideward

IX. THE DIPPER (Min. 6; Max. 15)

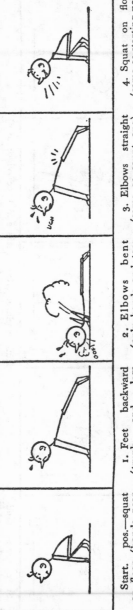

Start. pos.—squat on floor (hands near feet)

1. Feet backward (trunk and legs straight)

2. Elbows bent (only hands and toes touch floor)

3. Elbows straight (same as count one)

4. Squat on floor (same as starting position)

X. THE HIGH STEPPER (Min. 10 steps; Max. 20)

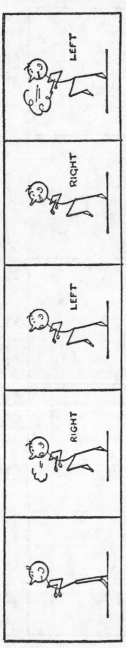

Start. pos.—standing erect, fists clenched

Run in place. (Raise arms and knees vigorously)

XI. THE EXPANDER (Min. 5; Max. 10)

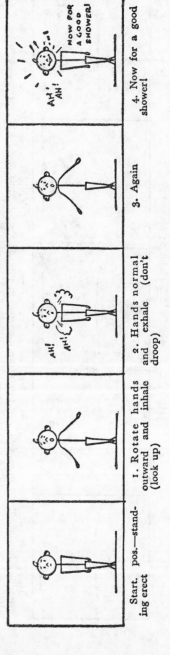

Start. pos.—standing erect

1. Rotate hands outward and inhale (look up)

2. Hands normal and exhale (don't droop)

3. Again

4. Now for a good shower!

CHAPTER XXXIII

YOUR VACATION

WHEN YOUR HEAD starts drooping about three o'clock in the afternoon, when you begin complaining of the heat, and when your work loses much of its usual interest, you are about ready for your vacation. You may think you are doing better to stay home and work. Scientific studies show, however, that a vacation is an asset from the financial point of view, because you do more productive work afterward than you did before.

Vacation cost of an average family in the United States with an income of from $8,000 to $10,000 a year varies from $8.00, spent by a worker who stays at home and goes to the ball game every afternoon, to hundreds of dollars, spent by families that take motor trips. Most people think that the cheapest vacation they can get is to visit their relatives, but even that costs money for entertaining and gifts. Sometimes the cheapest vacation is the best, and the most expensive vacation may be a total loss from the point of view of producing rest and health.

An old-time doctor was asked by a young assistant how to run his office successfully. The doctor gave him two suggestions for routine treatment. "First," he said, "ask your patients what they eat and order something else; second, find out where they are going on their vacations and send them some place else." The old doctor knew from common experience that most people do not pick their vacations properly for health and rest.

Any vacation should bring about a change from the routine of daily life, but rest is most important. In fact, hygienists have asserted that one of the greatest contributions of the biblical code to hygiene was its emphasis on one day of rest in every seven. With the coming of the machine age the pressure has so greatly increased that a four-day week is likely in many industries, which means the regular disposal of three days each week for recreation.

Many organizations have become interested in proper disposal of this time, from the point of view not only of recreation but also of adult education. Executives who work under high pressure with great responsibility are likely to take both winter and summer vacations. If we live twice as fast as we used to, we ought to rest twice as much and twice as often.

GET AWAY FROM YOUR
YEAR-ROUND HABITS

A long and healthy life depends largely on the type of body you inherit from your ancestors and your freedom from infection. It depends also on the speed with which you use up your vitality and the amount of time that you take for recreation. There are many records in medicine of men and women who pushed themselves to the breaking point and who developed nervous breakdowns simply because they refused to rest.

One of the greatest British doctors said that the best test of the necessity for a vacation is to try one. The type of vacation you choose should allow you to forget your usual occupation and habits. Desk workers should preferably spend their vacations in some occupation involving muscular exercise. The manual laborer will probably find his vacation most profitable with suitable amounts of time in rest flat on his back or perhaps in a hammock with a good book. The desk worker who spends his two-weeks' holiday playing bridge in a hotel room or attending theaters in a crowded city is not getting the kind of rest he ought to have.

There is nothing so sad as a vacation that goes sour. The worst vacation is that of the businessman who loads his family into a big car and drives away to some resort. The demands on him during travel and at the resort are greater than any single day in his office. He is forced not only to look after the family and to provide for them, but to amuse them as well. It is unfair to ask the mother of a family, whose full time is spent in looking after the children, to spend her vacation looking after them under conditions far more difficult than those at home.

A vacation always should mean a change from routine. It should be

238

a change not only from routine work but also from the routine of home and of recreation. It should be a change not only of surroundings but also of people. Everybody knows that some people get on one's nerves. That type of person is no help on a vacation.

VACATION FOOD AND DRINK

In picking a place for your vacation always consider questions of health. Pure water, good sanitation, pure milk and a good food supply are absolutely essential.

The motor vacation, which involves stops in numerous camps, demands particular watchfulness. The summer camp for children needs to be studied with these points in mind.

Any exposed drinking water is a possible source of danger. Seaside springs should be distrusted. Health authorities ought to cover them with concrete and arrange to discharge the flowing water into a river or a sewer. Any spring water properly filtered and treated with chlorine may be considered safe. Spring water in camps may be protected by suitable disposal of sewage. Water unfit for drinking is probably equally unfit for bathing, in most instances. It is always wise to take some drinking water with you when you go on a camping trip.

Dishes may be washed in water taken from springs or rivers, provided the water is first thoroughly boiled. Most people who live in cities are so used to drinking water as it comes from the faucet that they forget to watch the water supply when they travel.

Be certain also that the food supplies you buy from wayside vendors are fresh and cleanly handled. Particular precautions must be taken in regard to milk. It is better to drink no milk than to take a chance on milk bought from a farm which does not use pasteurization or does not determine whether the cattle that supply the milk are free from infection. Modern cities demand that cattle be tuberculin tested and free from streptococci infection. These facts are determined by inspectors. When you buy milk from any farmer along the roadside you cannot be sure even of ordinary cleanliness.

It is safer to eat canned vegetables and fruits than to take a chance on vegetables sold at a roadside stand, without proper equipment for cleaning them. Improper handling of vegetables may be responsible for many kinds of illness.

Flies around eating places are a constant menace. Eating places should be guarded from flies by use of mosquito netting or screening.

Some persons traveling on vacations try to get along with a diet of

239

bread, eggs, and coffee. Such diets are tiresome and lack the essentials of a well-balanced diet, which include fresh fruits, vegetables, and plenty of milk. A suitable diet is a great help to a healthful vacation. Many persons who go to American-plan hotels overeat and return from their vacations with digestion completely disordered by the extra strain they have borne during the weeks supposed to be given to rest. Your internal organs need a rest, as well as the muscles and the brain.

A HEALTHFUL VACATION

Chief factors of a healthful vacation can be listed as follows: first, change of occupation; second, sunshine and the open air; third, plenty of rest at night and during the day; fourth, congenial friends and surroundings; fifth, freedom from social routine.

This, for instance, was the type of vacation long taken by Henry Ford, Thomas Edison, Harvey Firestone, and John Burroughs—all noted for hard work, success, and long lives. These representative notables used to travel about in a motorcar, camping at night in the woods or in some convenient place. They were with congenial people who were not included in their usual environment. They had interesting conversation different from that of their daily lives. They spent much time in the sunshine and in the open air. They went to bed early at night and arose when they wished in the morning. They were not governed by any routine on their vacation. They did not have to dress for meals or for the evening but wore the most comfortable and roughest clothing that they had. Their vacations have become proverbial as representing the best type.

Your vacation always should be selected according to your build and your state of health. The real vacation for the average city dweller is one in which he can have comforts suitable to the conditions of his body. For a real rest, a real bed with a real mattress is a help to weary limbs. A hot bath with a rubdown by trained hands helps to soothe the tired muscles.

Instead of attaining these comforts, many a worker who has had fifty weeks of office routine tries mountain climbing or playing thirty-six holes of golf daily, putting terrific stress on his blood vessels and his heart. Thereafter, instead of sleeping in a comfortable bed, he finds a strange bed with a mattress concocted from cotton, straw, or corncobs. Then he wonders why his back and his thighs hurt so much when he gets up the next morning.

Many a vacationist has been heard moaning for his own bed, his own hot bath, coffee cooked the way he likes it, and the morning paper with the news that interests him. Under such circumstances, there is no place like home!

TOURING AND CAMPING

The people who really have to worry most about their vacations are those who take to the road. It is astounding how much wreckage a family vacation in a motorcar can bring about, from a health point of view. Driving all day means that the calls of nature are ignored. Cinders fly in the eye; elbows and knees are bumped and rubbed. The digestion is disturbed and the muscles are cramped by hours of sitting in contorted positions. Children suffer from the glare of the sun, the dust of the road, the impossibility of getting the right kind of food, insect bites, bad meals and water. A baby should never be taken on such a vacation, and even children from two to six years of age are likely to suffer from such performances.

Fortunately, most of our states have taken over control of motor camps, so that you can be reasonably sure in such camps of suitable water and milk supplies. Smart tourists nowadays carry along twenty or thirty yards of mosquito netting to fend off insects. There is little fear of infection from the average mosquitoes in the northern part of the United States, but a mosquito bite that itches or bleeds can spoil any vacation. A weak solution of camphor or a one-per-cent solution of menthol in a suitable lotion will stop the itching and give comfort.

Every camper ought to take along a spade and a first-aid kit. The spade is used to bury remnants of food, empty tin cans, and bottles. These always should be buried twenty-five feet from any running stream or body of water. The spade also is used to cover fires.

The first-aid kit should contain, at least, a bottle of tincture of iodine, a cake of soap, two rolls of gauze, some cotton, and adhesive plaster. It should also carry some of the family's favorite laxative, vaseline or petrolatum, and a simple ointment for abrasions, chafing, and sunburn. Any ordinary zinc-oxide ointment serves this purpose. There should be cold cream for use on dry, chapped lips and perhaps a small amount of some antiseptic solution that is really antiseptic and will not act as a caustic on a burn.

Such a first-aid kit may save a life, and is of great help in securing comfort and relief from pain in emergencies. Manufacturers now make such kits for use of motorists.

241

NERVOUS EXHAUSTION

There seems to be an idea that anyone who suffers from nervous exhaustion or nervous breakdown will be benefited by a sea voyage. Such voyages do have the advantage of taking people away from their usual surroundings. But certain precautions must be taken.

If depression is a prominent symptom the intervals between ports should be short. People who are melancholic become more and more depressed by the sight of nothing but water for several days. People who have been ill and get seasick easily should not take a sea voyage for convalescence. A person who has had a nervous breakdown should never travel alone.

After all, the choice of a vacation is a relatively simple matter if you are reasonable, but it does demand a good deal of foresight. A good vacation is one during which you enjoy yourself thoroughly, in which you are rested when you return, and in which your mind selects a new groove. A good vacation is one without undue exposure to the sun, the rain or the cold, or bad weather generally, particularly if you suffer from coughs or colds, hay fever or asthma.

A good vacation is one in which the persons who surround you are so congenial that you never lose your temper. A good vacation is one in which your health is benefited, as determined by effects on your digestion, your blood pressure, your circulation, and your nervous system. A good vacation is one taken in a place where there is pure water, pure milk, and a good food supply. A good vacation is one in which the muscles are exercised, but not to the point of exhaustion or danger to the tissue beyond repair. A good vacation is one in which you think of your business, but do not worry about it. A man who thinks so little of his business that he can forget it completely while on a vacation is not in the right business.

CHAPTER XXXIV

FIRST AID AND
COMMON COMPLAINTS

Accidents are fourth in the list of causes of death in the United States. Motorcar accidents constitute one-fourth of all that occur. Under such circumstances, people ought to be aware of the immediate steps that need to be taken whenever anyone is involved in an accident, far-removed from any contact with a doctor or a hospital. People who frequently drive the country roads will be well advised to provide their cars with a first-aid kit containing at least some adhesive tape, bandages, cotton, tourniquets, and the other essentials that are helpful in stopping hemorrhage and thus saving a life.

Remember that the immediate services of a competent doctor are better than any amount of first aid by those not specially trained in care of wounds and injuries.

FIRST AID

In attending an injured person:

1. Keep the injured person lying down in a comfortable position, his head level with his body, until you know whether the injury is serious.

2. Look for hemorrhage, stoppage of breathing, poisoning, wounds, burns, fractures, and dislocations. Be sure you locate every injury. Remove enough clothing to determine the extent of the injury. Rip the seams if necessary. Attempts to remove the clothes in the usual manner may cause unnecessary suffering or may aggravate injury. Serious bleeding, stoppage of breathing, and poisoning must be treated immediately before anything else is done.

3. Keep the injured person warm.

4. Send someone to call a physician or an ambulance.

5. Keep calm and do not be hurried into moving an injured person unless absolutely necessary.

6. Never give water or other liquid to an unconscious person.

7. Keep onlookers away from the injured.

8. Make the patient comfortable and keep him cheerful, if possible.

9. Don't let the patient see his own injury.

SHOCK

Any person severely injured may develop shock, and treatment must be started immediately to prevent shock, if possible. This involves:

1. Prevention of hemorrhage by application of pressure.

2. Maintaining body temperature by covering the patient with a blanket but not applying heat.

3. Increasing the flow of blood to vital organs by tilting the body so that the blood tends to flow to the upper portions, raising the foot of the stretcher or bed from twelve to eighteen inches.

4. Except when there is abdominal injury, giving fluids in small amounts and frequently, preferably as hot as can be taken comfortably.

5. Administering artificial respiration as described later, if necessary, to restore breathing.

DRESSINGS AND BANDAGES

Do not use absorbent cotton directly over a wound or burn because it sticks and is hard to remove. Do not use adhesive tape, electrician's tape, collodion, or similar materials directly on a wound. Apply sterilized gauze squares or bandage compresses to wounds. Bandages are not applied directly over wounds, which should always be covered first with a dressing.

WOUNDS AND THEIR CARE

Do not touch any wound with the hand, mouth, clothing, or any unclean material. Apply a sterile dressing or compress and bandage snugly in place. When bleeding is present, apply a dressing as soon as available; press firmly. Make sure that bleeding is stopped before moving the patient. Tourniquets are dangerous, and should not be used if bleeding can be checked readily otherwise. Whenever there is serious bleeding get a physician as soon as possible to take responsibility for care of the patient.

PUNCTURING WOUNDS

Always secure a physician, who will not only treat the wound itself but may give tetanus antitoxin for prevention of lockjaw.

POWDER BURNS

Explosion of gunpowder usually carries burned powder and dirt into the skin. Make sure that the patient is seen by a physician. The value of tetanus antitoxin in such cases cannot be overemphasized.

INFECTED WOUNDS

Apply wet dressings, consisting of three heaping tablespoonfuls of ordinary salt, or twice this amount of Epsom salts, in each quart of water. Change wet dressing often enough to keep hot, and apply continuously for an hour. Repeat every three to four hours until the patient is turned over to a physician.

WOUNDS OF ABDOMEN

Keep the patient lying quietly on his back. Keep him warm. Give him nothing by mouth, neither water nor stimulants. Cover the wound with a sterile dressing and a binder. Move patients with wounds of the abdomen carefully. When intestines protrude from wound, keep patient on back with a coat or pillow under the knees. Don't try to push the intestine back in. Cover with a sterile dressing and keep moist.

ANIMAL BITES

Wash the wound thoroughly to remove saliva. Use a gauze compress and a thick solution of soap and water to scrub the wound. Rinse it

245

with clean running water and apply a sterile dressing. Consult a physician at once. Do not kill the biting animal except to protect others from danger. Have biting animals examined by competent veterinarians to determine whether or not they have rabies.

SNAKE BITES

Make the victim lie down and keep quiet. Tie a constricting band firmly around the limb just above the bite, to restrict the spread of the poison. Sterilize a sharp knife or razor blade with a match flame, iodine, or alcohol. Make a crosscut incision about one-quarter-inch long through each fang mark. Apply suction with a suction cup or syringe; apply suction by mouth if a mechanical device is not available. Call a doctor as promptly as possible. Antivenin serum should be given by someone experienced, if it is available.

FOREIGN BODIES IN WOUNDS

If a foreign body like a splinter, a piece of glass or metal is near the surface, apply an antiseptic to the skin. Sterilize a knife, needle, or tweezers by passing through a flame; use this to remove foreign body. Encourage a little bleeding by gentle pressure on the wound. After bleeding has stopped apply a sterile compress.

FOREIGN BODY IN THE EYE

Never rub the eye. Never touch it until you have washed your hands thoroughly. Never be rough with the eye. Never try to remove a foreign body from the eye with a toothpick, match, knife blade, or any instrument. Pull down the lower eyelid and see if the foreign substance is on the surface of the lower lid. If visible, it can be removed by touching it with a corner of a clean handkerchief. Grasp the eyelashes of the upper lid gently between the thumb and forefinger. Have the patient look upward, and pull the upper eyelid upward and downward over the lower eyelid. This may dislodge a foreign body, so that it will be washed away by the tears. Wash the eye with a solution of boric acid (a half teaspoonful to a drinking glass of boiled water). If foreign bodies are still present, make sure that the patient has attention from a physician.

NOSEBLEED

Have patient sit up with head thrown slightly back, breathing through mouth. Apply cold wet compresses over the nose. Tell person with nosebleed not to blow nose for a few hours. Press the nostril on the bleeding side firmly against the middle portion for four or five minutes. If these measures do not stop the bleeding in a few minutes, call a physician. Try putting sterile gauze pack back in the nostril, leaving the end out so it can be easily removed.

INTERNAL BLEEDING

Keep the patient lying on his back as flat as possible. Turn the head to one side for vomiting or coughing. Keep the patient warm. Get a physician at the earliest possible moment.

ARTIFICIAL RESPIRATION

The foremost method recommended today by leading authorities, including the American Red Cross, is mouth-to-mouth resuscitation. Following are the steps in the mouth-to-mouth technique:

1. Place the person on his back and check whether there is any foreign matter in the mouth. If there is, turn his head to one side and clear the mouth with your fingers or a piece of cloth.

2. Tilt the head back so that the chin is pointing upwards. Kneel close beside the head to do this.

3. Using the thumb of one hand, open the person's mouth and grasp the lower jaw (quickly wrap your thumb first, for protection). Lift the jaw upward and forward, so that it "juts out."

4. Close the person's nose with your other hand. Take a deep breath, place your mouth firmly over his, and blow hard. Watch his chest, and when it rises, take your mouth off his and let him breathe out. Then repeat your blowing and letting him exhale, giving between 12 and 20 breaths a minute.

Note: If the mouth-to-mouth technique is used on a baby or very small child, what might be called the mouth-to-mouth-and-nose technique is used. Follow Steps 1 through 3. Then place your mouth over the child's mouth *and* nose, making a relatively leakproof seal, and blow in. Blow fairly gently with small children, and use only puffs from the cheeks for a baby. Give up to 20 breaths a minute. Follow the cycle of blowing and exhaling as described in Step 4.

247

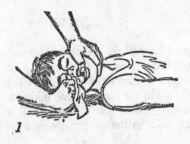
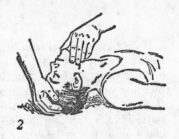

Figure 1: Place the person on his back and, if necessary, turn his head to one side to clear the mouth of foreign matter (Step 1). Figure 2: Tilt the head so that the chin is pointing upward (Step 2).

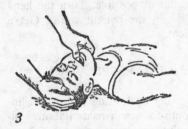
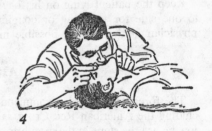

Figure 3: Open the person's mouth with your thumb, grasp the lower jaw, and lift it upward and forward (Step 3). Figure 4: Close the person's nose with your other hand. After taking a deep breath, place your mouth firmly over his and blow forcefully (Step 4).

DROWNING

Remove the victim from the water and place him in a prone position with his head lower than the rest of his body. Make a quick inspection of his mouth and remove any sand, muck, or weeds. Pull the lower jaw forward. This brings the tongue forward and helps to keep it from plugging the upper air passages. Start artificial respiration. The preliminary steps should not take more than ten seconds.

Don't attempt to remove water from the lungs. There is usually a little in them, but that is readily expelled by the action of artificial respiration. Rolling a person to get the water out is a waste of precious time.

Remember, the conservation of body heat is important. A person rescued from the water under normal conditions loses body heat rapidly. Even on a hot day water evaporation from wet clothing has the effect of cooling the body at a dangerous rate.

HANGING

Cut the rope holding the person suspended. Loosen it immediately from around the neck. Start artificial respiration at once.

POISONS

Give immediately four to seven glassfuls of soap suds, salt water, soda water, lukewarm water or milk. After the patient has had several glassfuls, tickle the back of the throat to induce vomiting. This washes out the stomach.

For acid poison, neutralize with alkalis like magnesium, chalk, baking soda, or lime water. Keep the patient warm.

For alkaline poison, neutralize with weak acids such as lemon juice or vinegar, and keep the patient warm.

For poisoning by opium, morphine, barbituric acid derivatives, or sleeping tablets, keep the patient awake, give strong coffee—a cup every half hour or so. Call a physician.

FRACTURES

Avoid handling the injured part. Control shock by methods already mentioned. Learn about fractures in the *American Red Cross First Aid Textbook* and never attempt to apply splints or traction without first having had full instructions in the technic.

BURNS

Shock and infection are the chief dangers from burns. For small burns apply sterile petrolatum ointment or burn ointment over the burned area. Cover with fine-mesh gauze. For extensive burns keep the patient lying down with the head down and avoid exposure or cold. Remove all loose clothing from the burned area, but not if it sticks to the burned area, cut around it, and leave the clothing that has stuck to the wound for the doctor to remove. Dip strips of clean, freshly laundered sheeting into a solution made of warm water, one quart containing three tablespoonfuls of baking soda, and apply to burned area. Do not use absorbent cotton directly on a burn. Immersing the burned area in cold water stops pain.

SERIOUS SUNBURNS

Calamine lotion is soothing and does not stain clothing. Wet dressings of baking soda or Epsom salts prevent pain. For severe blisters apply a dressing of sterile, petrolatum-coated gauze.

SUNSTROKE

Get the victim into the shade and into as cool a place as possible. Remove the clothing. Lay the patient on his back, with the head and shoulders somewhat elevated. Start treatment immediately. Apply cold to the head—wet cloths, ice bag, ice. The brain withstands heat least. Cool the body by one of these methods:

1. Wrap the patient's body in a sheet and pour on cold water. This method is probably best. Don't cool the body too much at a time. Continue treatment for several minutes, then stop and observe the patient. If the skin becomes hot again, the treatment must be renewed. Rubbing the limbs toward the heart aids the circulation, and it is important. Rub through the wet sheet. Give no stimulants. Call a doctor at once. Give cool drinks after consciousness returns.

2. Give a cool bath, up to twenty minutes long, with brisk rubbing of the limbs and trunk to stimulate circulation. One of the most effective ways of cooling the body is an ice-water tub bath.

3. Apply cold, wet cloths or ice bags, with rubbing.

If the patient is taken to a hospital in an ambulance, treatment should be continued during transportation.

FROSTBITE

1. Put the frozen person in a warm room. Give a warm drink, preferably coffee.

2. The frozen limb should be gently massaged, starting at its junc-

tion with the trunk and moving toward the tip; rub with a coarse, dry towel, taking care not to injure the skin.

3. When a joint is passed, subject it to slight passive movement without force, followed by active motions.

4. Frost blisters should not be disturbed.

COMMON EMERGENCIES

Brain Hemorrhage

Lay the patient on his back with the head and shoulders slightly raised. Apply cold cloths or ice bag to the head. Insist on absolute quiet. Use great care in moving the patient. Do not use stimulants.

Drunkenness

Patient will usually sleep off the condition in a few hours. If the patient can be aroused, make him vomit and then give coffee. Apply artificial respiration if patient stops breathing.

Fainting

If a person feels faint make him lie down with his body level. Keep him lying down, and lower his head. If he is in a chair tilt the chair backward. If it is impossible to lower his head, elevate his legs. Loosen tight clothing. Smelling salts inhaled may be helpful, but do not use ammonia. Sprinkle the face with cold water. After consciousness returns, give stimulant by mouth.

Heart Failure

Keep the patient absolutely quiet, lying down. Never give stimulants or drugs, unless prescribed by the doctor. Keep the patient warm and quiet. Reassurance will prevent fear.

Convulsions

Prevent the patient from injuring himself. Place a pencil wrapped in cloth or a folded cloth or other suitable material between the teeth to prevent the tongue from being bitten. Put a pillow, coat, or any other soft material under the head. Do not try to hold the patient rigid to prevent convulsive movements. Do not give stimulants. Convulsions are usually followed by sleep or quiet unconsciousness. Do not disturb the patient.

251

Convulsions in Children

Loosen constricting clothing. If the convulsions do not stop promptly, apply hot packs, wrapping the child in a blanket or in large heavy towels wrung out of warm water, not hot water. Following the pack, put the child to bed between warm blankets.

Earaches

Any earache that persists for even a short time demands the attention of a doctor. Apply a hot water bottle to the painful ear. Cold may give relief in cases not relieved by heat. Early puncture of the eardrum when there is internal pressure is important in preventing secondary infection in the mastoid.

Hiccups

Try holding the breath as long as possible, or drink a glass of cold water slowly. Breathe in and out of a paper bag that fits tightly over the face.

Foreign Bodies in Ear or Nose

Never push any pin or piece of wire or instrument into the ear or nose. Try syringing the ear with warm water. Leave removal of foreign bodies in the ear or nose to the doctor.

Insect Bites

Remove the sting if it is still present. Apply a paste made of baking soda and cold cream or a compress moistened with ammonia water. Cold applications help relieve pain. Calamine lotion with 1 per cent menthol relieves itching of mosquito and chigger bites.

HALITOSIS, OR BAD BREATH

Bad breath, now politely referred to as "halitosis," is offensive. There is little excuse for permitting oneself to become obnoxious for this reason to everyone around him, since it is possible to prevent the presence of such odors. The most frequent cause is related to the teeth, which may be subject to cavities or which may simply be surrounded with accumulations of decaying food particles. Cavities should be filled and tartar deposits should be removed at least once every six months. The teeth may be kept clean by the use of dental floss and by the regular use, after eating, of a toothbrush with proper powder or paste. A high-fat diet may be related to halitosis.

There are innumerable mouthwashes containing antiseptics, alkalis, or acids, that may be used after the teeth have been brushed. Weak hydrogen peroxide solutions are sometimes of value. Use strong solutions only on the advice of a competent physician or dentist.

After the teeth have been eliminated as the cause of bad breath, the tonsils must be examined for infection. Another frequent cause of bad breath is infection in the nose or in the space behind the nose. The formation of crusts and of accumulations of infected material is bound to produce foul odor of the breath. Halitosis may also result from chronic disturbances of the stomach and of the intestines. If the tongue is constantly coated, if there is eruction of sour material from the stomach, consult a physician.

SEASICKNESS

Recent discoveries in the control of seasickness mean that almost anyone may now take a voyage on an ocean or a lake and, even when the boat rocks, still not be too sick to enjoy the voyage. Many a person used to get sick even before the ship left the dock.

Experience has shown that people who get on a ship or a boat in good health are less likely to have trouble than others. Avoid heavy meals, going-away dinners, and indigestible food. If you start out free from difficulty with your digestion and with a stomach that is reasonably empty, you are less likely to be sick.

When confronted with sickness lie down; do not try to make everybody believe that you are feeling wonderful, because, actually, you will look green and everybody will wonder why you are up anyway. People who lie down are much less affected by rocking of the boat or rolling of the ship.

Good air is important, and that means plenty of air. However, do not get chilled. Put on a warm coat, cover yourself with a rug, lie back, inhale good air, and be comfortable. Now and then a short, brisk walk will be helpful. Do not, however, spend your time watching the waves, because this tends to produce eructation or vomiting.

The stewards know that a little weak tea or a warm drink and a dry biscuit helps to settle a queasy stomach. Usually, on board the larger vessels tea is served each morning around eleven, each afternoon around three, in addition to the usual meals.

The older seasickness remedies depended on hyoscine and scopolamine, which have for many years been known to be helpful. Most recent are such preventive drugs as Dramamine and Merazine and Bonamine. Successful use in thousands of cases on all sorts of ocean voyages has proved that the vast majority of people, with a good routine of life aboard ship and helped by these remedies, can take a sea voyage without the slightest trouble.

NEURALGIA AND SCIATICA

Neuralgia is probably just another word for pain. Pain is something that you feel. You may have pain because of pressure on a nerve. On the other hand, pains may come from emotional exhaustion or similar disturbances. Experts in nerve surgery say that neuralgia occurs only when there are intermittent pains passing along the nerves of the brain or the spine without any loss of function or evidence of damage to the nerves. As new studies are made the number of neuralgias is constantly diminished, since specific causes are found —such as the slipping of disks between the bones of the spine or pressure on other large nerves where they cross bones. Neuralgia is a symptom and not a disease. Whenever it occurs the most careful investigation needs to be made as to what may be behind the condition.

TRIGEMINAL NEURALGIA

Dr. Winchell McK. Craig says that there are three major neuralgias. The first is the pain in the face called trigeminal neuralgia; second, the pain in the ear and throat which is known as glossopharyngeal neuralgia because of the nerves involved; and third, the pain over the lower portion of the back of the neck known as occipital neuralgia because it is at the occiput or back of the skull. Other neuralgias are related to nerves elsewhere in the body, such as pains in the arm, called brachial neuralgia, pains in the side of the chest, called intercostal neuralgia, and, of course, also sciatic neuralgia. Among the most serious is trigeminal neuralgia, or neuralgia of the facial nerve, which was given the French name of *tic douloureux*. In this condition there is severe paroxysmal pain in the various portions of the face to which the nerve from the brain reaches. The pain is sharp and usually lasts less than a minute. The pain can be caused by pressure on the angle of the mouth, the cheek, or a tooth, by eating, drinking, washing, shaving, or even by blowing on the face. Physicians have found that the injection of alcohol into the nerve will stop the pain, and a surgical operation has been developed for cutting the nerve away from the ganglion cell. This operation, which is done by specialists called neurologic surgeons, has now been proved to be successful in many instances. Physicians now have available excellent analgesic drugs to relieve pain. Aspirin may be purchased without a doctor's prescription. Others more potent must be prescribed by the doctor.

GLOSSOPHARYNGEAL NEURALGIA

Glossopharyngeal neuralgia is the result of stimuli to nerves coming off what is known as the ninth cranial nerve, which goes to the area around the tonsils, back of the tongue, the pharynx, the ear, and the eardrum. This neuralgia is like facial-nerve neuralgia, except that it affects the throat, the back of the tongue, and the ear. The pain often spreads to the back of the jaw. Patients may not actually complain of pain in the ear but during an attack will point toward the point where they are feeling the pain. The exact cause of this neuralgia is not known, but obviously is some irritant factor reaching the nerve.

OCCIPITAL NEURALGIA

Pain at the back of the neck, called occipital neuralgia, brings on severe tenderness, and the skin may be so sensitive to touch that it is impossible even to brush the hair. Since there are other causes of pain in this portion of the body, the doctor has to make a most careful investigation to determine that it is the involvement of two nerves coming from the spine to this area that is responsible.

Obviously, any inflammation, new growth, poisoning, or other irritant factor that can reach a nerve can cause severe pain that persists and that demands medical attention. Pain involving the shoulder and arm may occur from arthritis, from inflammation of a bursa, from a job involving constant arm use, such as telegraphy. Whenever the pain is diffuse and involves the muscles and joints it is unlikely to be neuralgia, and more likely to be some of the other conditions that have been mentioned.

SCIATIC NEURALGIA

Sciatic neuralgia is any pain that follows the distribution of the sciatic nerve. The pain is made worse by coughing, sneezing, and straining

THE HANDY HOME MEDICAL ADVISER

or by bending forward. The examination may be unable to reveal any specific changes in the tissues.

The doctor, however, traces the course of the nerve and the areas into which the roots of the nerve travel, and is thus able to define the painful areas as those definitely associated with the nerves. If any specific cause can be found, such as pressure on the nerve at any point or a disk that has slipped in the lower part of the spine, operative procedures will eliminate the cause and control the condition.

PART TWO

CONCISE
MEDICAL ENCYCLOPEDIA

HERE, IN SIMPLE LANGUAGE, are considerations of the most important symptoms and diseases that affect human beings; also hints as to prevention and treatment. This is a section for reference, not intended to substitute in any way for care by a doctor. Dosages and methods of use of drugs are not given. Self-diagnosis is dangerous and any treatment that is effective when used properly may do harm if used incorrectly. The best advice for anyone who is ill is to consult the doctor as soon as possible.

A

ABDOMINAL PAIN A colic or griping pain in the abdomen. It may come from overeating or from foods that are irritating or from sensitivity to foods. Occasionally a pain in the abdomen is reflected from elsewhere in the body, as from the lungs. Pain may also be associated with excess acid in the stomach and with ulcers or with tumors. A pain on the right side of the abdomen in the lower third is most often due to appendicitis but may be associated with a blocking of the tube from the kidney to the bladder. Swelling of the gall bladder or a blocking of its tubes by stones produces severe pain. A sudden blocking of the bowel either by something inside the bowel or by the drawing of one part of the bowel into another can cause excruciating and agonizing pain. Excessive gas or air in the bowel brings a feeling of fullness which may be painful. Occasionally inflammation of the spine is a cause of pain. Most common is ordinary stomach-ache—"belly-ache."

Do not try to get rid of pain by taking large doses of cathartics or laxatives. This is dangerous and may cause a pus-filled appendix to break and thus produce peritonitis. Get a doctor and find the cause of the abdominal pain as soon as possible. (*See also* ADHESIONS; AMEBIASIS; APPENDICITIS; CHOLECYSTITIS; COLIC; GALLSTONES; GASTRITIS; HER-NIAS; INDIGESTION; PANCREAS; *and also* CHAPTERS II, VII, XVIII, XXIV.)

ABORTION Premature expulsion of the human foetus. Abortions occur most frequently in the eighth to the twelfth week of pregnancy. Any cause that brings about death of the unborn child results in an emptying of the womb or uterus. Chief signs of a threatened spontaneous miscarriage or abortion are pain in the womb, bleeding, and expulsion of all or parts of the unborn child. Severe pain and bleeding of a pregnant woman is a threatening sign. She should go to bed at once and secure immediate attention of a doctor.

ABRASION Any spot from which the skin, mucous membrane or the upper layer has been removed by rubbing or scraping. If someone has rubbed the surface of the eye, for example, and removed tissue it is a corneal abrasion, since the cornea is the outer membrane covering the eye. The tissue that has been damaged is usually covered by a flow of serum or of blood. If it is the skin that is concerned, the best treatment is thoroughly to wash the abrasion with soap and water and then to cover it with a sterile protective bandage. An abrasion of the eye or of one of the mucous surfaces may demand medical attention.

ABSCESS A collection of pus or of infected material anywhere in the body. Empyema is the name of an abscess in the chest cavity. The germs which form pus are chiefly the staphylococci and the streptococci, but other germs may also produce infected material like pus or may become contaminated with the pus-forming germs. If the wall of an abscess, formed by the defensive material of the body, breaks down, the abscess bursts. Thus a boil may come to a head and burst. The safest method is to have a surgeon open the boil, in order to keep the pus under control and thus prevent spread of the infection to the adjacent tissues or to other parts of the body.

ABSTINENCE Whenever one voluntarily gives up food, alcohol, sex relations, or other appetites, he is practicing abstinence.

ACARIASIS Infestation of the body with acaries or mites. (*See also* CHAPTER XXIX.)

ACCIDENT An unfortunate or unexpected occurrence of an injurious nature which may complicate any condition. Thus the term a cerebral accident is commonly used to describe a brain hemorrhage or apoplexy. Accidents resulting from falls, motorcars, or from contact with foreign substances constitute a major cause of illness or death and have sometimes risen as high as fourth or fifth place in the causes of death in adults and first in causes of death in children. (*See also* CHAPTER XXXIV.)

ACCOMMODATION When one looks at a near object or a far object, the eye adjusts itself to accommodate for the difference in distance. Both eyes must be able to accommodate to have binocular vi-

sion. When the eye accommodates, the muscles contract, adjusting the size of the lens and the curvature of the surface of the lens.

ACETIC ACID The chemical substance of vinegar is a characteristic form. Other forms of acetic acid are caustic and are used to destroy warts, corns or other horny tissue growths.

ACHE A constant or fixed pain, usually modified by the portion of the body, such as *head*ache, *stomach*-ache, or *ear*ache. (*See also* CHAPTER II.)

ACHLORHYDRIA The inability of the wall of the stomach to produce hydrochloric acid, which is a constituent of the gastric juice. The absence of acid in the gastric juice is rare, but does occur in about 10 per cent of people, and cases of decreased acid are more frequent. The condition is often associated with anemia. Doctors can prescribe acid to take the place of that which is not secreted by the stomach. (*See also* ANEMIA, PERNICIOUS.)

ACHONDROPLASIA A deformity of growth which results in dwarfism. The difficulty is in the growth of the bones. It begins before the child is born, when the ends of the bones unite and become ossified too soon. The mental condition of such dwarfs is usually normal and they are often used as comedians with acrobatic or musical troupes. (*See also* GLANDS; *and also* CHAPTER XVII.)

ACHYLIA The complete absence of gastric juice. This is exceedingly rare; achlorhydria, previously described, is more common. The term may also refer to absence of the pancreatic juice, which results in intestinal indigestion and the appearance of much fat in the feces. (*See also* PANCREAS.)

ACIDOSIS A tendency to produce excess acid or to diminish the alkali of the blood is present in certain diseases. Loss of fluid from vomiting or diarrhea results in acidosis. The obvious symptoms are headache, weakness, rapid breathing, and a fruity odor of the breath. Frequently soda or sodium bicarbonate is used to overcome acidosis. The treatment is to replace loss of fluid and to hinder production of acid by giving water, salt and glucose. This can be taken by mouth or injected directly into the blood. Diabetes is the chief disease accompanied by acidosis. The condition also develops in some diseases of the kidney. Excessive secretion of acid by the stomach may be related to work, worry or mental processes affecting the stomach. There are few foods that have an acid tendency, although people fear tomatoes or meat. Estimates indicate that one would have to eat four and a half pounds of lean beef in a single meal to produce even a slight shift toward the acid side. Citrus fruits have been recommended to overcome acidosis but tremendous quantities would be required for that effect, whereas bicarbonate of soda is much more effective. (*See also* DIABETES.)

ACNE A condition of the skin of which blackheads and pimples are the significant signs. It occurs most often in boys and girls between ages 12 and 25. Specialists in conditions affecting the skin relate the acne to the constitutional structure of the person, causing his skin to secrete much oil, also to secondary infections by germs, the eating of large amounts of sugars, and occasional disturbances of the secretions of the glands, especially the sex glands. Sometimes the taking of certain drugs produces an acne, as is particularly the case with iodine. Various kinds of acne are defined, the most common being *acne vulgaris,* which merely means the common kind of acne.

Successful treatment depends on determining definitely the nature of the condition and on encouraging the function of the skin, through perspiration, and stretching aided often by some light or ultraviolet rays. The spots of infection at the blackheads may be removed, and the doctor prescribe ointments, pastes or lotions which will cause mild peeling of the skin. The sugars in the diet are restricted, and if special hormones are needed they also are prescribed by the doctor. Since outbursts of acne follow mental excitement, it is well to practice good psychotherapy in such cases. (*See also* CHAPTER XXIII.)

ACQUIRED Conditions may be either congenital, meaning present at birth, or acquired, as those resulting from infection.

ACRODYNIA A condition affecting the soles and palms, with rheumatoid pains and a brilliant red eruption. The technical name is *erythredema polyneuropathy,* which means simply a red and swelling condition with multiple disturbances of the nerves. The condition has been associated with a deficiency of some vitamins, particularly A and B, and occurs chiefly in children. (*See also* VITAMINS; *and also* CHAPTER XV.)

ACROMEGALY Giantism, resulting usually from excessive functioning of the cells of the pituitary gland. The condition is marked by enlargement of the hands, feet, jaws, lips, nose and tongue. Usually the great size of the person is associated with a tremendous appetite. Giants seldom reach a height greater than 7 feet, although a few cases are known of giants 8 feet tall (*See also* GLANDS; *and also* CHAPTER XVI.)

ACROPHOBIA The fear of being at great height.

ACTH The adrenocorticotropic hormone—a substance from the pituitary gland that stimulates production of Cortisone by the adrenal gland.

ACTINOMYCOSIS A parasitic, infectious disease caused by a fungus called actinomyces which infects people and also cattle. It grows like a star, which gives it its name. This condition in cattle is called lumpy jaw. People sometimes get it from chewing grass, straw or grain infected with the organism.

ACUPUNCTURE For three thousand years the Chinese and people in some other Asian countries have treated a variety of disorders, some of unknown cause like essential hypertension, some of glandular basis, also chronic disorders like diabetes and rheumatism, also peptic ulcer, asthma, and some skin diseases, with a system called acupuncture. The method is also used for temporary anesthesia. The method has been tested and not proved of any value in cancer. Scientifically the neurologists have known for years of a condition called referred pains which are painful areas related to difficulties elsewhere in the body. The neurologists have found areas of the brain associated with other areas in the body, such as the skin. The glands of internal secretion, such as the thyroid, adrenal glands, and sex glands, are influenced by hormones coming from the pituitary which, in turn, has nerve tracts traced to the area of the brain called the hypothalamus. This means that the body's resistance is stimulated by impulses which reach the central nervous system and are then transmitted to such structures as the glands and the autonomic nervous system.

The ability of acupuncture to produce anesthesia in some instances is not understood. Several explanations have been offered but have not been accepted as scientific. The theory has been offered that the response to acupuncture is a form of enhancement of the power of suggestion as occurs in hypnotism and in direct psychic suggestion.

In acupuncture, as seen in China, needles are inserted at specific areas in the body according to a chart used in teaching the method. Sometimes the needles are rotated, sometimes a mild electronic stimulation is applied. For anesthesia, occasionally a sedative drug is given before the acupuncture is used.

Because of opening of relations

with the Chinese government, medical attention has been focused on acupuncture. Much experimentation may result in learning more about how it works, if it really does.

ADDICTION, DRUG Legally, addiction is defined as a state of periodic or chronic intoxication detrimental to the individual and to society, produced by the repeated consumption of a drug. Stimulants include such drugs as cocaine, amphetamine, benzedrine and mescoline. Depressants include all of the opium, morphine, heroin, codeine and similar substances; also chloral, bromides, barbituric derivatives, marihuana and alcohol. The essential step in curing an addiction is to withdraw contact with the drug. (*See also* ALCOHOLISM; *and also* CHAPTER XVIII.)

ADDISON'S DISEASE Insufficient action of the adrenal glands (also called suprarenal glands) which lie above the kidney. The symptoms include progressive loss of salt and of water, shock, loss of weight, vomiting, muscle weakness (which is the most important symptom) and bronzing of the skin. Addison's disease is treated by the administration of these hormones. (*See also* GLANDS; *and also* CHAPTER XVI.)

ADENOIDS Lymphoid tissue in the back of the nose that picks up infectious germs, and helps the body get rid of them. When overgrown or infected, the adenoids interfere with breathing and should be removed. The doctor can feel the adenoids with his finger or see them, using a mirror which he passes into the throat. Large or infected adenoids

may produce frequent earache. People often ask whether or not the adenoids can be treated by drugs or X-ray or radium. In some cases this is attempted. The operation for adenoids is not serious or difficult, and usually yields a perfect result. (*See also* LYMPH; *and also* CHAPTER XXVI.)

ADENOMA A tumor which is made up of glandular material.

ADHESIONS Fibrous scars formed when tissues heal, causing adjacent organs to stick to each other. Adhesions in the abdomen may result in pain, upon pulling or stretching, because fibrous tissue is not elastic. Surgeons do an operation called adhesiotomy, which is simply the surgical cutting or division of adhesions.

ADIPOSIS This is another word for obesity or corpulence. It represents an excessive accumulation of fat in the body. (*See also* WEIGHT, OVER-; *and also* CHAPTER XIV.)

ADJUSTMENT Manipulation of the body is called adjustment. This manipulation forms the basis of osteopathic and chiropractic treatment.

ADOLESCENCE That period of youth which extends from puberty to maturity—roughly from the ages of 12 to 21—is adolescence. Important changes take place in the body and the mind. These distinguish the adult from the child. During adolescence growth is more rapid than at any time except during the first two years of life. During adolescence the male assumes the typical form and grows a beard. The female develops hips, breasts and other characteristics. During this period, children need advice as to the problems that confront them. The first appearance of interest in sex, the changes in the voice, and the mental attitudes that develop are important, because they may mark the entire life of the person concerned.

AEROPHOBIA A morbid fear of drafts of air; also a morbid fear of being high up in the air.

AFTERBIRTH The material that comes from the womb of the woman following the birth of a child. It includes the placenta and the membrane. The placenta forms the connection between the child and the mother which provides food and oxygen for growth during the period of pregnancy.

AFTEREFFECTS The symptoms or conditions which appear following a disease, and which may remain permanently. For example, the loss of hearing following an infection of the ear.

AGUE A name formerly given to malaria; used also to describe chills. The shakes or fits.

AIR CONDITIONING Air is the most necessary of all substances for sustaining life. One can live forty days without food, about four days without water, about four minutes without air. Air contains oxygen and nitrogen, and in our large cities is frequently mingled with gases, smoke, dust, pollens, germs and other extraneous substances. All air contains some moisture unless specifically dried. The humidity reflects the moisture in the air. The best temperature for a room is from 65 to 68 degrees, with sufficient moisture to produce a humidity of from 30 to 60 per cent. Few diseases are due to bad ventilation, but the other ingredients—such as dust, germs and pollens—may produce a variety of illnesses. With ordinary temperatures, the average home can easily be ventilated by opening the windows occasionally. Mechanical systems of air conditioning are valuable in crowded places, as factories, theaters and halls. The air conditioning provides a high degree of comfort. However, sudden changes in temperature from cold to warm or warm to cold put stress on the automatic mechanisms of the human body. One of the big advantages of air conditioning is that it removes pollens and dusts. Old people usually require a higher temperature for comfort than do young people.

AIRSICKNESS Airsickness is usually the result of high altitude accompanied by the effects of motion. This means nausea and vomiting, as the result of deficient oxygen and of pressure. It is seldom noticed below 10,000 feet. Air travel is usually forbidden to people who are anemic, psychotic, asthmatic or tuberculous; also to those with infections of the nose and throat, heart disease or injuries to the chest. Pregnant women preferably should not fly during the last month of the pregnancy or during the first two weeks after the child is born. Seriously ill patients should invariably be flown in pressurized cabins. The drugs called

Dramamine and Bonamine are the most recent developments for controlling airsickness. Hyoscine hydrobromide is an old standard remedy. During ascent and descent the effect of pressure, particularly in the ears, is decreased by chewing gum, swallowing, yawning, or drinking. Carbonated beverages taken during or just before a trip lead to air in the bowel, with a tendency to belch and to pass gas. (*See also* SEASICKNESS.)

ALBINO A person born without pigment in the skin. The condition is called albinism. This is distinguished from the condition called vitiligo, which merely refers to small patches of skin without pigmentation. Albinos are found all over the world. Scientists believe that a hormone from the pituitary gland known as the melano-stimulating hormone or MSH is the substance that controls pigmentation; obviously a deficiency there might be the basis of albinism.

ALBUMINURIA The appearance of albumin in the urine. Frequently this is a sign of damage to the kidney, but may be associated with albumin derived from other portions of the urinary tract. The symptom is easily detected by heating urine or by adding a strong acid to it, in which case a flocculent precipitate forms. (*See also* KIDNEYS; *and also* CHAPTER VIII.)

ALCOHOLISM Addiction to alcohol. Alcohol is used for destroying germs or for bathing the skin to reduce temperature, but chiefly as a fluid for dissolving drugs and as a beverage. Alcoholic drinks include beer, ale, wine, and liquors of the type of whiskey, gin and rum. Alcohol taken in excess produces serious damage to the human body. The symptoms are loss of command of judgment, loss of control over ordinary inhibitions, and frequently mental confusion. If used properly, alcohol may yield pleasure. The majority of people are not drunkards. Addiction to alcohol may occur as described under addiction. The taking of alcohol produces dilation of the blood vessels of the skin, with warmth and redness of the face. Serious addiction to alcohol is best treated in a hospital or sanitarium under the care of an expert. Arrangements may be made with such groups as the National Committee on Alcoholism or Alcoholics Anonymous for assistance and for the recommendation of suitable institutions. A new drug called Antabuse is valuable in creating a dislike for alcohol but cannot, of course, be taken permanently. (*See also* ADDICTION, DRUG; *and also* CHAPTER XVIII.)

ALEXIA Inability to read because of word blindness. Also includes inability to read aloud, even though the person understands what he reads. Musical alexia is the inability to read music.

ALIMENTATION The act of giving or receiving nutritional material into the body.

ALKALOSIS An amount of alkali or basic substances in the blood beyond what is normal. This is the opposite of acidosis. The condition is

265

occasionally seen in persons with ulcer who have taken too much sodium bicarbonate.

ALLERGY A reaction in which the cells or tissues of the body develop defenses against particular substances to which it is sensitive, accompanied by the pouring out of a substance called histamine; also known as hypersensitiveness, sensitivity, idiosyncrasy, atopy, and anaphylaxis. The condition gives rise to many symptoms beside the usual difficulties of breathing, running nose, pouring of tears from the eyes, or eruptions on the skin commonly recognized as allergic.

Emotional states may predispose or precipitate an allergic condition. These include tensions, conflicts, anxieties, and emotional stresses. The substances ("allergens") most frequently producing allergy include pollens, plants, germs, animal tissues, cosmetics, drugs, serums, dyes, chemical substances, and physical forces like heat, cold, and sunlight.

The first step in treatment is to detect the offending substance and eliminate contact with it. (Specialists frequently detect the offending substance by the use of a patch test, which consists of placing some of the material on a patch of adhesive and sticking it to the patient's skin to see whether there will be a reaction.) It is also possible to desensitize a person to an allergen by injecting increasing doses of the offending substance. Drugs called antihistamines are also now used to prevent the histamine reaction. (*See also* ASTHMA; HAY FEVER; HIVES; *and also* CHAPTER XII.)

ALOES A cathartic substance derived from a plant of the same name.

ALOPECIA (*See* BALDNESS, *under* HAIR.)

AMAUROSIS Blindness that results from a disease of the optic nerve, the retina or that portion of the nervous tissue of the spinal cord and brain associated with vision.

AMBLYOPIA Dimness or loss of vision especially due to toxic causes rather than to errors of refraction or organic changes.

AMEBIASIS An infection caused by *Endamoeba histolytica*. About 30,000,000 Americans are said to carry this organism in their bowels. Most have no symptoms; others apparently more sensitive to the infestation develop fatigue, fail to gain weight, have difficulty in sleeping, may occasionally become nauseated and vomit, suffer from abdominal pain or tenderness and often a low-grade fever. The diagnosis depends on finding the organism in the material excreted by the bowel. This is examined with special stains and observed under the microscope. The condition, once thought to be a tropical disease, is now recognized rather generally throughout the world. A number of drugs have been developed which are quite effective in destroying the amebae and removing them from the body. The one most widely used throughout the world is emetine, but others, such as aralin, chiniofon, fumadil, and milibis are widely used. The patient must be watched carefully to see that he has enough fluids in the body. Signs of abscess-formation in the liver—a most serious complication—must be detected promptly to prevent fatality. Quite commonly used for mild cases is terramycin. For the prevention of the diarrhea, ordinary paregoric may be helpful. The diet should include soft foods, and vitamins are usually given, because the person who is having severe diarrhea with loss of appetite is quite certain not to get sufficient vitamins. (*See also* DYSENTERY; *and also* CHAPTER VII.)

AMENORRHEA Absence or abnormal cessation of menstruation.

AMINO ACIDS Some twenty amino acids have been defined and at least eight, possibly ten, are necessary for health. The eight amino acids now considered essential for health include isolucine, lucine, lysine, methionine, phenyllalanine, threonine, tryptophane, and valine. Preparations of combined amino acids are now available as drugs for those who need them. Lack of essential amino acids results in the collecting of water in the tissues, with swelling.

AMNESIA Loss of memory, especially inability to remember the proper words.

AMNIOCENTESIS Puncture of the amniotic sac inside the uterus to obtain fluid or cells for examination, which permits diagnosis of Mongolism, Tay-Sachs disease or other potential birth defects.

AMYOTROPHIC LATERAL SCLEROSIS This complicated term refers to degeneration and hardening of portions of the spinal cord, which results in weakness and paralysis. This is the disease that killed Lou Gehrig, famous baseball player, and it is sometimes popularly called Gehrig's Disease. The chief symptoms are a progressive twitching of the muscles with increasing weakness and a wasting away. The condition is progressive and does not tend to improve. Treatment is given to maintain the tone of the muscles and to establish a proper mental attitude toward the condition.

ANALGESIA Absence of response to pain, loss of the feeling of pain, sometimes brought on by the use of drugs and anesthetics and sometimes by damage to nerves.

ANCYLOSTOMIASIS (*See* WORMS.)

ANEMIA A condition caused by a loss of blood, or from the red blood cells being destroyed more rapidly than new blood cells can be produced. Sometimes the production of cells falls below the rate of destruction of cells. Sometimes the red coloring matter in the blood falls below normal. Following hemorrhage, the red blood cells and red coloring matter usually return to normal within two months, if the patient lives. If one-third of the blood is lost suddenly, death may follow immediately unless blood is given by transfusion.

Anemia may result from defective

formation of the blood, due to a deficiency in nutrition. The lack of iron, proteins and some vitamins may produce what is known as an iron-deficiency anemia. The production of blood cells depends on a number of factors, involving various organs of the body. The bone marrow is especially important in producing red blood cells. Iron may be deficient when there is loss of blood, when it is not taken into the body in sufficient amounts or when it is not properly absorbed from the bowel. Women may lose so much blood during menstruation as to become anemic. The symptoms include a feeling of weakness, tiring easily, a shortness of breath on exertion, occasionally a swelling of the legs. If the anemia develops gradually, the number of red blood cells may fall as low as 1,000,000, instead of the normal 6,000,000.

In recovery from anemia, diet is important. Patients should have a nourishing diet containing spinach, meat, liver, eggs, apricots, peaches —foods rich in vitamins and proteins. Extra iron should be prescribed, in order to produce more hemoglobin, more red coloring matter and more red blood cells by speeding up the function of the bone marrow. Customary also is the taking of liver or lamb kidneys, which contain much of the necessary blood-stimulating material. Physicians may prescribe drugs if necessary, such as: folic acid, vitamin B_{12} or various liver extracts. Once the cause of blood-destruction is removed or the bone marrow properly stimulated, if that is needed, the ability of the body to grow blood cells is improved. (*See also* VITAMINS.)

ANEMIA, COOLEY'S Also called thalassanemia and Mediterranean anemia. A hereditary anemia occurring principally in Italians, Greeks, and Chinese. The red cells do not incorporate sufficient iron or hemoglobin. Treatment involves transfusion of blood and of red blood cells. When the spleen enlarges, it may be removed. Iron treatment is to be avoided.

ANEMIA, PERNICIOUS (Also called primary anemia, Addisonian anemia.) A condition that is due to a deficiency of secretions from the lining of the stomach wall and from the liver which are necessary for the building of blood cells. The diagnosis is made by examining the bood with microscopic and other tests. The rate of improvement also is determined by counting the newly-formed blood cells under the microscope. Frequently in this condition the stomach lacks hydrochloric acid in its secretions, or there may be a complete lack of secretion from the wall of the stomach. Pernicious anemia, which rarely occurs under 30 years of age, was formerly considered invariably fatal. The condition is now treated by administering the missing factors, with recovery in the vast majority of cases; often, however, patients need to continue taking these substitutes for body secretions throughout life. Vitamin B_{12} and/or liver extracts are injected into the muscles, in order to secure the most prompt results. The vitamin B_{12} is especially necessary to prevent complications affecting the nervous system in this disease. (*See also* LIVER EXTRACTS; VITAMINS.)

ANESTHESIA Loss of sensation, produced by anesthetic substances such as ether, chloroform, ethylene, cyclopropane, nitrous oxide, oxygen gas mixtures, and many other substances. Local anesthetics include derivatives of cocaine, such as procaine; also butyn and novocain. By injection of such local anesthetics into nerve areas, the passage of pain is prohibited. Injections of anesthetics are also made directly into the spinal column to block the nerves as they come from the spine. Injections are made into the lower portions of the spinal column to prevent pain in childbirth. Sedative drugs may be injected directly into the blood, and produce profound anesthesia for rather short periods of time.

ANEURYSM A dilation in the wall of a blood vessel caused when the pressure of the blood stretches a weak area, causing it to swell out like a similar place in a tube of a tire or like a rubber balloon. This may be caused by a physical injury, as when the side of a blood vessel is scraped by a bullet, or from an infection which attacks the wall of the blood vessel. Obviously, the bursting of an aneurysm is a serious accident, which may result in death. Now surgical methods have been developed for repairing aneurysms of blood vessels, using sometimes blood vessel walls from blood vessel banks.

ANGINA The word angina means choking or strangling, a condition which may occur in a variety of infections. The word is also taken occasionally to mean a sore throat and even any kind of spasmodic, cramplike pain. Thus one may speak of an "angina of the throat" or angina from diphtheria or, most frequently, of angina pectoris. Especially prevalent is the use of the term in connection with an infection of the mouth and throat called *Vincent's angina*, which is also commonly called trench mouth.

ANGINA PECTORIS A pain—continuous, aching, burning, or with a feeling of constriction—behind the breastbone, sometimes over the heart, radiating to the arm, the neck or the jaws. The pain becomes worse upon walking or upon association with any emotional strain or other stimulus that increases the work of the heart. Immediate rest stops the pain. Immediate relief from stress also stops the pain. It is most important to be certain that the pain is that of angina pectoris. Associated with it is a feeling of impending death which is frightening. The cause of the pain is believed to be a deficiency of the supply of oxygen to the muscle of the heart. The muscle needs oxygen in order to function. An increased demand for oxygen is therefore associated with exercise, emotional strain or anything that causes the heart to beat faster. High blood pressure or constriction of the blood vessels to the heart will also lessen its blood supply. Experts say that the underlying cause of angina pectoris in the vast majority of cases is a constriction of the coronary arteries which impedes the flow of blood into the muscles of the heart. Obviously, in such cases there is always the danger of a sudden complete blocking of these blood vessels,

269

as occurs in coronary thrombosis. When people who have had angina pectoris for a long time develop such attacks while at rest, there is a possibility that coronary thrombosis is threatening. An operation involves connecting a new supply to the heart by using a vein taken from the thigh and transplanting it from the aorta to the heart.

Here are ten commandments for people who have angina pectoris:

1. Do not subject your heart to sudden, strenuous, or prolonged physical activity.
2. Eat regularly, slowly, and temperately.
3. If you are excessively overweight, seek sound counsel as to how best dispense with this form of heart handicap.
4. Try to avoid physical activity for at least thirty minutes after eating, particularly after the heaviest meal of the day.
5. Avoid emotional stress and strain. Worry is an important factor in relation to heart strain.
6. By appropriate measures, keep your body as free as possible from so-called foci of infection.
7. Remember that regular intestinal elimination is highly important.
8. Average not less than eight hours of sleep in a room abundantly supplied with fresh air.
9. Remember that perennial health demands a proper balance between work, play, and rest.
10. Have periodic medical exam-

inations, in order to uncover defects of which you may be unaware.

People with angina pectoris can now get relief by various drugs. There are small glass bottles or ampules which contain amyl nitrite. Inhaling this drug brings prompt relief. Some people do well with nitroglycerin tablets which are dissolved under the tongue. Relief of the acute attack is not difficult but the doctor must regulate the life of the person with angina pectoris to minimize attacks, both as to frequency and severity, as much as possible. (*See also* HEART; *and also* CHAPTERS III, VI.)

ANGIOMA A tumor composed of blood vessels, most frequently seen as collections of swollen blood vessels in blue-like masses on the skin.

ANISEIKONIA A disturbance of vision in which the image seen by one eye is different from that seen by the other eye. A person with aniseikonia may think that a table is level when it is actually tipped, or vice versa. If he will move the table until it seems to him level, one then can judge the extent of the distortion. About 2 per cent of people have this condition in a state correctable by the prescription of proper eyeglasses.

ANOREXIA This term is used to describe a loss of desire for food. (*See also* APPETITE; *and also* CHAPTERS IX, XIV.)

ANTHRAX Infections and malignant boils, as well as serious infections of the lungs, are caused by the germ of anthrax. The condition affects particularly people working with cattle, wool sorters, or persons working with hides. The condition was commonly called wool-sorters disease. Prevention depends on most careful avoidance of contact with animals suspected of having this infection. The condition is rare. Serums have been developed which are effective. The condition is also successfully treated with the newer antibiotic drugs appropriate to the infection.

ANTIBIOTICS Substances derived from various living materials which have the power to act against other living organisms. The leading antibiotics now in common use include penicillin, streptomycin, aureomycin, chloromycetin or chloramphenicol, tetracycline, erthromycin, bacitracin, neomycin, polymyxin, cycloserine, puromycin, and many modifications. Several thousand other sources of antibiotics are under investigation. Some of the newer products are cathomycin, albamycin, and spiramycin.

ANTIHISTAMINES Drugs which act to oppose the release into the tissues of the body of a substance called histamine which is associated with various allergies. Thus antihistamines are used chiefly against hay fever, asthma, food allergies, urticaria and migraine. The most prominent antihistamines are Pyribenzamine, Benadryl, Neohetramine, Chlortrimeton, but there are at least 25 others.

ANTITOXIN Among the antibodies that are developed in the blood are the antitoxins, which act specifically against poisons from various germs. Antibodies may include those that agglutinate the germs, those that dissolve them or those that precipitate them. The antibodies are usually associated with the *gamma globulin,* about which so much has been heard, as a container for the antisubstances against measles, hepatitis and infantile paralysis. Antitoxins are sometimes prepared by injecting germs into animals such as the horse; the horse then develops in its serum the antitoxic substances. The antitoxins now recognized as among the most useful in medicine include those against botulism, diphtheria, lockjaw, scarlet fever, snake bite, and staphylococcus infections. Antitoxins have also been tried in erysipelas, epidemic sore throat, and meningitis. The developments in modern antibiotic drugs like penicillin, terramycin, aureomycin and chloromycetin are so effective that in many instances antitoxins are used only for severe and resistant cases. Scarlet fever antitoxin was greatly used but is now never used in such conditions, until antibiotics seem to fail. (*See also* CHAPTER XXII.)

ANTRUM Most frequently this term is used to refer to the maxillary antrum or maxillary sinuses, which are spaces within the jaw bones on each side of the nose. The mastoid antrum is the area infected in mastoiditis. (*See also* CHAPTER XXVI.)

ANUS This is the termination of the rectum at the lower end of the bowel.

271

ANXIETY A state of apprehension and fear, associated with restlessness and uncertainty. Modern psychoanalysis places the blame for many conditions of illness on anxieties, sometimes referred to as anxiety neuroses. (*See also* CHAPTER XXX.)

AORTA The large blood vessel that comes from the left ventricle of the heart and then branches off into arteries is called the "aorta." It may be affected by the deposit of plaques in its walls or by inflammations, or it may be congenitally misformed, a condition now susceptible to surgical operation. The valve between the heart and the aorta is called the aortic valve. (*See also* CHAPTER VI.)

APHASIA When a person loses the capacity to use words to convey ideas, the condition is called aphasia. It is usually due to damage to the portion of the brain involved in carrying on this function. Thus aphasia is not a problem of hearing or speaking but is involved in the use of language to translate thought.

APHONIA The loss of speech due either to a physical or a mental condition.

APHRODISIAC Any drug, thought or substance that can stimulate sexual desire is called an aphrodisiac.

APOPLEXY When a blood vessel in the brain breaks so that bleeding occurs into or onto the brain, or when a blood vessel to the brain is suddenly blocked so as to produce paralysis and unconsciousness, the condition is commonly called apoplexy. When an apoplexy or stroke

occurs, the first step is to put the person at rest, allowing him to lie flat on his side while unconscious in order to prevent the tongue from falling back and producing choking. After the first recovery from a stroke, certain parts of the body may be found to be paralyzed. As the person recovers, the blood vessels work their way through the clot, and a return of function to some of the paralyzed parts may occur. People who are unconscious for long periods of time are sometimes unable to drink or swallow. Fluids must then be put into the body according to the method suggested by the doctor. Feeding of such people may also be difficult. Proper attention should always be given to the skin to prevent bedsores, which includes a daily bath with soap and water, the use of powder, and the prevention of continuous contact of the skin at any one portion of the body with the bedclothing, since continuous pressure of the body on any one portion of it where the bones are near the surface will break the skin and result in a bedsore or ulcer. (*See also* CHAPTER III.)

APPENDICITIS Infection and inflammation of the appendix, a little tube from the "cecum," a large portion of the bowel in the lower part of the abdomen on the right side. Symptoms include a sudden onset of pain, with nausea, vomiting, fever, tenderness and rigidity. The vomiting may be of the projectile type. If the doctor examines the blood, he finds the number of white blood cells greatly increased. If the condition does not receive prompt attention, gangrene may occur or the abscess may burst and spread peritonitis through the abdomen. The operation is now perfected, and death rarely results. Unattended, appendicitis may cause death. The use of antibiotic drugs may diminish infection but is not considered by the vast majority of doctors a dependable method of treating appendicitis. If the diagnosis is made promptly and the appendix is removed, the patients frequently get up by the second day and leave the hospital within a week. (*See also* CHAPTER II.)

APPETITE People who eat regularly and in fair amounts seldom feel hunger. The desire to eat is not the same as hunger. Appetite is a longing for food. Some people always have a good appetite; others seldom crave food. The appetite may be perverted so as to produce excessive craving for unusual foods. Overweight is not often due to excessive appetite but to careless eating of vast amounts of food. It is sometimes associated with boredom, sometimes as a substitute for other desires. Appetite is a complex phenomenon involving the mind and the nervous system. Complete loss of appetite and failure to eat is called *anorexia nervosa,* and is usually associated with some emotional instability. (*See also* CHAPTERS IX, XIV.)

ARACHNODACTALY Spider fingers is a term used to characterize people with fingers and toes that are unusually long and thin. The condition apparently is transmitted through heredity.

ARTERIOSCLEROSIS Hardening of the walls of the arteries. The blood

vessels, which are usually elastic, fairly thin and soft, become rigid, thickened and hardened in many people as they grow older. Hardening of the arteries is one of the leading causes of death. The exact cause is not known.

Hardening of the walls of the arteries is frequently associated with high blood pressure, buy may not be itself the cause of high blood pressure. The current theory of the cause of hardening of the arteries is a congenital disposition toward the condition associated with the overeating of fatty foods and the taking-in of excessive amounts of cholesterol. Specific treatment for hardening of the arteries is not established. Doctors generally recommend good hygiene, the avoidance of excesses of all kinds, and particularly freedom from stress and worry. Usually more attention is paid to controlling the manifestations of high blood pressure than to the hardening of the blood vessels.

Most of the symptoms of hardening of the arteries are related to the high blood pressure. These include occasional attacks of dizziness, drowsiness and ringing in the ears; sometimes changes in the blood vessels of the legs and interference with the circulation produce cramping, blueness of the tissues, and other signs of a lack of sufficient circulation.

People who advocate cholesterol-free diets eliminate milk, butter, cream, cheese, ice cream and other dairy products, mayonnaise, fried foods, gravies, pastries and many other substances. Incidentally, it is practically impossible to maintain a completely fat-free and cholesterol-free diet. Especially recommended

273

are vegetable oils like corn oil, peanut oil, cottonseed and safflower oil which are polyunsaturated fats. (*See also* BLOOD PRESSURE, HIGH; *and also* CHAPTER V.)

ARTHRITIS Arthritis means, strictly, inflammation of the joints. The condition occurs in many different forms. Sometimes germs get into joints, such as the germs of scarlet fever, gonorrhea, tuberculosis, or the streptococci. These definite infections of joints should be distinguished from what is called rheumatoid arthritis. The exact cause of rheumatoid arthritis is not known. Among factors related to it are fatigue, shock, injury, exposure to cold and dampness. People with chronic rheumatism feel better on nice warm days than on cold rainy days. The amount of pain in the joints varies. Usually the pain is accompanied by swelling and sometimes by severe inflammation. In rheumatoid arthritis nodules may appear under the skin, around the elbows, wrists and fingers, and occasionally on the ankles.

Rheumatoid arthritis must be differentiated from the degenerative type. Usually rheumatoid arthritis comes on before 40 years of age, whereas the degenerative type comes on after 50. Unfortunately, specific forms of treatment that will definitely prevent the advancement of rheumatoid arthritis have not been developed. However, an approach to a better understanding of the condition and to relief from it are frequently obtained by the use of products like ACTH and Cortisone. The control of rheumatoid arthritis may involve co-operation between a general physician, a physical therapist,

and an orthopedic surgeon, and occasionally also the physician who specializes in psychosomatic diseases. Rest is one of the most important factors in treatment, and this includes emotional rest. The diet should not be restricted, and modern physicians no longer stop the patients from using citrus fruits or pork. The diet should be rich in proteins, calories and iron and adequate in vitamins. More recently meticorten has been developed as a replacement for Cortisone, so that restriction on salt is not severe. Pain is now relieved by such drugs as aspirin and other salicylates; butazolidine, Indocin[R], and other analgesics, and by proper use of ACTH and Cortisone. Individual patients are given physical treatment with heat and water, such as bathing and whirlpools, and other methods which an expert physiotherapist may utilize.

Patients do not die of rheumatoid arthritis, but rather with it. The condition persists. In a large group of cases followed for many years, using the methods that have been mentioned, more than 50 per cent, definitely improved, about 12 per cent remained stationary and something over 35 per cent gradually grew worse. (*See also* RHEUMATIC FEVER; *and also* CHAPTER XIII.)

ASBESTOSIS People who inhale dust or other materials associated with the manufacture or use of asbestos may have inflammations of the lungs, called asbestosis. Development of this condition means removal from that type of work. Protection is to be had by the wearing of appropriate face masks and by the installation of suitable dust-prevention devices in such plants.

ASCITES An abnormal accumulation of fluid in the abdominal cavity, also called dropsy.

ASCORBIC ACID The scientific name for vitamin C, found in fresh green vegetables, citrus fruits and acerola juice. (*See also* VITAMINS; *and also* CHAPTER XV.)

ASPHYXIA Asphyxia is suffocation resulting from loss of air. When people are deprived of oxygen, the damage to the tissues is almost immediate, and death may result. Babies sometimes are asphyxiated in their cribs by bedclothing, or by people lying upon them when sleeping with an adult. People who are shocked by electricity may become asphyxiated; and death results from the inhalation of carbon monoxide gas, which is the chief ingredient of illuminating gas. People also become asphyxiated from inhaling automobile exhaust gas. Finally, suffocation occurs during drowning. Nobody can live whose lungs have been without a change of air for a matter of from five to ten minutes. However, resuscitation should always be attempted, with the hope that the period during which the person has been without air is less than was originally estimated. The usual method of restoring breathing to a person who has been drowned or shocked by electricity is artificial respiration by the use of the Holger-Nielson method or the mouth-to-mouth breathing technic. (*See also* CHAPTER III.)

ASTHENIA Absence or loss of

strength. (*See also* EXHAUSTION; *and also* CHAPTER III.)

ASTHMA A condition of constriction of the bronchial tubes due to sensitivity to various substances such as are listed under allergy. The term comes from a Greek word meaning panting or gasping for breath. The condition occurs at any age. The most frequent causes are sensitivities to dust, which is found in various occupations, to dandruff, germs or chemicals. The tendency to sensitivity resulting in asthma seems to run in families. Among the most common causes of asthma in children are sensitivities to foods. The attack begins with a strong desire to sneeze; a struggling for air with a feeling of suffocation; the breath may come and go with a high-pitched sound; the muscles of the chest are strained. In asthma the difficulty in breathing may eventually produce changes in the chest formation, also loss of weight due to difficulty in eating, and perhaps damage to the heart from the strain placed on that organ.

Asthma is prevented by detecting the substances to which the person is sensitive and eliminating these items from his surroundings. Allergists can detect these substances by tests specifically for the purpose. They also can practice, in some instances, desensitization.

In acute attacks the doctor may get immediate relief for the patient by injecting epinephrine or adrenalin which relieves the bronchial spasms. The amount to be given and the manner of giving depend on the decision of the doctor for the individual person. The drugs may be taken by inhalation. People with asthma sometimes obtain relief by wearing masks to protect themselves against dusts, and by the use of air-conditioned rooms. People who are sensitive to dusts from down or feathers may use pillows or mattresses filled with air. Usually the person with asthma should sleep alone in a well-aired room in which the temperature and humidity are under control. All upholstered furniture, rugs, and other dust catchers should be removed from the bedroom. The person should eat little at night, since a full stomach makes breathing more difficult. (*See also* ALLERGY; *and also* CHAPTER XII.)

ASTIGMATISM This is a disturbance of vision due to a faulty formation of the shape of the eye. (*See also* EYE; *and also* CHAPTER XXV.)

ATAXIA Loss of co-ordination in motion, which reflects disturbances of the nervous system.

ATELECTASIS The loss of air from the small air chambers in the lungs gives the lungs a contracted, solid appearance as they are viewed in X-ray plates. (*See also* CHAPTER IV.)

ATHEROSCLEROSIS Deposits of fibrous tissue and fat in the lining of the arteries which may block them or slow the flow of blood.

ATHLETE'S FOOT (*See* RINGWORM; *and also* CHAPTER XXIII.)

AUSCULTATION The, use of hearing for signs of changes within the body. Auscultation is best done with the stethoscope. The doctor can

hear the valves of the heart opening and closing, detect the presence of fluid in the lungs, and even hear excessive motion of other organs. (*See also* CHAPTER I.)

AUTONOMIC NERVOUS SYSTEM (*See* SYMPATHETIC NERVOUS SYSTEM.)

AUTOSENSITIZATION Proof has been developed that people may become sensitized to their own tissues. Certain disorders of the blood and possibly multiple sclerosis may be disorders of this type.

AUTOPSY Postmortem examination of the body is called autopsy.

B

BABINSKI TEST This is a test in which a doctor scrapes the bottom of the foot, causing extension of the great toe to determine the integrity of the spinal cord.

BACKACHE Pain in the back is among the most frequent of all symptoms affecting human beings. A woman was once defined as "a two-legged animal with a pain in the back." Man has been declared by mechanical experts "a mechanical misfit." The backbone is shaped like a spring curved like the letter "S." The spinal column is composed of small bones between which are cushions of cartilage known as disks. The bones are bound together by strong tissues called ligaments. The nerves come out in little notches between the bones. Any inflammation or infection of any of these tissues may cause a pain in the back. A sudden stress or a long-continued strain may throw any of the joints into a wrong position. Diseases may injure the cartilage or bone and result in pain. People who do heavy lifting or who stand long on their feet are especially likely to have pains in the back.

The common name for backache is lumbago; scientifically doctors speak of it as low back pain since it is the lower portion of the spine that is most frequently affected. In determining the cause of the pain in the back, X-ray pictures are a necessity. The use of such pictures and of other tests will reveal whether or not damage has been done to a disk, or whether or not it has slipped out of position. Sometimes an inequality in the length of the legs, even of a tiny amount, may throw a strain on some portion of the back and bring about pain. Tumors also affect the back, as they do any other portion of the body.

Sometimes backache is incidental to gout, gall bladder disease, ulcer of the stomach, or childbirth. The pain in the back which women often have after childbirth is sometimes related to the organs of childbirth, but at other times to disturbances of the intestines and kidneys. Sometimes the stress comes from sleeping in a bed which does not properly support the spine. For this reason, the doctor who handles such cases will want to know about the bed. He may consider the patient's obtaining relief by wearing proper braces or supports. He will treat any

detectable infection. He will measure the length of the legs, examine the patient for overweight or flat feet, and of course prescribe drugs, to relieve the pain while he is making his studies. He will also recommend the application of heat and sometimes of massage or manipulation to bring about relief. (*See also* CHAPTER II.)

BACITRACIN One of the important antibiotic drugs, it is used frequently in treating localized infections, rarely used internally. (*See also* CHAPTER XXI.)

BACTERIA Any of the microorganisms. People who do not say germs often use the word bacteria to describe the microorganisms that can infect human beings and animals. Some bacteria are seriously damaging varieties, others are less important. Modern sanitary experts demand that food, clothing and other environmental substances of man be free from dangerous germs. (*See also* CHAPTER XXII.)

BAKING SODA Common name for sodium bicarbonate. Often used in ulcers to overcome acid.

BAL This word is an abbreviation for a substance called "British anti-lewisite" which was developed during World War II for the treatment of poisoning by arsenic in war gases, also for poisoning by arsenic derived from any other source; now used as an antidote against poisoning from any of the metallic substances like mercury. (*See also* CHAPTER XVIII.)

BALDNESS (Also called *alopecia*). (*See also* HAIR; *and also* CHAPTER X.)

BANDAGE Any strip of gauze, muslin, flannel or similar material used to cover a wound, to hold dressings in place, to immobilize a part of the body, or even to stop hemorrhage may be called a bandage. There are many kinds of bandages and methods of applying them, which are part of the doctor's training.

BARBER'S ITCH Infection of the skin of the face following irritation of an ingrown hair or the use of an infected razor, shaving brush or towels, by a common pus-forming germ called a staphylococcus. Some such infections are also related to ringworm contamination. Occasionally the trouble begins on the back of the neck, due to rubbing by a rough collar. Such infections are associated with bleeding and crusting. The condition is curable by the application of proper remedies, but control of such remedies—which are potent—must be left to the physician. Many states have laws regulating the sanitation of barber shops and the sterilization of implements following their use on each customer. The antibiotic drugs have proved most efficient in relieving barber's itch but there is always the danger of sensitization to the antibiotic through its effect on the skin. The technical name for barber's itch is sycosis which is not related to nor to be confused with the term psychosis, referring to a mental disturbance.

BARBITURATES Derivatives of barbituric acid, used in medicine as hypnotic and sedative drugs. There are many different varieties, and all of them have different names. They are properly used for producing relaxation and sleep but people may sometimes become sensitive to them and have as a result rashes of the skin, and occasionally changes in the blood. Among the commonly used barbiturates are nembutal, sedormid, veronal, and phenobarbital.

BASAL METABOLISM The relationship between the taking of materials into the body and their consumption. The normal person produces heat through the chemical changes which go on in the body. Several methods are known for measuring the basal metabolic rate, which is done by complicated apparatus. Measurement of protein-bound iodine is one way of determining the basal metabolic rate, called the PBI test. Anger and fear speed the rate; sleep lessens; and undernutrition is associated with a lowered basal metabolic rate.

BATHS AND BATHING Water is essential to the human body inside and out. It participates in every chemical reaction, aids absorption and digestion of food, and the passage of waste material from the body.

Bathing habits differ throughout the world but cleanliness is highly regarded everywhere. The habit of bathing may vary from once a season to twice or more daily. The routine use of soap is recent. Soap cleanses the skin by emulsifying the oils and dissolving them, making easy the removal of grease and dirt. Shower baths are more stimulating than tub baths. Warm tub baths are relaxing and sedative. People who are sensitive to soap may wash the soap away thoroughly, or try various detergents. The temperature of water most agreeable to the skin is from 95° to 100° Fahrenheit.

Baths can be harmful when they emacerate the skin. For older people with sensitive skin the application of oils or greases may be helpful. Cool baths conduct heat away and lower temperatures. The tonic bath usually is a quick cold shower or sponge taken, preferably, in the morning. Evidence has not shown that cold baths help people to resist catching cold.

BEDSORES Pressure of the bones on the skin of people who have to lie long in one position may result in damage to the tissue and the formation of ulcers or bedsores. Inflated rubber cushions help to avoid such sores; also the shifting of the position of the body by the use of soft pillows or similar material. Undersheets and clothing should be pulled smooth. Bedclothing should not be too tight.

A moist skin macerates more easily than a dry one. Hence nurses who wish to prevent bedsores will wash the skin, dry it properly by absorbing excess water with a towel instead of rubbing, treat it with alcohol applications, and use powder to decrease the possibility of maceration.

BED WETTING (*See* ENURESIS.)

BELLADONNA A commonly used drug derived from a plant, used as an antispasmodic and to check secretions. The drug is much used in such spasmodic disorders as *paralysis agitans;* also used to prevent excessive secretions by the stomach.

BELL'S PALSY Paralysis of the muscles of the face, usually on only one side at a time. Has been called Bell's palsy because first described by a British doctor named Bell. The condition has been associated with long exposure of one side of the face to cold, such as occurs when one is driving next to an open window or sleeping in the draft from a ventilator on a train. Most investigators now believe this condition is due to an attack by a virus on a portion of the facial nerve which controls the muscles of the face. The condition comes on suddenly; it may cause the mouth to be drawn to one side by the muscles that are not affected; it may interfere with closing the eye, so that tears run down the cheek. In mild cases, patients recover in two or three weeks or less. An exceedingly small percentage of people may be permanently affected. The condition has been treated with Cortisone derivatives, with good results. Splints are applied to the muscles, to hold them so that they are not stretched until the nerve recovers.

BENADRYL The trademark name of a compound which is classed with antihistamines.

BENIGN The opposite of malignant; usually applied to tumors which are not cancerous.

BERIBERI A condition of inflammation of the nerves due to a lack of thiamin or vitamin B_1, widely known in the tropical countries where people depend primarily on rice, following the eating of polished rice, from which the thiamin has been removed. Among the symptoms of thiamin deficiency which in beriberi go on to do serious damage to the tissues of the body are inflammation of the nerves, collection of fluids in the legs and in the tissues of the glands. Symptoms include tingling and numbness of the portions of the body reached by the affected nerves. The treatment requires administration of large doses of thiamin, which cause the symptoms and the defect to disappear. (*See also* VITAMINS; *and also* CHAPTER XV.)

BILE The secretion which passes from the liver into the gall bladder and then into the duodenum. It aids in emulsifying, digesting and absorbing fat. Failure of the gall bladder to eliminate the bile because of blocking by stones results in gall bladder inflammation called cholecystitis. (*See also* CHOLECYSTITIS; *and also* CHAPTER VII.)

BILIOUSNESS Popular name for general malaise, headache, loss of appetite, indigestion and a coated tongue formerly thought to be caused by absorption of bile into the blood. The condition now recognized by this name is probably better known as indigestion. Biliousness occurs more commonly in men than in women. Among the dietary substances frequently associated with it are chocolates, cream cake, yolks of eggs, excessive amounts of fat and fried foods. (*See also* CHAPTER VII.)

BIOPSY Study of a living person, as opposed to necropsy which is the postmortem examination of a dead body. When tissue is cut from the living person in order to make an examination under the microscope, usually for cancer, the process is called biopsy. (*See also* CHAPTER I.)

BIRTH CONTROL Any method for preventing or regulating the conception of a child is called birth control. Scientifically, these methods are known as contraception. (*See also* CONTRACEPTION.)

BIRTHMARK Birthmarks are usually colored spots on the skin which are collections of blood vessels, deposit of pigment, or other blemishes. The strawberry birthmark is a mass of blood vessels collected in a knot on the surface. Often birthmarks, if not too permanent or large, disappear with growth.

The port-wine birthmark is a collection of small blood vessels, with a certain amount of pigment deposited from the blood into the skin.

Birthmarks may be treated with the method known as freezing with carbon-dioxide snow, by coagulation with the electric needle, by exposure to radium or X-rays and, preferably, by carefully done surgery.

BITTERS Medicines which have a bitter taste and which act as stimulants to the appetite are called bitters. These may be aromatic or astringent and they seem to stimulate the gastrointestinal tract, without being absorbed into the body.

BLACKOUT Sudden temporary loss of vision and even of consciousness due to a sudden diminution of the flow of blood to the brain. This may result simply from sudden increases of speed or sudden ascent to higher altitudes. (*See also* CHAPTER XIX.)

BLADDER DISEASES Diseases affecting the two chief bladders in the body, the gall bladder and the urinary bladder. The gall bladder conditions are discussed under CHOLECYSTITIS.

Two tubes called ureters pass from the kidneys a distance of about a foot and carry the urine to the urinary bladder. This is an elastic storage receptacle which is emptied from time to time. It has an average capacity of something less than a pint but can stretch considerably when the flow of urine out of the bladder is subjected to interference. Inflammation of the bladder follows infections which result from contamination by various germs. Among the chief ones that affect the bladder are the colon bacilli, but almost any type of germ can upon occasion infect and inflame the bladder. Inflammation of the bladder is called cystitis. Old people or those who remain in bed practically all the time are more likely to have such conditions than those who are active. Enlargement of the prostate gland in men interferes with the flow of urine from the bladder and thus aids contamination and infection. Many tests are used by doctors in diagnosing such conditions. These include looking into the bladder with a cystoscope; feeling the prostate gland with a finger placed in the rectum; using dye substances that are excreted by the kidneys; giving the patient substances which are opaque to the X-ray, then taking X-ray pictures. Many methods have been developed for treating inflammation and infection of the bladder and there are now drugs such as the sulfonamides, the furadantin derivatives, the antibiotics, and mandelic acid, which act to control such infections.

Stones may form in the urinary bladder itself or may get there from the kidney by passing down the ureters. Stones in the urinary bladder occur about twenty times as often among men as among women. If the stone causes symptoms by blocking the flow of urine, it should be removed with the instruments which doctors have for this purpose.

A tumor of the bladder may be exceedingly serious because it causes bleeding, difficulties in urinating and other disturbances. By the use of the cystoscope for looking into the bladder and the X-ray for detecting changes in the bladder, diagnosis may be made certain, and with modern techniques, treatment and cure are possible. (*See also* KIDNEY; *and also* CHAPTER VIII.)

BLAST INJURY Serious harm is done to the human body by exposure to high explosives. The pressure of the blast on the body can cause hemorrhages in the lungs or tearing of abdominal organs.

BLASTOMYCOSIS A fungous disease like ACTINOMYCOSIS but produced by a different organism and found in various countries. Infection with this organism produces tumorous growths which may involve not only the skin, but also the organs and even the bones of the body. (*See also* ACTINOMYCOSIS.)

281

BLEB A blister on the skin, filled with serum or blood.

BLEPHARITIS Inflammation of the eyelid is called blepharitis. Rapid winking and blinking is called blepharospasm; swelling, blepharedema. Any of these conditions affecting the eyelids must be diagnosed as to cause and treated according to what is found.

BLINDNESS The causes of blindness are discussed under the heading *Eye. (See also* EYE; *and also* CHAPTER XXV.)

BLOOD Most important fluid in the human body. The normal blood contains from about five million red blood cells to six million, in each cubic millimeter. The blood of women contains slightly less than that of men. The body of a woman is smaller and needs fewer red blood cells. Red blood cells grow in the bone marrow. The blood contains fluid matter called plasma which contains some solid substances that settle out, leaving the serum. An examination of the blood is a vital part of any complete physical examination. The doctor may obtain the blood from a puncture of the ear or finger or by putting a needle into a vein. He counts the red blood cells, the white blood cells and the blood platelets; he may determine the amount of sugar or protein in the blood as a whole; he detects the amount of hemoglobin, or red coloring matter. The blood carries the anti-substances against infections, it provides the tissues with oxygen and nutrients and it carries waste matter to the kidneys, where such

waste matter is eliminated. It is also responsible for carrying the hormones, or substances of the glands of internal secretion, to various parts of the body. The total amount of blood is equal to about one-thirteenth of the body weight. Of this 78 per cent is water and 22 per cent solid. (*See also* CHAPTER IV.)

BLOOD POISONING A common term used for infections of the blood known as *septicemia. (See also* SEPTICEMIA.)

BLOOD PRESSURE—high (Hypertension) Blood pressure above the normal is hypertensive disease, now one of the chief causes of death. The cause of hypertensive disease is not known positively, but contributing causes are the stresses and strains of modern life, the effect of psychic and emotional activities of the brain, the results of infections and poisonings and, conceivably, glandular and structural causes. A constant high blood pressure may be associated with headaches and a variety of pains. Such common symptoms as ringing in the ears have been attributed to high blood pressure. The danger from an exceedingly high blood pressure lies in the possible breaking of a blood vessel, particularly in the brain, which results in apoplexy or stroke. Overweight is considered by insurance companies to be a frequent associate of high blood pressure. A high salt diet has perhaps not been incriminated but a low salt diet is believed to be helpful in cases of high blood pressure. People suffering from high blood pressure should not indulge in exercises such as running or lifting heavy weights or in any type of activity which produces shortness of breath. Mild exercise and massage tend to produce relaxation. Emotional excitement, particularly anger, is to be avoided. Suitable sedative drugs may be prescribed to control excessive excitement. Up to the age of fifty, the blood pressure rises slowly from 120 with the heart contracted and 80 with the heart relaxed, to 130 with the heart contracted and 85 with the heart relaxed. The blood pressure may be higher in older people. Extensive studies have shown that higher blood pressures, even up to 160 or 165, may be carried without harm by some people. Actually, the exact relationship of high blood pressure to the length of life and the aging process has not been fully established. Many new drugs are now available for use in high blood pressure, including Diuril[R], Guanethidine[R] and Alpha-Dopa. (*See also* APOPLEXY; WEIGHT, OVER-; *and also* CHAPTERS V, XXXII.)

BLOOD PRESSURE—low (Hypotension) Blood pressure below the normal. When a person is nauseated or faint or has a severe hemorrhage, the blood pressure falls. Low blood pressure is associated with weakness. Low blood pressure may follow acute or long-continued infection. Certain diseases that attack the glands of internal secretion which are concerned with keeping the blood pressure normal may produce a continuous low blood pressure. In general, low blood pressure favors long life but is not likely to be associated with physical vigor. (*See also* CHAPTER V.)

BLOOD TYPES Human beings can be divided into groups according to certain factors in the blood which react with factors of a different type in other blood. The blood of some groups may be mixed without danger. In some cases, the fluid matter in the blood of one person will coagulate the red blood cells of another. This is of the greatest importance in blood transfusion. By testing the blood of one person with that of another, in many thousands of people, the groups were divided, and it is now known that group "O" blood can be mixed without any danger. The other classifications have been made to indicate when transfusions are safe and when they are not.

More recently, the Rh factor has been discovered, and it is known that an Rh negative and an Rh positive together may produce a child that suffers promptly after birth with a condition that destroys the red blood cells. Under such circumstances, life is saved by transfusion into the child of a blood that is safe. In legal cases, the presence of the blood groups has been found useful because it can be shown that a certain man could not possibly be the father of a certain child. (*See also* RH FACTOR.)

BODY ODOR Occasionally the perspiration of a person will have a strong odor. The condition is called "bromidrosis." Such people should bathe every day or twice daily using a good soap, preferably one without an offensive odor of its own.

Under the arms, under the breasts, and in other places where perspiration may be excessive, preparations may be applied that prevent excessive perspiration. These usually contain salts of aluminum. The stopping of the perspiration in small areas is not harmful. Afterward a powder may be put on the skin.

Excessive perspiration of the feet has been related by some investigations to the wearing of woolen stockings, and such persons do better with stockings of another textile. The regular bathing of the feet with suitable solutions of an astringent character will limit the amount of perspiration of the feet. Another new investigation has definitely related offensive odors under the arms to the presence of bacteria which get into the fatty material of the perspiration and increase the odor. In severe cases, mild applications of X-ray are helpful.

BOILS A boil is an infection of the skin which follows, usually, maceration or breaking of the skin. Boils occur particularly in the portions of the skin covered by hair. These little openings offer exceptional opportunity for the invasion of germs.

Certain diseases such as diabetes weaken the ability of the skin to resist infection. Boils occur with greater frequency in diabetics than in others. Persons who frequently have boils must try to keep the body in the best possible state by practicing cleanliness, by a diet containing vitamins and adequate protein, and by getting plenty of fresh air. All infections must be attended to promptly, to avoid their spreading.

In the treatment of boils, heat may be applied because it brings a good supply of blood, which aids in destroying germs. Opening a boil should be considered a serious sur-

gical procedure and should not be attempted except by those trained in this work. In some cases X-ray or ultraviolet rays have been applied to persistent boils and have helped. Vaccines have been prepared from germs, and these have helped to build resistance. Most recently, the sulfonamide and antibiotic drugs applied in cases of infections of this type have been curative.

A carbuncle is, usually, a group of boils close together, and because of its size may be especially serious. Boils and carbuncles are dangerous when they are around the lip or the nose, where the infected material may pass easily into the blood.

BONES The bones compose the basic structure of the human body. They are connected by joints and, with the ligaments, are held in approximation to each other. The shafts of the bones are solid. The marrow, which is spongy, is concerned in building blood cells. Bones suffer from congenital defects, from deficiencies of growth, from infections like osteomyelitis, from changes such as the loss of calcium in Paget's disease, from tumors, and from breaks or fractures. Modern progress has developed the use of bone banks in which bony material is stored for use in repairing bones by surgery.

BORBORYGMUS A rumbling noise caused by air or gas in the intestines.

BORIC ACID A mild antiseptic substance sometimes used as a dressing for mild infections of the skin. Internally, it may be poisonous, particularly to little children.

BOTULISM Food poisoning is due to several different infectious organisms. The most dangerous is the one called *Clostridium botulinum*. Foods improperly canned and contaminated by this organism develop serious poisons which can cause death if taken in sufficient amounts. The nature of the food, whether acid or alkaline, the amount of sugar present or the extent of the heating during preserving will definitely affect the amount of botulinum present and the amount of the toxin that may be developed. Commercially canned foods are seldom or practically never infected with botulinum. Home canning is not as safe as commercial canning. Home-preserved foods should be boiled for six minutes before they are tasted or served.

The symptoms of botulism are weakness and paralysis, sometimes beginning with double vision. Eventually the people who have been poisoned with the toxin develop difficulty in talking and in swallowing. Doctors will do their best to keep the patient alive until the anti-botulism serum can be secured and administered. (*See also* FOOD POISONING.)

BRADYCARDIA Slowness of the heart is called by this term. It describes a heartbeat of less than 60 per minute. The prefix "brady" refers to slowness. (*See also* CHAPTER VI.)

BRAIN The brain of an average man weighs between three and four pounds. The size of the brain is not an indication of the intellect. The brain chiefly distinguishes man from animals. In the brain are the centers of special functions of the body such as seeing, hearing and smelling, also the transmission system for putting into action the parts of the body that are under voluntary control. The thinking portion of the brain is thought to be the outside or cortex. The brain may get tired, exactly as any other organ of the body may become fatigued. The gray matter comprises about 40 per cent of the brain. Investigators have localized certain functions in certain portions of the brain. Damage to these portions is reflected in failure of the parts concerned. In difficulties with words, something is usually wrong in the front part of the brain. The motor-controlling sections are about halfway back on each side, a left leg being controlled by the right side of the brain, and vice versa.

In cases of disordered function of any portion of the body a neurologist can localize the portion of the brain or nervous system that is concerned. (*See also* CHAPTER II.)

BREATHING The lungs conduct the breathing of the body. Air is taken into the lungs, which take the oxygen out of the air and release carbon dioxide. The lungs are like a sponge organized into little individual cells which communicate with larger tubes and these with still larger tubes, passing them from the air spaces to the bronchial tubes and then into the trachea, or windpipe. The air changes in the lungs at about the rate of four quarts per minute. The average human being breathes from twelve to fifteen times per minute. We breathe more rapidly when we exercise because then we need more oxygen. The capacity of the chest differs in different people, also the ability to hold the breath. Shortness of the breath is a serious symptom, sometimes related to heart disease, on other occasions to deficiencies in the blood. From the small cells of the lungs the air passes into small tubes which carry it to the windpipe. These tubes are called bronchi. Inflammation of or around these tubes causes distressing cough and expectoration of material. Breathing becomes difficult. Obviously, it is important to get the infected material out of the body. When detected early, the use of an antibiotic drug will stop the infection. Other remedies are given to lessen the cough. Inhalations of steam will loosen the material and permit it to be expectorated more easily. Great care must be taken not to burn the patient by tipping over the kettle or basin which is creating the steam. The chief danger from bronchitis is secondary pneumonia. Children who have had bronchitis after measles or other infectious diseases may improve greatly in sunny climates. Rest, fresh air, sunshine and nutritious food will help build the body and create increased resistance. A persistent cough means there is continuing infection. Chronic bronchitis produces constant coughing, which may be noticed particularly during the night.

Bronchiectasis is an infection in the lungs and must be relieved by resting the lungs; sometimes such infections become so serious and damaging that surgical removal of a portion of the lung is necessary. People with bronchiectasis are helped by plenty of rest. Drainage is encouraged by allowing the head to lean over the edge of the bed or by bending it over a chair. Nowadays inhalations of antibiotic drugs are given. A device has been developed to encourage coughing and thus to permit the lung to eliminate infectious material more easily. (*See also* TRACHEA; OXYGEN; COUGHING; *and also* CHAPTERS III, IV, XII, XXXII.)

BROMIDES Bromides are salts derived from a chemical called bromine. The bromides are used medicinally to stop convulsions, to relieve pain, to relax people and to help them to sleep. (*See also* CHAPTER XVIII.)

BRUISES An injury to the surface of the body that does not break the skin may be sufficient to cause a bruise. Bruising may result from blows with blunt objects such as clubs, a rubber hose or a whip. Bruises may result from bumping into the corners of chairs or tables or from falls. The black-and-blue marks which characterize prize fighters are the results of bruising with the glove. A bruise of the scalp is particularly important because there may be hemorrhage under the scalp or a broken bone in the skull. Ruptures of the liver have occurred following a bruise which seemed at first merely to be an injury to the surface of the body.

Some people bruise much more easily than others, because of conditions of the blood or of the capillary blood vessels, which may be fragile. Women frequently bruise easily around the time of menstruation and may not bruise easily at other times. The change in the color of bruised skin, from black to blue to yellow, is a reflection of the gradual absorption of the extravasated material by the blood. The first blood in the bruise is represented by a clot which appears black. As the pigment is absorbed, this changes to blue, to brown, to yellow, and finally disappears. A severe bruise may be painful because of the stretching of the tissues and may require application of heat and rest.

BUERGER'S DISEASE A condition in which the lining of the blood vessels is inflamed, the passage of the blood is slowed, the legs get cold, and gangrene may result. The disease was named for the New York physician called Buerger who first described the condition. Buerger's disease affects chiefly men from twenty to fifty years of age. A definite relationship seems to be established between the occurrence of Buerger's disease and excessive smoking. Because of the danger of gangrene in Buerger's disease, with a necessary amputation, people with this condition are urged particularly to watch carefully the care of the feet, to keep the feet clean, warm and dry. Use loose-fitting bed socks instead of hot-water bottles. Wear properly fitted shoes. Do not cut the toenails too close. Do not attempt to cut corns or calluses. Do not use strong antiseptic drugs on the feet. Do not use tobacco in any form if threatened with Buerger's disease.

BUNIONS (*See* FEET; *and also* CHAPTER XXVIII.)

BURNS Burns are among the most frequent of all injuries. When a serious burn occurs, the first attention should be paid to enabling the person to recover from the shock. Blood plasma or blood transfusion may be used promptly. Seldom does anyone recover who has had as much as one-half of the surface of the body burned.

To prevent burns, stoves, grates, hot water, and matches should be kept from contact with children. In early childhood, hot water is the leading cause of accidental burns. Electric burns are about the same in their effects as burns from direct heat. For an ordinary burn, the best first aid is simply to cover the area with a sterile bandage at once, and give the person fluids. If necessary, drugs may be given to control pain. More serious burns should come promptly to the attention of a physician, preferably in a hospital. (*See also* CHAPTER XXXIV.)

BURSITIS Inflammation of a bursa, a shock-absorbing sac of fluid which helps to lubricate friction points. Most frequently bursas become inflamed at the top of the shoulder, back of the shoulder blades, and occasionally at the elbow and at the hip. When a bursa is bruised, irritated or infected, it is filled with excess fluid and may become exceedingly painful, particularly on motion.

Housemaid's knee is a form of bursitis which results from pressure on the kneecap from kneeling on the floor.

Deltoid bursitis occurs most frequently in men who play golf or

287

tennis or who swing the arms. Calcium is deposited in the bursa, may cause disability, may become so constantly painful as to interfere with sleep. Nowadays, bursas are treated by placing a needle in the sac to remove excess fluid. Heat and rest are used to permit absorption of the excess fluid. The application of X-ray has been helpful. Most recent is the injection of hydrocortisone directly into the bursa, to lessen the inflammation and relieve pain.

C

CACHEXIA Weakness and emaciation caused by a serious disease.

CAFFEINE A primary ingredient of coffee, tea and cola drinks which has a stimulating effect on the body as a whole and which can increase the flow of urine. It stimulates the mind also.

CALAMINE Calamine is a mixture of zinc oxide with a small amount of ferric or iron oxide. It occurs as a pink powder and is used, mixed with water, glycerin or other substances, in the treatment of skin diseases. (*See also* CHAPTER XXIII.)

CALCIUM A substance which is the main ingredient of bones, and which acts chemically in the human body to diminish spasmodic irritations. It is necessary in the growth of bones and teeth and of the blood. It may be immobilized in the body

by vitamin D. Calcium combined with many other chemicals is used for various conditions. (*See also* CHAPTERS XV, XVII.)

CALCULUS A stony formation or one made principally of calcium is called a calculus. Such stones can occur anywhere in the body but particularly in the gall bladder, the kidneys, and in nodules such as occur under the skin in the ear or around the jaw. (*See also* BLADDER DISEASES; *and also* CHAPTER VIII.)

CALLUS Any area of hardened and thickened skin, usually on the palm of the hand or the sole of the foot, is a callus. Calluses are formed by thickening of the upper layers of the skin in response to pressure and friction. Special files have been developed for removing calluses. They should not be torn away or cut away except by an expert. Sometimes changing the weight-bearing area of the foot will stop the formation of calluses.

The term callus is also used to describe the formation of new tissue when a bone heals after a fracture. (*See also* FEET; *and also* CHAPTER XXVIII.)

CALOMEL This is a compound of mercury that was formerly much used as a cathartic and laxative. The product has fallen into disuse in the face of new discoveries in this field which are far more preferable. (*See also* CONSTIPATION.)

CALORIES The energy intake of the body is measured by calories. The usual calorie is the amount of heat required to raise one cubic centimeter of water one degree centigrade. The average person uses approximately 2,500 to 3,000 calories daily in food. The overweight should use under 1,200 calories daily in order to lose weight. Tables are available showing the number of calories in an ordinary portion of all common foodstuffs. (*See also* WEIGHT, OVER- AND UNDER-; *and also* CHAPTER XIV.)

CAMPHOR A drug used in preparations designed to stop inflammation of the mucous membranes and the skin. Occasionally, camphor is injected to stimulate the circulation of the blood.

CANCER Any malignant growth. Other names for cancer are *car-cin*oma, *sarc*oma; and occasionally there are special types of cancer such as *epitheli*oma. The term "oma" is used to refer to a new growth. Cancer is also referred to by the term neoplasm, which means new growth. Occasionally, cancers are called malignancies, because of their malignant growth character. The exact causes which initiate the sudden, rapid growth of cells and their migration into other parts of the body are not known. We know that irritation from broken teeth or the constant heat and pressure associated with smoking, particularly of pipes, may start the cancer on the mouth or lip. Irritations anywhere in the body may start a cancer. Early recognition of cancer is of utmost importance. Any sore on the mouth of more than two days' duration should be regarded with suspicion. Hoarseness which lasts more than a few days should arouse suspicion

of some chronic condition affecting the vocal cords.

Any discomfort, pain, thickening or lump in the breast of a man or woman or any discharge from the nipple, particularly a bloody discharge, should mean an immediate examination.

Difficulty in swallowing, loss of appetite, constant discomfort, nausea, diarrhea or the appearance of blood in the bowel movement should demand thorough investigation, including study with the X-ray.

Persistent pain in the bones in people of any age means either a serious infection or a growth. Immediate use of the X-ray will help determine the nature of the trouble.

Slight bleeding at irregular intervals from the female sex organs is a dangerous sign. Every woman beyond the age of 35 should have an examination once every year by the doctor to determine whether or not any changes have occurred. The Papanicolaou or "Pap" test involves taking a scraping from the cervix or mouth of the uterus and examining under the microscope.

Many new developments have been made in detecting cancer and in treating it. Still of primary importance are the application of surgery, X-ray and radium. For cancers related to the blood, such as leukemia, new drugs have been found which can reduce the number of white blood cells. New types of irradiation involving the cobalt bomb and high voltage have been applied for special forms of cancer.

Cancer of the brain is diagnosed by the neurologist, and special radioactive dye substances have been found which localize in cancer tissue.

Radioactive isotopes are being used in the treatment of cancer, including isotopes of gold and strontium, and radioactive iodine is used in treating cancer of the thyroid.

Discoveries have been made relating to control of cancer, particularly of the breast and of the prostate, by hormone substances. The male sex hormone is used in cancer of the breast and the female sex hormone in cancer of the prostate gland.

A new operative procedure has been tried, consisting of the removal of the adrenal glands and also removal of the pituitary gland, to control rapidly growing cancers.

Cancerophobia, the morbid fear of acquiring a cancer, is not unwarranted. (*See also* CHAPTER XXIV.)

CANKER Canker sores are ulcerations and blisters in the mouth and lips, usually associated with sensitivity to various food substances. Occasionally blisters form from slight irritation, particularly in persons with conditions affecting the blood. These sores tend to heal promptly. When they persist and ulcerate, studies should be made by allergists, and examination of the blood should be made to determine the presence of proper numbers of blood cells.

CAPILLARIES These are the smallest terminations of the blood vessels in the skin and elsewhere in the body. When they are fragile and break easily, the person bruises readily.

CARBOHYDRATE The compounds like sugars, dextrins, starches and celluloses are classified as carbohydrates. They are important in developing energy for the human body. However, they are not quite as significant as proteins in health and growth. (*See also* CHAPTER XIV.)

CARBON MONOXIDE POISONING Carbon monoxide is a gas which is one of the most important toxic ingredients of illuminating gas and of automobile exhaust gas. This gas is odorless and colorless. In the blood it unites with red coloring matter and prevents the carrying of oxygen. A person who has been poisoned by carbon monoxide should be put immediately at rest and given inhalations of oxygen with carbon dioxide, which stimulates breathing and replaces the damaged blood about four times as rapidly as would the inhalation of air. A person with serious carbon monoxide poisoning should be taken at once to a hospital, where proper medication and blood transfusions may be used. (*See also* CHAPTER XVIII.)

CARBUNCLE (*See* BOILS.)

CARCINOMA (*See* CANCER.)

CARDIAC Related to the heart. (*See also* HEART.)

CARDIAC ARREST Complete standstill of the heartbeat, requiring prompt resuscitation.

CARRIERS OF DISEASE Much confusion exists between what is contagious and what is infectious. For all practical purposes any disease spread by germs is either contagious or infectious. A better term is communicable disease, which means that it can be passed from one person to another.

When a person has disease germs in his body, as in the nose, throat, skin or interior of the body and can pass these germs on to other persons, he is known as a disease carrier. People may become infected from contact with germs that come from secretions or excretions from any portion of the body. Sometimes animals are carriers of disease, including cats, dogs, birds and other pets. (*See also* CHAPTER XXII.)

CASCARA This substance has been used as a laxative for habitual constipation, usually prescribed as an aromatic extract of cascara. Although widely used in the past, this laxative has been replaced by other more modern methods, including regulation of the diet and various new drugs.

CASTOR OIL An oil obtained from the seed of a plant known as the castor plant, is a strong cathartic. (*See also* CATHARTICS AND LAXATIVES; CONSTIPATION.)

CATARACT When the lens of the eye becomes opaque, so that light does not pass through, the condition is called cataract. This usually affects people between fifty and sixty years of age but does occur occasionally in young people. All sorts of quack treatments have been offered. The operation is now done by ophthalmologic surgeons or eye surgeons, with great success in the vast majority of cases. When a cataract is removed, the effect is the same as the defrosting of a window or the removing of a shade that prevents the passing of light. After a cataract

is removed, suitable glasses are provided, which will yield good vision. (*See also* EYE; *and also* CHAPTER XXV.)

CATARRH The word catarrh is an old word meaning a flow. Therefore any condition in which there was an excess of mucus or fluid was called a catarrh—of the nose, of the stomach or of the bowel. The term no longer has any standing in scientific medicine. (*See also* COLDS; RHINITIS.)

CATHARTICS AND LAXATIVES Modern methods of controlling difficulty of elimination from the bowel involve study to determine the cause and a regulation of the hygiene and diet to make such drugs, if possible, unnecessary. Mildest among modern cathartics is mineral oil. Also much used are substances to provide bulk, such as agar and cellulose. Among the laxatives now widely popular is phenolphthalein. These laxatives are taken in combination with controlled diets so as to establish regularity. (*See also* CONSTIPATION; *and also* CHAPTER VII.)

CECUM The large portion of the large bowel occupying the position in the lower third of the abdomen on the right side. From the cecum the appendix juts off.

CELIAC DISEASE A chronic disturbance of nutrition, which is seen most often in children two to three years old, characterized by a distended abdomen, diarrhea, and eliminations of large amounts of frothy, vile-smelling material from the

291

bowel. Recently the condition has been determined to be associated with sensitivity to certain food products, and related to that is a difficulty which keeps the child from digesting and using properly starches and fats. Elimination from the diet of the food substances which cause the trouble, principally wheat products, brings about relief from the disease. For a while it was thought that bananas had a specific effect but this is now recognized to be the substitution of the banana for the offending food. During celiac disease, the baby must avoid butter, creams, fats, fried foods and pastries.

CELLULITIS This term is used in reference to deep inflammation or infection of fibrous tissue just under the outer skin. It may, however, refer to connective tissue elsewhere in the body.

CEREBELLUM The lower portion of the brain at the back, chiefly concerned with the co-ordination of movements. (*See also* BRAIN.)

CEREBRAL EMBOLISM Blocking of an artery in the brain by some substance in the circulation, frequently a small blood clot.

CEREBRAL PALSY A condition which results from a defect in the brain usually following a hemorrhage during childbirth and is a situation that is not amenable to any kind of radical cure. Such children are helped by training, by orthopedic surgery and by psychological studies leading to making the most of what they have. When cerebral palsy is accompanied by deviations, defects of sensation, or convulsions, procedures are necessary to overcome these difficulties. Sometimes during growth developmental changes take place which lead to improvement in the capacity of the child. This improvement is sometimes erroneously ascribed to the treatment that happens to be given at the time. Careful study of each case enables the physician to know what are the primary disturbances and to determine what is best done for improvement.

Psychiatrists have discovered that the motor defects which such children have influence their entire personality and development. Such children become objects of anxiety rather than joy to their parents. As a result the children fail to learn many of the things which other children do. They hear language about them referring to things or actions which they have never seen or experienced and thus their development is hindered. Defects of hearing may be found; visual defects, ability to feel or perceive may be greatly hampered, and all of this interferes with development. However, much help can be given when these conditions are determined. The authorities believe that long-time planning for cerebral palsy must change from exclusive emphasis on defects of motion to greater consideration of what can be accomplished by training and to greater interest in supplying emotional and sensory experiences out of which stability and knowledge may arise. Direct operation on the brain is not recommended except for intolerable convulsions. Neither does any drug treatment seem to be useful except for control of convulsions.

CEREBRUM The brain, particularly the large portion of the front of the brain which is divided into two parts or hemispheres. The term cerebral hemorrhage means a stroke or bleeding into the brain. (*See also* BRAIN.)

CERVICITIS Inflammation of the lower portion of the uterus which is the neck of the uterus.

CERVIX Cervix means the neck. The term can also be used to refer to the cervix of the uterus, which is the lower portion at the front that projects into the vagina.

CESAREAN OPERATION Whenever it becomes necessary, because of a difficult childbirth, to open the abdomen and the uterus, the operation is called the Cesarean operation. Modifications of the operation are also known, in which the operation is done from below. With the development of new forms of anesthesia, new techniques for controlling hemorrhage and infection, and the use of the X-ray to determine the position of the child, the operation has a high degree of safety, when done in a proper hospital by a qualified gynecologist, obstetrician or surgeon.

CHAFING Irritation of the skin by rubbing is called chafing. The inflammation that results from contact of two surfaces of the skin which rub together, as between the thighs, under the breasts, between the buttocks, and in the folds of the skin of people who are very fat, can be irritating and can result in secondary infections. The scientific name is *erythema intertrigo*. The condition is prevented by methods which keep the surfaces from rubbing together. Proper supports for the breasts and the use of underwear that intervenes between the skin folds may be useful. The skin may be protected by powders and other medicaments, which the doctor may prescribe after observing the condition of the skin.

CHANCRE The chancre is the sore which appears as the first sign of syphilis. Another infection also causes a form of chancre not due to syphilis. Any suspected sore should be carefully examined by the doctor with the apparatus and techniques available, to determine its exact character. (*See also* SYPHILIS; *and also* CHAPTER XXVII.)

CHAPPING The skin responds to physical irritation by dry air, cold air and lack of proper moisture with an irritated condition called chapping. Lack of sufficient fat from the skin secretions will also contribute to producing this condition. When skin is chapped, soap and water should be used in great moderation. Caustic soaps are irritating and should not be used on chapped skin. Cold cream or other ointments may be put on thickly at night and allowed to remain on the skin. These help to take the place of missing fat. Humidity of the air indoors may increase in winter. Gloves should be worn for chapped hands. If the skin breaks or becomes infected, special attention will be required.

CHICKEN POX One of the most contagious of infectious diseases, chicken pox, begins twelve to fourteen days or fourteen to sixteen days after contact with another case of the disease. The cause is a virus. Most cases occur in children from five to fifteen years old. The only known way to aid prevention is to keep the child away from others who have chicken pox. Blisters usually appear in groups. The only treatment necessary is to make certain that the blisters are not broken and infected. The child should have the fingernails cut short to keep him from damaging the skin by scratching. After a few hours the blisters break, dry and form crusts. The crusts disappear in from two to four days. Chicken pox leaves few scars unless the spots become secondarily infected. (*See also* CHAPTER XXII.)

CHIGGERS Insect mites whose bite causes inflammatory lesions that itch. Red blotches appear, and blisters form. Infestation can be prevented by putting flour of sulphur on the stockings and underclothing when going into tall grass or weeds. If seriously bitten, wash the skin thoroughly with soap and water and allow some of the lather to remain on the skin about ten minutes. Then apply any of the well-known preparations for insect bites or itching. Sometimes antihistamine ointments are helpful. A mixture of one per cent menthol with calamine lotion will control the itching. (*See also* CHAPTER XXIX.)

CHILBLAINS Poor circulation in the skin and exposure to cold brings on painful redness and swelling called chilblains. The spots are bluish red. Proper warmth and protection will prevent chilblains. Those with a tend-

ency to react to cold should wear woolen socks in cold weather and keep the hands warm by the use of gloves. In treatment, paraffin-wax baths are useful. Bathing in warm water is helpful. (*See also* CHAPTER XIX.)

CHILLS A sensation of cold accompanied by shivering is the form in which many infectious diseases begin. Chills, are, however, especially likely to appear in malaria. Actually, a chill is the reaction of the body to cold; the shivering produces heat. One of the methods of controlling chills is to apply heat, with blankets, warm bedclothing, hot-water bottles and electric pads.

CHIROPRACTIC This is a method of healing which aims at restoring health by finding misplaced bones in the spine and adjusting them by hand. Many states license chiropractors for this special method, and chiropractors in many places endeavor to use all the different methods of healing, including drugs.

CHLOASMA Deposits of pigment in the skin may occur in patches of various sizes and shapes colored yellow, brown or black. They are frequently called liver spots. New drugs have been discovered for bringing about removal of pigment from the skin. Among them is benoquin. The drugs are potent and should be used only under medical control.

CHLORAL A chemical substance which has a profound effect in producing unconsciousness. Chloral has been the basis of knockout drops. (*See also* ANESTHESIA.)

CHLOROSIS This condition has been popularly called green sickness. It is a form of secondary anemia which has practically disappeared among the young women now who live an outdoor life and have adequate nutrition.

CHOLECYSTITIS AND CHOLE-LITHIASIS Diseases of the gall bladder, a pear-shaped sac located on the lower side of the liver, from which tubes carry the bile which has come to the gall bladder from the liver. The gall bladder stores the bile and concentrates it. Anything that blocks the tubes will cause symptoms of obstruction, with pain. Infection may also attack the gall bladder. Gallstones form in the bile, and quite often block the tubes. The person with gallstones is usually said to be a woman who is fair, fat and forty years old.

Inflammation of the gall bladder is accompanied by severe pain and rigidity of the upper part of the abdomen on the right side. Jaundice may occur from absorption of bile into the blood. Severe attacks demand surgical operation, with removal of the gall bladder. These operations are not considered dangerous under modern conditions, with good surgery and the use of antibiotic drugs.

Gallstones are detected by the use of dye substances such as iodophthalein, which when taken into the body either by mouth or by injection goes to the liver and is passed with the bile into the gall bladder. Then an X-ray picture will show the presence of the stones in the gall bladder.

The symptoms of gall bladder disease and inflammation with or without gallstones include a sense of fullness, which comes on usually after eating and is worse when greasy or fatty foods are eaten. Associated with the sense of fullness may be a dull aching pain below the ribs, aggravated by stooping over. Heartburn is quite common in such conditions. Jaundice is not necessarily a symptom unless there is blocking of the flow of bile. Many people live for years and have rather good health with chronic diseases of the gall bladder—particularly if they avoid large meals and heavy or fatty foods. But the threat of a serious complication is always present. (*See also* GALL; GALLSTONES; JAUNDICE; *and also* CHAPTER VII.)

CHOLERA This is a serious intestinal disease which occurs principally in the tropics, where sanitation is poor and water and other food materials are constantly contaminated. Characteristics include severe diarrhea, vomiting, collapse, muscular cramps and suppression of urine. Cholera is an exceedingly serious disease. People who are going to travel in the Orient, particularly in India, should be vaccinated against cholera. Protection lasts for some months.

CHOLESTEROL A constituent of all animal fats and oils and of egg yolk. It has been related to the occurrence of hardening of the arteries.

CHOREA In this condition, unusual twitching movements occur which have caused the condition to be called St. Vitus' dance. The condition is now definitely related to streptococcal infections and to rheumatic fever. Girls suffer with chorea about twice as often as do boys. Almost all of the cases occur in childhood. Frequently the condition begins with a streptococcus sore throat, with headache, vomiting and fever. Certainly any child with a streptococcus infection should have careful study and attention. Nowadays the sulfonamide drugs and penicillin, used promptly in cases of streptococcal infections of the throat, have greatly diminished the incidence of chorea.

CHOREA, HUNTINGTON'S A hereditary condition called chronic, progressive hereditary chorea syndrome, which develops principally in people between 30 and 45 years of age who have involuntary dancelike motions. Any child in a family in which the condition has occurred has a one-in-two chance of having it. About 100 cases appeared in a family in Minnesota, all descendants of one man who had it in 1831. No specific treatment is known.

CIRCUMCISION Cutting the foreskin from the male sex organ; a procedure originally established as a religious rite among Jews, Mohammedans and South Sea Islanders. The operation is also performed as a preventive operation against infection. Inflammation and irritation under the foreskin not infrequently create illnesses among little boys. The operation of circumcision is frequently done with a local anesthetic. It can, however, be done as any other surgical operation, with anesthesia and with the strictest surgical precautions.

CIRRHOSIS This means hardening

of any tissue, but mostly refers to hardening of the liver, called cirrhosis of the liver. The condition has been associated with excessive use of alcohol but is now believed more likely to be related to a deficiency of thiamin which not infrequently occurs in alcoholics. The condition may follow also hepatitis or inflammation of the liver. The treatment involves also the use of large doses of protein substances in the form of amino acids. (*See also* LIVER.)

CLAUDICATION Cramplike pain and weaknesses in the legs, particularly in the calves, is associated with conditions like Buerger's disease; also with inflammation of the blood vessels. The condition has been associated with smoking, and with hardening of the arteries.

CLEFT PALATE A child is sometimes born in whom the tissues of the head have not come properly together, so that there is an opening in the palate or the roof of the mouth. If the lips have failed to come together, the condition is called harelip. If surgical operation does not bring the separated parts sufficiently close together special apparatus is available to aid in holding a covering over the opening; and persons are taught to speak properly regardless of the defect.

CLIMACTERIC As the person passes from middle age to old age, the functions of the body change often as radically as they do at puberty. The term climacteric has come to be synonymous with the menopause, and nowadays men are supposed to suffer similar symptoms when the activities of the sex glands become weak or disappear. (*See also* MENOPAUSE.)

CLUBFOOT Children are sometimes born with twisted feet. If detected sufficiently soon, by repeated manipulations and the application of suitable bandages, the foot can be held properly in place until it assumes a normal appearance. The exact cause of such distortion is not known.

COBALT This metallic substance was detected many years ago, and was recognized as a constituent of substances which produced blue colors. Its salts were known to be irritant and capable of producing an emetic effect. Now cobalt is recognized as a fundamental constituent of vitamin B_{12}. It is also important in the making of cobalt bombs with radioactivity of great power.

COCAINE A drug which has tremendous stimulant effects, and when applied to mucous membranes, has a pain-controlling effect. It produces addiction and is never used nowadays unless in the related forms of procaine, for local anesthesia. (*See also* ANESTHESIA.)

COCCIDIOSIS A respiratory disease, with occasional overgrowth of tissue, produced by a parisitic organism which gets into the tissues by inhalation. It occurs particularly in the Far West. So frequent was it in one area in California, that it became known as San Joaquin Valley fever.

COCCYX The small bone at the

lowermost extent of the spine. Frequently this bone becomes bruised or broken by falls.

COD-LIVER OIL An oil derived from the liver of the codfish, rich in vitamins A and D, and given to babies chiefly to prevent and to cure rickets. Through the preventive use of this oil and related products of vitamins A and D such as halibut-liver oil and percomorph, rickets is becoming a rare and seldom-seen disease. (*See also* VITAMINS; *and also* CHAPTER XVI.)

COFFEE Coffee has long been used as a stimulating and pleasant drink. A cup of coffee made with a tablespoonful of coffee contains from one and one half to three grains of caffeine, a drug which stimulates the nervous system. People who have used coffee regularly seldom get overstimulated. Some people claim that coffee interferes with sleep. For them, coffees are available which have had the caffeine greatly reduced or well-nigh eliminated. Caffeine appears also in tea, and similar substances in cocoa.

COITUS The scientific term used, among others, for sexual intercourse.

COLCHICINE A drug derived from a plant, which has a specific action against gout. (*See also* GOUT.)

COLDS A highly contagious condition now believed to be due to viruses associated with other common germs. Colds are most prevalent in the United States during midwinter, early spring and early fall. Some people have more colds than do others. The methods of building resistance against colds frequently advocated, which include the taking of vitamins, of citrus drinks, of various drugs and of vaccines, have all proved without any real merit. A cold itself does not immunize or build resistance to such infections for more than a short time. Avoidance of exposure to colds includes washing the hands before eating, and avoiding direct contact with people who have colds. Once the cold has developed, relief is secured more promptly by rest and by taking care of the ordinary symptoms as they develop. Certain drugs have good effects in reducing the fever, the running of the nose and similar symptoms. Combinations are available which include pain relievers like aspirin and phenacetin, antiallergic drugs like the antihistamines, and preparations for the nose which may contain ephedrine or other drugs which contract the blood vessels and the mucous membranes. The antibiotic drugs sometimes applied are useful, not against the cold itself but against the secondary infecting organisms. (*See also* CHAPTER XXII.)

COLD SORES A common name for *herpes simplex* or fever blisters. New drugs have been found which are specific against herpes of the eye and the lips.

COLIC This refers to an acute pain in the abdomen due to a variety of causes. Cramps is the common public name for it. With babies, the cause is sometimes the swallowing of air by rapid eating. In adults, colic may be associated with a stone caught in

a tube like the gall ducts or the ureters from the kidneys. Occasionally the pain of colic is related to infections, with the salmonella or staphylococci that produce food poisoning. A special form of colic related to the bowel is associated with spasm of the muscles of the bowel. Obviously, repeated attacks of severe colic demand medical study, including the use of X-rays as to the motility of the bowel and the extent to which an actual cramping or spasm of the bowel muscles occurs.

COLITIS An inflammation of the large bowel. The human bowel is a long tube which begins immediately following the stomach and continues some thirty to thirty-two feet to its lower end. The food passes along the bowel and materials are absorbed from the bowel. The waste matter, or indigestible residue, passes along until it is eliminated. It may be accompanied by the secretion of large amounts of mucus, occasionally by an actual infection; sometimes the condition would appear to be purely psychosomatic. Diets have been prescribed for patients with this condition. The diets vary according to the nature of the colitis. Enemas which produce washing of the bowel may be as harmful as they are helpful, and should be tried only with the recommendation of the doctor. (*See also* CHAPTERS VII, XIV.)

COLOR BLINDNESS The inability to detect red from green, yellow from blue, or similar color difficulties; it is a fairly common condition, often inherited. The condition is more common among boys than among girls. No specific cure for it is known. Obviously, color blindness may bar a person from the Army, Navy or the Air Force.

COMA A complete loss of consciousness, from which the person cannot be aroused even by powerful stimulation. Coma may be associated with alcoholic intoxication or with diabetes. (*See also* CHAPTER III.)

COMEDONES The scientific name for blackheads. (*See* ACNE; *see also* CHAPTER XXIII.)

COMEDONES The scientific name of the conjunctiva, the lining of the eyelid and the covering of the eyeball. Symptoms include burning and smarting of the eyelids, formation of pus, and reddened eyelids.

Pink eye is a common type of conjunctivitis, caused by germs frequently spread by the use of the common towel. The eyes may also be inflamed with strong chemical substances. In allergic conditions, sensitivity of the eye may cause an inflammatory response which will affect the conjunctiva. To prevent inflammatory conditions, never use towels to wipe the eyes which have been used by other people. Such conditions nowadays are frequently controlled by antibiotic solutions and ointments. (*See also* EYE; *and also* CHAPTER XXV.)

CONSTIPATION Failure to excrete the residue from food after forty-eight hours. Failure to have one bowel movement a day is not necessarily constipation. Normal babies have three or four actions of the bowels in twenty-four hours.

Most modern physicians treat constipation by diets including stewed fruits, the taking of plenty of water, and other control of food. Constipation may result simply from bad habits of attention to this necessary function of elimination. Older people may develop constipation through gradual breakdown of the tissues involved in moving the bowels. For people who have not become too severely addicted to bad habits, a good mixed diet with proper proteins, carbohydrates, minerals and fats, as well as vitamins and enough indigestible residue, will provide regular action of the bowel.

Among the drugs most commonly used to stir action are saline and vegetable cathartics, organic and mineral preparations, mechanically-acting substances, and water. Strong salts cause a pulling of fluid into the bowel and may produce inflammation. The vegetable cathartics like cascara, senna, rhubarb and jalap act by irritating the lining of the bowel, which makes it empty itself. The mechanically-acting substances include mineral oil or liquid petrolatum, agar, psyllium seeds, flax seeds, bran and cellulose. Other substances frequently used are based on phenolphthalein, which is known to be an inert chemical substance with a specific action in causing motion of the bowel. (*See also* CATHARTICS AND LAXATIVES; *and also* CHAPTER VII.)

CONTACT LENSES For actors, public speakers, and others who may be concerned with sports, eyeglasses can be provided which consist of a lens put under the eyelid in contact with the eye. These are contact lenses.

CONTRACEPTION This term is used for birth control. Methods consist of devices which retain the male sperm or the female egg cell and prevent contact. Also there is the natural method, which depends on the fact that the female ovum is ordinarily available for contact with the male sperm over a period of from forty-eight to seventy-two hours, this so-called "safe" period can be determined by a variety of techniques. Finally, there are substances in the form of suppositories, creams and solutions which destroy the male sperm when it enters the female canal.

CONVALESCENCE This is the period following an acute disease, during which the person is recovering. Convalescence should be guided by the doctor exactly as the care of the patient is guided during illness. The regulation of diet, exercise and rest and the going back to work is a matter for the doctor to determine. The patient who has been long in bed should not try to get up all at once, but gradually over a period of a few days.

CONVULSIONS In ordinary convulsions, consciousness is lost, and there may be rigidity associated with spasmodic jerking of the face, the arms and the legs. Epileptic convulsions are of a special type. Important is prompt determination of the cause of the convulsions. Sometimes acute inflammations of the brain following infectious diseases like measles may be responsible. Warmth

is sedative and a hot bath is often used to control mild convulsions. A baby may be wrapped in blankets and kept warm.

Parents have found that convulsions are sometimes associated with specific foods or with constipation. Parents have felt that convulsions might be concomitant of teething. However, these have not been definitely established as common causes of convulsions. A deficiency of calcium in the body produces a type of convulsive disorder called "tetany," which is controlled by calcium and vitamin D. (*See also* CHAPTER III.)

CORNS Corns, like calluses, are horny thickenings of portions of the feet. They may be removed by cutting, or softened by the application of mild salicylic acid, or prevented by changes in shoes and stockings and by removing the cause of rubbing and changing the weight-bearing areas of the feet. (*See also* FEET; *and also* CHAPTER XXVIII.)

CORONARY THROMBOSIS A blocking of the blood vessels known as the coronary arteries, which supply the heart with blood. (*See also* HEART; *and also* CHAPTER VI.)

CORTISONE A hormone secreted by the adrenal glands which also secrete a number of other hormones including adrenalin, desoxycorticosterone, and perhaps many others not yet isolated. Cortisone is now available in several forms, of which the latest is called prednisone which comes as Meticorten, Sterane, Deltra, etc. The primary action of the Cortisone is against inflammation. Another hormone called aldosterone modifies water and salt balance in the body.

CORYZA A term sometimes used to describe head colds.

COUGHING Coughing is not a disease but a symptom of irritation in the breathing tract of the body or interference with the free passing of air in and out of the lungs. Coughing may be due to foreign substances like fishbones or feathers or hairs which have gotten into the breathing tract. Perhaps coughing is due to a collection of dust or broken-down tissue or mucus in the breathing passages. The cough serves the purpose of removing the secretions or the obstructing materials and removing infectious germs at the same time. Certain diseases are especially likely to produce coughing, particularly whooping cough. Whooping cough may develop a habit of coughing which will persist. If any obstruction is detected, it of course must be removed or suitably controlled. The inhalation of steam loosens secretions so that they can be coughed out.

Because of the danger of coughing, one of the means of spreading disease, health officers recommend that people wear gauze face masks in times of epidemic, to stop the spread of infectious material by coughing. (*See also* BREATHING AND BRONCHIECTASIS; WHOOPING COUGH; *and also* CHAPTERS III, XXII.)

CRAMPS (*See* COLIC; COLITIS.)

CROSS-EYES Strabismus is the scientific name given to this condition in which the two eyes do not focus on the same point. This is frequently due to the presence of lengthened, relaxed or weak muscles. Every case should have careful study by a specialist, since crossed eyes can be controlled early, sometimes by the prescription of proper lenses, sometimes with the aid of suitable exercises for strengthening muscles, and almost certainly in every case by an appropriate surgical procedure. (*See also* CHAPTER XXV.)

CROUP A harsh brassy cough, with difficult breathing and a crowing sound occurring in children. This is usually due to an inflammation and swelling of the membranes of the throat and may occur with streptococcus sore throat, with diphtheria, or with other infections in the larynx. Important is the distinction between croup as a symptom and actually infection with germs like the streptococci or diphtheria. The inhalation of steam, medicated sometimes with balsam or tincture of benzoin, relieves the inflammation so that the croup disappears. (*See also* CHAPTERS XXI, XXVI.)

CRYING Crying is natural to babies, and even weak premature babies will moan with a low feeble whine that sounds like the mewing of a cat. The baby uses crying to show anger or fear. It is the voicing of an emotional reaction.

Crying can help to ventilate the baby's lungs by forcing out air and replacing it with fresh air which is drawn in by the deep breathing associated with crying.

Some children cry more often than others; some of them develop the practice of holding the breath

301

until they get attention. Children cry because they are not comfortable, as, for instance, when the sharp end of a pin penetrates the skin. Children are not comfortable in winter if they become wet and cold in bed. If they are uncomfortable because of digestive disturbances or cramps, they will cry. When a baby cries, remember that it may be from hunger, from extremes of temperature, from colic or other pains or from fear. Children particularly fear loud noises, such as doors slamming and pans banging. When the baby is angry, it will stiffen its body and cry aloud. Anger may follow the too-tight wrapping of the baby in clothing. Study the baby, and if you can detect the cause of the crying and eliminate it everyone, including the baby, will be more happy.

CYANOSIS When the skin looks blue, it is said to be cyanotic, from the Greek word meaning "blue." The chief cause of cyanosis is a lack of oxygen in the blood. This may result from insufficient air coming into the lungs, a weakness of the heart which prevents the forcing of the blood through the lungs, sometimes from poisoning by illuminating gas or automobile exhaust gas. In some cases of congenital heart disease the heart is wrongly constructed, so that the blood passes directly from the veins to the arteries without circulating through the lungs. These blue babies are now cured by a suitable surgical operation. (*See also* HEART; *and also* CHAPTERS IV, VI.)

CYST Any sac or small cavity in the body which contains fluid surrounded by a bag of tissue. Cysts

may occur wherever there are glands that secrete fluid, particularly when the outlet or normal emptying spot for the gland is blocked.

CYSTOSCOPY Examination of the interior of the human urinary bladder by looking through a special instrument with reflected light. (*See also* BLADDER DISEASES.)

D

DANDRUFF Dandruff results from a condition called *seborrheic dermatitis*. This is the most common of all skin diseases. The dandruff may be drying and scaly or moist and greasy, depending on the amount of oil secreted from the oil glands. Suggestion has been made that this condition is controllable by eliminating or limiting fats in the diet, although this is doubtful. Thorough washing of the scalp will remove dandruff which, however, usually returns. Various antiseptic substances have been tried. More recently a derivative of the chemical called selenium has been developed into a drug product called Selsun which seems to have the specific power of controlling dandruff. Many of the common treatments used in barber and beauty shops for the control of dandruff depend on the presence of alcohol and salicylic acid. (*See also* HAIR.)

DEAFNESS Loss or impairment of the sense of hearing. Within the internal ear is a special mechanism which picks up vibrations from the eardrum and transmits them to the small bones in contact with the eardrum which is in the middle ear to the hearing mechanism in the internal ear. Any infection that destroys tissues or inflames any portion of this mechanism will produce hardness of hearing. Most dangerous are the infectious diseases like measles, meningitis, scarlet fever, and the streptococcus infections, also the infections of the adenoids and tonsils, colds in the head and sinuses.

From the throat or back of the nose there passes to the ear a tube known as the Eustachian tube. This is also concerned with good hearing. Inflammation or blocking of the Eustachian tube will interfere with hearing.

Deafness or impaired hearing may result from accidents like a blow on the head, from rupture of the eardrum, from a foreign substance getting into the ear and blocking the transmission of sound to the eardrum. Certain diseases definitely damage the nerve that is responsible for conveying stimulation from the internal ear to the brain. Damage to this nerve will produce permanent deafness. As people grow older, there sometimes comes on a condition of progressive loss of hearing, which may be due to inflammations that harden the connections between the tissues involved in hearing. This disease is called otosclerosis.

Devices have been invented for measuring loss of hearing and helping the doctor to detect the nature of the condition responsible. Nowadays hearing aids have been developed of two types—those which act by air conduction and those which act by bone conduction. The specialist can determine the nature of the loss of hearing and thus prescribe the device best suited to the condition.

In a new operation called fenestration, a window is made into the internal ear, and by this technic many cases of what seemed to be permanent deafness have been cured. (*See also* EAR; OTOSCLEROSIS; *and also* CHAPTER XXVI.)

DEBILITY A term like biliousness, which simply refers to general weakness without a specific cause.

DEFECATION The act of evacuating the bowel.

DEGENERATION A term used to describe the deterioration and breaking-down of the tissues which usually comes on with increasing years. It may assume various forms and attack various tissues. (*See also* CHAPTER X.)

DELIRIUM TREMENS People who have been long addicted to alcohol and who are suddenly deprived of it may develop disturbances of the nervous system which are represented by the disease delirium tremens. An ordinary case lasts from two to ten days, during which time the victim displays disorientation as to time and place, great fear, disturbances of vision and hearing, sensations of pain, and crawling sensations on the skin. This condition is controlled by the use of sedative drugs and the administration of the vitamin B complex, including, particularly, nicotinic acid. In some cases of delirium tremens, Cortisone products have seemed to be especially helpful.

DENGUE A tropical disease caused by a virus; also known as breakbone fever. Its symptoms include backache and prostration, with high fever, painful joints, sometimes a rash, and frequently enlargement of the glands. The condition is carried by infected mosquitoes.

DENTIFRICES At least fifty different mouth washes are available, containing various antiseptic substances, flavorings, colorings, and other materials. People who like a mouth wash can select according to their taste either peppermint, lemon or orange flavors. Most mouth washes and gargles are not exceedingly effective, because potent antibiotics and antiseptics are not usually permissible in mouth washes.

DEPILATORIES Any substances that will remove hair. There are chemicals that dissolve hair; waxes that are put on, allowed to harden and then pulled off; the X-ray may be used to remove hair; certain glandular substances may be used as antagonists to glands that cause an excess growth of hair.

DERMATITIS An inflammation of the skin.

DESENSITIZATION A method of producing resistance to allergy by injection of gradually increasing doses of the substance to which the person is sensitive. (*See also* AL-LERGY; PATCH TEST; *and also* CHAPTER XII.)

DEXTROSE A form of sugar prepared by the digestion of starch. Dextrose is an essential constituent of the blood and supplies energy to the body, entering also into the metabolism of fats. The glycogen which is stored in the liver is manufactured from the dextrose brought by the blood. Dextrose, used as a solution, is administered by injection into the veins to combat shock and for its food value. The product is often called glucose.

DIABETES The word diabetes comes from a Greek word meaning fountain, so-named because the striking symptom of the disease is the pouring from the body of considerable amounts of urine containing sugar. Diabetes is not infectious. To some extent it is inherited, but it is a recessive and tends to breed out of the family. If a person with diabetes marries one who does not have the disease and whose family shows no record of the disease, there is no reason to expect that the children will have diabetes. If two people who are diabetic marry and their histories show a considerable number of cases among the ancestors, it is quite likely that their children will have this disease. Nowadays, a diabetic person who follows instructions as to hygiene and who is in contact with a physician who controls his diet and the use of insulin, can have a normal life expectancy. He must, however, avoid overeating, avoid infections, test the urine for sugar frequently (at least twice a week) to make sure that the status of the disease is not progressing and take the necessary measures to avoid acidosis or coma. New drugs have been discovered which, taken by mouth, will lower blood sugar.

Juvenile diabetes was once invariably fatal. Children now have a normal life expectancy, with proper treatment. (*See also* CHAPTER XVI.)

DIABETES INSIPIDUS A condition due to a disorder of a structure of the brain called the hypothalamus. This is characterized by the passing of large quantities of dilute urine, and is associated with intense thirst and dehydration. Patients are relieved by taking extracts of the posterior pituitary lobe. (*See also* CHAPTER XVI.)

DIAPER RASH (*See* CHAFING.)

DIAPHRAGM The large muscle between the abdominal chest cavity is known as the diaphragm. It is essential to normal breathing. Inflammation of the muscle of the diaphragm may constitute a serious symptom which shortens the breath, causes pain, pressure over the lower part of the chest, and hiccups. Paralysis of the diaphragm, due to injury of its nerves, is a serious condition.

By use of the X-ray, rupture of the tissues through the diaphragm with pinching, known as *diaphragmatic hernia,* may be discovered. This condition is controllable by surgical operation. (*See also* CHAPTER III.)

DIARRHEA The too-rapid evacuation of too-fluid material from the bowel is called diarrhea. The condition may result from an infection or from irritating materials or from

overdosing with cathartics of irritating character. Most frequent causes of diarrhea are those related to food and, secondarily, those related to infection. Nervous and emotional causes are important.

Ulcerative colitis and cancer, which are not nearly so frequent, may also be associated with diarrhea.

The occurrence of diarrhea repeatedly after eating certain foods suggests the possibility of an allergy. Too much roughage like bran, cabbage or celery, and the excess taking of certain alcoholic beverages may also precipitate diarrhea.

Treatment related to the cause is effective, and excellent drugs may be prescribed that will have a sedative action on the irritated bowel. (*See also* CHAPTER VII.)

DIET (*See* WEIGHT, OVER- AND UNDER-; VITAMINS; *and also* CHAPTERS XIV, XV.)

DIGITALIS The most important drug for controlling heart action, slowing and strengthening the beat, is digitalis. This drug is toxic, and should never be taken except when and if the dosage is prescribed by the doctor. (*See also* HEART.)

DIPHTHERIA Once the most serious of all infectious diseases, diphtheria is now known to be a wholly controllable disease. Many of our larger cities have not had a death from diphtheria in many years. The condition is caused by a special germ which is usually in the body through contact with someone who has had the disease, and who may be carry-

305

ing the germ in the throat. From two to five days after exposure to the germ, the child who is infected will develop a slight fever which may become severe, sore throat, general illness and weakness. Examination of the throat shows a thin grayish membrane which thickens. This is the diphtheric membrane and was responsible in the past for death, due to interference with breathing. Technics have now been discovered for overcoming this hazard. Diphtheria antitoxin is effective in controlling the disease. More important, however, is inoculation of children against diphtheria with diphtheria toxoid. This has proved most effective in stamping out the infection. (*See also* CHAPTER XXII.)

DISINFECTION After any infectious disease, the contents of the room which has been used by the patient must be thoroughly cleaned. All the windows of the room should be thrown wide open to admit fresh air and sunshine. In certain serious infectious disorders, everything associated with the patient must be sterilized by boiling. Clothing and material that cannot be boiled should be put out of doors and exposed to direct sunlight for at least twenty-four hours, which will destroy the germs. Disinfection involves also the treating of material from the body, including sputum, urine and feces, so that the germs in this material are destroyed or disposed of in such a manner as to prevent secondary infection from contact with them.

DIURESIS Excessive action of the kidneys. Drugs have been discov-

ered, such as various compounds of mercury and Diuril, which can hasten elimination of fluid from the body. (*See also* KIDNEYS; *and also* CHAPTER VIII.)

DIVERTICULITIS Inflammation of diverticuli, little projections from the intestines. These may be demonstrated with the X-ray after the person has swallowed a mixture which contains a substance opaque to the X-ray. When these little pouches or tubes come off from the walls of the intestine, they may be irritated or infected and may cause symptoms. Old people particularly may suffer from this condition, and from chronic irritation of a diverticulum, cancer may develop. If the doctor finds the diverticuli inflamed, he prescribes a soft diet, the use of rest, enemas when necessary to help clean the bowel and mineral oil for a laxative effect. If there is persistent obstruction as a result of diverticuli, or constant inflammation and pain, a surgical operation may be necessary.

DIZZINESS Like a cough or a pain, dizziness is a symptom that needs attention. It occurs in all kinds of illnesses and may be associated with poisoning or with insufficient supply of blood to the brain. Anything that interferes with the working of the semicircular canals inside the ear will produce attacks of dizziness. If the sensation is temporary and goes away, the condition need not give concern; if, however, dizziness occurs often or persists, a most careful study must be made to determine the cause. Sometimes attacks of dizziness coming on in the later years of life produce a condition called Ménière's disease which is associated with dizziness that may seriously interfere with life. New drugs that have been developed, such as Dramamine and Bonamine, have been especially helpful in dizziness. (*See also* MÉNIÈRE'S DISEASE.)

DROPSY (*See* ASCITES; EDEMA.)

DUODENAL ULCER (*See* STOMACH ULCER.)

DUSTS Dusts arise from industrial processes involving grinding or drilling. Most dusts contain some carbon and other materials of animal and plant origin. Wood dusts are also frequently found in air. Coal dust produces a blackening of the lungs. Silica dust is an irritating substance which, in the lung, can cause fibrous changes leading to silicosis. Asbestos produces similar changes, and a condition called asbestosis. Dusts in industry are preventable by the use of exhaust systems or suction devices which trap the dust. Spraying with water or oil will keep dusts down. People working in exceedingly dusty occupations wear helmets or breathing devices to prevent access of dust. In houses, dust known as house dust may produce sensitization, and allergy to house dust is one of the most frequent forms. (*See also* ALLERGY; *and also* CHAPTERS XII, XX.)

DWARFISM (*See* ACHONDROPLASIA; GLANDS; *and also* CHAPTER XVI.)

DYSCRASIA Any abnormal state of the body.

DYSENTERY Inflammation of the bowel, with pain, intense diarrhea and the frequent passage of small amounts of mucus and blood, and associated with that a severe illness. Scientifically, different forms are diagnosed according to the organisms which infect the bowel—sometimes bacilli, sometimes amebae, and sometimes other organisms. In the tropics, dysentery spread by the use of contaminated food and water affects millions of people. In dysentery the lining of the large bowel is swollen and red. The prevention of dysentery depends on the sanitary disposal of material from the bowel; the prevention of contamination of food and water by flies, filthy hands and other contacts with the infected material. The new drugs include the sulfa drugs and antibiotics, which are capable of controlling dysentery. Even amebic dysentery (discussed elsewhere, under AMEBIASIS) is now controllable through several new drugs.

DYSKESIA (*See* CONSTIPATION.)

DYSMENORRHEA Painful menstruation. In the United States, girls usually begin to menstruate between twelve and sixteen years of age. The average interval between periods is twenty-eight days, and in the vast majority of instances the condition is not painful.

Whenever it is sufficient to interfere with ordinary living, the doctor should be consulted. Most often, mental factors seem to be responsible. In mild cases, ordinary sedatives and pain-relieving substances can relieve the pain. Most young girls simply go to bed, apply a hot-water bottle and, with a correct mental attitude, are better within a few days. Sometimes the prescribing of glandular products specifically related to menstruation brings prompt relief. (*See also* MENSTRUATION.)

DYSPEPSIA (*See* INDIGESTION.)

DYSPNEA A scientific term for shortness of breath. (*See also* BREATHING; *and also* CHAPTER III.)

DYSTROPHY Defective or abnormal development or degeneration. This may refer to any one of a variety of conditions, some of them beginning in childbirth, many of them progressive and hereditary. The one most common and disturbing is progressive muscular dystrophy, a primary wasting disease of the muscles, in which weakness begins and becomes steadily worse. The condition is associated with degeneration in the nervous system. While it is believed to be related in some way to an inability of the body to use certain chemical materials, the exact cause is not yet known.

E

EAR The ear includes the external ear, the middle ear, and the internal ear, or the labyrinth. The outer visible portion is called the external ear. The middle ear includes the eardrum and the little bones which are in contact with the eardrum, and the mastoid cells. The internal ear includes the organs which are primarily concerned with hearing and with maintaining balance, hence the necessity for examinations of the ear in hardness of hearing and in dizziness. The conditions that affect the external ear are bruises, abrasions and infections. The "tin" ear of the prize fighter is a thickened ear due to hemorrhage. An infection or a boil in the ear canal can be most painful. People should avoid putting anything in the ears smaller than their elbow, because toothpicks or metallic instruments will scratch the surface and make possible easy infection. Insect organisms and fungi can invade the external ear and cause trouble. The ear is best cleaned by syringing with warm water. Remedies are available, which the doctor can supply, to control the infection and irritation. Blocking of the ear by too much ear wax is best treated by the use of the syringe, and not by trying to dig it out. (*See also* OTITIS; *and also* CHAPTER XXVI.)

EARACHE Pain in the ear is usually the result of infection with formation of pus. Puncture of the eardrum relieves the pressure and the pain, and prevents extension of the infection to the mastoid. (*See* OTITIS MEDIA.)

ECCHYMOSIS When blood gets under the skin, the spot is called an ecchymosis. Such spots appear after bruises and are associated also with purpura and easy bleeding.

ECLAMPSIA Convulsive seizures coming on during pregnancy. They frequently follow severe nausea and vomiting of pregnancy and toxemia. The first danger signal is usually headache or failing vision. The doctor finds that the blood pressure has risen and that the kidneys are inflamed and are putting out albumin. Anyone with threatened eclampsia should be put immediately into a hospital; the diet of salt should be restricted, and everything possible done to prevent any extra burden on the kidneys; drugs should be prescribed to diminish the stimulation and the convulsion. Eclampsia can occur to a woman of any age.

The cause of this condition is not known but much research is being devoted to nutrition in pregnancy and to glandular factors, as perhaps having some responsibility. Certainly in prenatal care there should be regular measurements of the blood pressure, checks of any increase in weight, and examinations of the urine.

-ECTOMY This is a term which, when added to the name of an area or organ of the body, means a surgical removal. For example: *append*ectomy, *tonsill*ectomy, *adenoid*ectomy.

ECTOPIC Any abnormality of position of an organ or part of the body. For example: an ectopic pregnancy, when the infant is in the Fallopian tube.

ECZEMA The common, old name for this condition was tetter or salt rheum. The word means simply a breaking-out. The word is now used to describe an acute or chronic, noncontagious, inflammatory, itching disease of the skin, in which there are swellings, blisters, scaling areas and sometimes a pouring out of serum. The exact cause of eczema is not known but the condition is generally believed to be related to sensitivity or allergy, with the difficulty of determining in each instance the substance that may be responsible. Other conditions like eczema result from contact with irritating substances, and these conditions, when the cause is definitely known, are called contact dermatitis. Eczemas are said to form from 20 to 40 per cent of all the cases that come to the offices of specialists in diseases affecting the skin. Obviously, the first step in eczema is to determine, if possible, the exciting agent. In infants, the food must be examined and tests made to determine which foods are least often followed by reactions. Among adults, shellfish, cheese, pastry, hot breads, pork and pickled meats are sometimes responsible. Specialists treat eczema by eliminating sensitivities; powders, lotions, ointments or creams may be used, depending on the nature of the inflammation. Remedies are applied to control itching, others to control infection, others to dry lesions that are overmoist. Some preparations are used to overcome thickening of the skin.

EDEMA Excessive accumulation of fluid in the tissue spaces; from the Greek word meaning "swelling." The terms dropsy and ascites are interchangeable. When the swelling is due to failure of the heart, the condition is called cardiac edema. Swelling caused by fluid in the brain is edema of the brain, and this may be related to toxic causes or to vitamin deficiencies, particularly deficiency of protein and thiamin. Swelling of the hands and feet occurs during hot weather, due to increased volume of the blood and dilation of the capillary blood vessels. This is called heat edema, and is mild. The people in countries that are starving, who develop swelling due to fluid, are said to have nutritional edema.

The prevention and treatment of edema depends on diagnosis of the cause; the treatment is given to eliminate fluid and to prevent its collecting again. The symptom is serious, and a proper diagnosis is of great importance to afford prompt relief. Fluid in the legs disappears when the person rests elevating the legs. Sometimes failure of the heart is helped by a proper posture. Several drugs are known which aid in eliminating fluid, but correction of the cause is more important than a quick elimination of the fluid. (*See also* DROPSY; ASCITES; *and also* CHAPTER VIII.)

ELBOW The elbow joint is in the middle of the arm where three bones come together—the humerus, which is the large bone of the upper arm, and the radius and ulna, which are the smaller bones of the forearm. The elbow joint suffers from any of the serious conditions that affect other joints. Specifically, it is sometimes dislocated, and under the X-ray it may be properly returned to its correct position. Sometimes splints or plaster casts are necessary to hold tissues in place until healing occurs. The conditions around the joint are important, as in the case of so-called tennis elbow, which is

a strain on ligaments associated with overactivity. At the end of the elbow joint is a structure commonly called "the funny bone." Pressure of the bone against nerves causes considerable pain. Cortisone products have been found especially useful in inflammations of the elbow joint. (*See also* ARTHRITIS; *and also* CHAPTER XIII.)

ELECTRICAL INJURIES The majority of fatal electrical accidents are due to industrial accidents affecting workmen, and household accidents involving faulty equipment or careless handling of electrical equipment.

People may be electrocuted by lightning or by accidental contact with high-voltage electricity. The first step is to restore breathing and movement of the heart.

A person who has been struck by lightning falls as if he had just received a stunning blow on the head; the skin may be burned; areas occur in which the clothing is torn from the body, particularly where metallic objects have been carried. After the shock, pain in various portions of the body and visual hallucinations may appear. The first step is to remove the person from contact with the source of electricity, preferably by pulling a switch to cut off current, if this can be done. The doctor should be summoned immediately to take care of shock or injuries.

ELECTROCARDIOGRAPH This is a device which takes measurements of the movement of the wave of stimulation through the heart. Electrocardiograms furnish important aid in the diagnosis and management of heart diseases. (*See also* HEART; *and also* CHAPTERS I, VI.)

ELEPHANTIASIS   Inflammation and obstruction of the lymphatic glands, causing thickening and swelling of the tissues, which may assume gigantic proportions. One of the common causes of this condition is the blocking of the lymph ducts by an organism known as the filaria which gets into them. The condition affected some hundreds of our soldiers in the tropics. The legs and the scrotum are most commonly affected. (*See also* FILARIASIS.)

EMBOLISM   When a blood vessel is blocked by any small piece of material traveling in the blood, the condition is called embolism. An embolus is the term applied to the material which does the blocking. If an important blood vessel is blocked, life may be lost. This applies particularly to blood vessels in the brain, heart, kidney or lung. Emboli may be of germs, air, blood clots, or fat.

New methods have been found for attacking this condition, including immediate surgical operation to open the blood vessel, once the diagnosis has been made, and to release the flow of blood. Several drugs have been developed which prevent blood clotting, including heparin, tromexan, and dicumarol.

EMETIC   Any drug or technique which has the power to cause vomiting is called an emetic.

EMPHYSEMA   When the normal air spaces in the lungs are increased or when an abnormal presence of air or gas is found in any body tissues, the condition is called emphysema. Emphysema may be caused by obstructions to breathing such as asthma, chronic bronchitis, or by persistent coughing. Among the chief symptoms are breathlessness upon exertion, and coughing. Emphysema produces a large, barrel-shaped chest. When the doctor thumps the chest, the sound is like the thumping of an empty barrel contrasted to something full. X-ray pictures show the accumulation of air spaces. Old people have emphysema because of the gradual weakness of tissues associated with advancing age. Smokers have an increased risk of developing emphysema although postmortem examinations on some heavy smokers have failed to show any emphysema. The causal connection has not been definitely established.

EMPYEMA   A condition in which pus collects in a cavity, in a hollow organ or space. This is especially serious in the lower part of the lung and may follow any infection of the lung. Under such circumstances the doctor detects the presence of the pus by X-ray or physical examination. He relieves the empyema by putting in a needle and drawing out the pus. Treatment involves the use of antibiotic drugs which overcome the infection.

ENCEPHALITIS   Inflammation of the brain may accompany various infections as, for example, measles; or it may be a distinct disease caused by a virus; or may be associated with such conditions as meningitis or *paralysis agitans*. Some types of "encephalitis" have been named after the area in which they occurred, as for instance Japanese encephalitis or St. Louis encephalitis. The infection of the brain begins, like other infections, with fever, headache, dizziness, and pains in the trunk and limbs. Vomiting and hiccups may be early symptoms, also disturbances of vision like double vision, and lethargy or sleepiness. The most serious effect of encephalitis is the permanent changes that may occur in the nervous system, resulting eventually in the shaking palsy, involuntary movements, and in paralysis, sometimes in deterioration in intelligence and behavior. The death rate from encephalitis may be exceedingly high, as anything that injures the brain carries with it great danger. Physicians are working on vaccines against encephalitis and also studying a variety of antibiotic drugs, with a view to controlling the infection. (*See also* CHAPTER XXII.)

ENDOCARDITIS Inflammation of the lining of the heart. (*See also* HEART; *and also* CHAPTER VI.)

ENDOCRINE GLANDS These are glands which pour their secretion into the blood rather than into the stomach, the mouth, the intestines or other organs. Examples are the thyroid, the adrenal, the pituitary and the sex glands. (*See also* GLANDS; *and also* CHAPTER XVI.)

ENDOMETRITIS Inflammation of the wall of the uterus. (*See also* MENSTRUATION; UTERUS.)

ENEMA Injection through the rectum into the bowel. Enemas may be used to diagnose diseases, to give nutrition when it is impossible to give it through the stomach, and for the treatment of a variety of conditions. High enemas are injected higher up in the bowel through special equipment. For small babies, enemas are given through a pear-shaped, soft, rubber-tipped ear syringe. For little babies soft rubber tips are safer. Such syringes hold a wine glass of fluid, which can be injected without causing pain or injury. For adults the ordinary fountain syringe is used. Make sure that it is clean, and that the tips are boiled before being used on other people. The ordinary enemas contain plain water, mixtures of soap and water, glycerine and water, soap-suds and salts, or other materials. If the enema is planned merely to empty the lower part of the bowel, a pint of fluid injected rapidly will do the work. If a complete cleaning of the bowel is desirable, one or two quarts of water (preferably warm) may be introduced, with the patient either lying on his side or kneeling with the chest touching the bed. (*See also* CONSTIPATION; *and also* CHAPTER VII.)

ENOVID This hormone derivative taken in tablet form will prevent ovulation and is extensively used in planned parenthood.

ENTERITIS Inflammation of the intestines. (*See also* DYSENTERY; DIARRHEA; FOOD POISONING; *and also* CHAPTER VII.)

ENURESIS Bed wetting, one of the habits of early childhood most difficult to control. Most babies learn to control the urine during the first two years of life, some even within six months. If a child fails to learn by the end of the third year or if a child once trained relapses, special study by the doctor is desirable. Among the alleged causes for persistent bed wetting are nervousness, infection, malnutrition, inflammation or physical defects.

For training against bed wetting, here are some frequent suggestions:

1. Do not give fluids after 5 P.M. If the child complains of thirst, give him a piece of orange or apple.
2. Pick up the child at 10 o'clock at night, wake him thoroughly, and put him on the toilet.
3. Protect the bed well, but do not put on diapers at night after he has once begun to go without them during the day.
4. Take the baby up just as soon as he wakes. Many children wet the bed a few minutes after waking in the morning.
5. If notice is made of the time when the baby wets the bed, practice picking him up just beforehand and permitting him to release the urine and go back to sleep.

Several devices have been invented to condition the child against bed wetting, including one which is put under the mattress and which rings a bell and gives the child a slight electric shock, when the pad becomes moist.

EPHEDRINE A drug derived from a Chinese alkaloid called *ma huang*. It is a constrictor of smooth muscle and can constrict blood vessels, as in the nose when there is a cold or anywhere there is oozing of blood or hemorrhage. It is used particularly in hay fever and asthma, urticaria, surgical shock and for application to the mucous membranes of the nose in congestions such as colds or vasomotor rhinitis.

EPIDEMIC Whenever a disease becomes exceedingly prevalent, beyond its ordinary incidence, when it attacks large numbers of people and spreads over a wide area, the condition is called epidemic. The average number of cases occurring for an equivalent time during a period of five years is used to determine what is normal for the area; anything in excess is epidemic.

EPIDIDYMITIS Just above the testicle is a hooded structure known as the epididymis. Infection of this structure, as with gonorrhea, is called epididymitis. Obviously, treatment of the infection is necessary. Relief from the pain and swelling of the epididymis is frequently accomplished by applications of hot water or hot packs.

EPILEPSY The nervous system may give off stimuli with irregular seizures marked by attacks of unconsciousness, with or without convulsive movements. The condition is called epilepsy. The common classification is *petit mal*, which is characterized by short lapses of unconsciousness and sudden momentary pauses in conversation or movement, rarely lasting more than thirty seconds. Brain-wave machines show that this is minor and slow. *Grand*

313

mal epilepsy is a complete epileptic seizure, with a sudden loss of consciousness, convulsions, blueness, and dilated pupils, followed by spasms of all the voluntary muscles. The eyes rotate upward, the head may be extended, there may be some frothing of the mouth, sometimes loss of urine. Then the convulsions disappear; the patient may be temporarily confused and fall into a deep sleep. During an epileptic attack the electric rhythm, as shown by the brain wave, is of increased rate and high voltage. Nowadays, epilepsy is not feared as it was formerly because much more is understood about it. Only a small per cent of people with epilepsy have mental disturbance of any kind. Many drugs have been found which are capable of subduing or controlling the epilepsy, among them derivatives of phenobarbital. Especially valuable is Dilantin[R]. All these drugs must be prescribed by a doctor. Any such drugs should be chosen and prescribed by the doctor according to their successful use in the individual patient. In some cases convulsions are diminished by using a special diet, called the ketogenic diet, which produces an acid tendency in the blood. Any person with epilepsy should have a physician whom he sees at fairly regular intervals and who is familiar with his condition. Estimates indicate that about 500,000 people in the United States have epilepsy. (*See also* CHAPTER III.)

EPINEPHRINE The scientific name for the active principle of the interior portion of the adrenal gland, also called adrenalin. The word "su-

prarenalin" is also used. (*See also* GLANDS; *and also* CHAPTER XVI.)

EPISTAXIS The scientific term for nosebleed is epistaxis. When serious bleeding occurs from the nose, put the person flat on his back and apply cold. If the bleeding persists, sterile gauze packs may be put on to make pressure. Various drugs are helpful in stopping bleeding of the nose by constricting the blood vessels. The doctor will indicate the remedies after an examination which indicates the nature of the bleeding. Obviously, people with bleeding disorders will bleed frequently from the nose. (*See also* HEMORRHAGE.)

EPITHELIOMA A term used to describe cancers of the skin or other epithelial tissue. The epithelium constitutes the outer cells of the skin and the lining of hollow organs. (*See also* CANCER; *and also* CHAPTER XXIV.)

ERGOT A drug derived from the rye plant, taken from a fungus which develops on such plants. It causes powerful contractions of the uterus; it is used for hemorrhages from the uterus; because it can cause contractions of the uterus, is to be used with great caution.

ERGOTAMINE A substance developed from ergot used for contractions and also in migraine.

EROTICISM Sexual excitement or desire, and in psychoanalysis any manifestation of the sexual instinct.

ERYSIPELAS A brilliantly red,

rapidly spreading inflammation of the skin; known in the Middle Ages as St. Anthony's fire. The germs called streptococci get into little breaks in the skin and multiply. Once there were great epidemics of erysipelas in hospitals, but nowadays the condition is quickly controllable by antibiotic drugs and these, including sulfonamides, stop the infection, so that the temperature drops and the spreading is rapidly checked. Formerly it was customary to paint the skin with antiseptic substances, but control through the blood is far superior to the attempt to control such conditions by anything put on outside. People may have erysipelas over and over again, but the disease no longer occasions the fear that it did in the past.

ERYTHROCYTES The red blood cells are scientifically called erythrocytes. (*See also* ANEMIA; BLOOD.)

ESCAPE MECHANISM In psychiatry, a mode of adjustment to a difficult, unpleasant situation by finding something easier or more pleasant than might be required to solve the situation permanently. Thus an escape mechanism is an evasion of responsibility.

ESOPHAGUS Properly called the gullet. This is a canal about nine inches long, which passes from the throat to the stomach. If damaged by caustic solutions it may close and require careful treatment. The X-ray can reveal the extent to which this tube is open. Infections may attack the wall of the "esophagus" as they do other portions of the body.

People sometimes have psychological conditions which cause them to avoid food. Spasms at the lower end of the esophagus may occur; these are called cardiospasms. Instances are known in which people have been known eventually to starve to death, wholly because of their reaction against swallowing.

In the condition called hysterical dysphasis, there is a mental condition which brings about inability to swallow.

Obviously, varicose veins in the esophagus which may rupture, or tumors of the esophagus, or similar serious conditions affecting this tube demand most careful study and diagnosis. Fortunately, modern surgery affords means of reaching the esophagus and operating on it. This is done frequently with great success.

ESTROGENS Hormones or glandular substances secreted by the female sex glands. These hormones control menstruation and activities related to childbirth. They are important in the menopause. (*See also* OVARY; GLANDS; *and also* CHAPTER XVI.)

EUCALYPTUS The leaves of the Eucalyptus provide an oil which is pleasant and which is used in nasal solutions and mouth washes.

EUNUCH A man or boy deprived of the external genitals and sex glands is called a eunuch.

EXANTHEM Any eruption on the skin is an exanthem.

EXERCISE Exercise makes one feel good and aids the circulation of

315

blood in the muscles and tissues generally. One suggestion is that four hours of muscular activity are desirable at age five; five hours from ages seven to nine; six hours from nine to eleven; five hours from eleven to thirteen; four hours from thirteen to sixteen; three hours from sixteen to eighteen and two hours from eighteen to twenty. This refers to daily exercise during the time of body growth. The amount of exercise in those of advanced years, obviously, must be regulated by their physical condition. People do not live for muscles alone. Big muscles are not necessarily associated with good health. Everyone should have sufficient strength of muscle to carry on the ordinary activities of life, with a little extra for emergencies. The use of calisthenics and setting-up exercises, so-called "daily dozens," helps to develop muscles and ligaments but is not necessarily connected with long life. The regular use of enough exercise in moderate amounts to maintain health, rather than occasional overindulgence to the point of muscle strain and exhaustion, is desirable. Among muscular activities suitable at all ages are swimming, walking, golf, horseback riding, fishing and gardening. (*See also* CHAPTER XXXII.)

EXHAUSTION The human being should never become exhausted except in times of emergency. Exhaustion is an indication that the body has been strained beyond its ability. People who work too long and too hard get overtired. People who are tired or exhausted are irritable. Associated with exhaustion comes the fear and anxiety of breakdown. When the sugar in the

blood is greatly lowered or when the liver does not have enough extra material to meet the needs of energy, exhaustion follows. An insufficient intake of certain vitamins may be a part of the development of exhaustion. (*See also* FATIGUE; *and also* CHAPTER III.)

EXOPHTHALMOS Bulging or forward displacement of the eyes. Usually this condition is caused by changes which are associated with excess activity of the thyroid gland; the thyroid gland enlarges; the complete syndrome is called exophthalmic goiter. (*See also* GLANDS; *and also* CHAPTER XVI.)

EYE The organ of vision. Some of its parts are: the retina (the sensitive tissue at the back of the eye, which receives the image formed by the lens and is connected with the brain by the optic nerve); the optic nerve; the lens; the pupil (the opening in the iris, which contracts or dilates in reaction to light or drugs); the iris (the colored part of the eye; its color is determined by heredity); the conjunctiva (the outer covering of the eye).

The eyes are in almost constant use from the moment of birth until that of death, except for the hours spent in sleeping, and should receive meticulous care. Upon entering school, children should have an eye examination and any visual defects should be corrected. Anyone of any age exhibiting such signs of visual difficulty as a habit of keeping the eyelids slightly closed, a tendency to bend too close to his work or to twist his body in order to see better, or anyone who experiences blind spots or extraordinary flashes of light should also have an eye examination. Blocking of the tear ducts is a serious condition, since the eye will run over with fluid. Treatment of this condition demands the attention of a specialist.

Here are a few simple rules to help guard eyesight:

1. Be sure the light is good when reading or doing close work. Do not face glare or extreme brightness.
2. Never wipe the eyes with a towel used by others.
3. Be sure there are no hooks, doorstops, or other projections on walls at the level of adults' or children's eyes.

Some disturbances of the eye are secondary effects of disease in other parts of the body—for example, jaundice, anemia, brain tumor, diabetes, streptococcal infection, syphilis. In such cases clearing up of the condition depends on successful treatment of the primary cause.

Other difficulties are due to disorders of the eye itself. Among these are astigmatism, cataracts, color blindness, conjunctivitis, cross-eyes, glaucoma, myopa ("near-sightedness"). These are discussed under separate headings (*which see*).

Care should be taken to protect the eyes of workers in industries which, by their nature, present hazards to eyesight—e.g., ultraviolet rays in arc welding; industrial poisons; flying fragments of metals, stone, and grit; caustic substances such as lime or acids. Employers should provide exhaust fans, protective goggles, safety devices on machines, and facilities for frequent washing of the hands.

Here are some hints for first aid for eye injuries:

1. Bathe the eye with a suitable mild sterile solution, preferably a weak solution of boric acid in sterilized water.
2. Cover the eye with a sterile bandage moistened with the above solution.
3. Consult an eye doctor immediately.

Warning: Under no circumstances should an untrained person attempt to remove any foreign substance from the eye. (*See also* CATARACT; COLOR BLINDNESS; CONJUNCTIVITIS; *and also* CHAPTER XXV.)

F

FAINTING Fainting is a sudden attack of swooning in which there may be a feeling of shock or of weakness. Often diminution of the blood supply to the brain results in fainting. Warning symptoms usually precede fainting. The person who faints should be put down flat on the floor or on a couch. If he has fallen, he should be left lying flat. The legs may be raised to increase return of blood through the veins and increase the arterial blood pressure. When consciousness comes back, the person who fainted may sit up cautiously and get up only if there is no further faintness.

FALLOPIAN TUBES Female organs that lead from the ovary to the uterus and through which the female egg cell passes from the ovary to the uterus each month. If the tube is blocked, the woman cannot become pregnant. A block may occur from twisting or from infection. The physician may use various tests including the Rubin test, which involves inflation of the tubes and the taking of pictures with the X-ray to show whether or not there is blocking. For serious infections, surgical removal of the tubes is regularly practiced.

Occasionally a female egg cell is caught in the tubes and pregnancy in the tube results. This is called ectopic pregnancy. Once the condition is diagnosed, surgical operation is usually desirable, to prevent continued growth and ultimate rupture of the tube with the possibility of fatal hemorrhage.

FATIGUE Fatigue is a protection for the body of the person who has sense enough to rest when he feels fatigue. Excessive, prolonged and accumulated fatigue is dangerous to health. A lack of sufficient rest and sleep increases the tendency to fatigue and exhaustion.

Long-standing fatigue is accompanied by loss of appetite and weight and by increasing irritability. The best treatment for fatigue is rest. Stop physical or mental activity before exhaustion. Do not try to overcome such fatigue by taking coffee or benzedrine or so-called pep pills. Little is accomplished by whipping a tired horse. If you are fatigued and exhausted beyond what is reasonable, have a medical examination which will include particularly studies of the blood and studies of the glands. (*See also* EXHAUSTION.)

FECES The scientific name for the excrement discharged from the bowel. The material consists chiefly of the undigested residue from food, bacteria, and the juices secreted by the walls of the bowel.

FEEBLE-MINDEDNESS Mental deficiency. The symptoms vary according to the extent of the feebleness. An idiot is a person so deeply defective in mind from birth as to be unable to guard himself against common physical dangers. An imbecile has mental defectiveness from birth, not amounting to idiocy but yet so pronounced that that person cannot manage his own affairs. In the case of a child, the child cannot be taught to take care of itself. Morons are feeble-minded persons in whom there exists from birth mental defectiveness not reaching imbecility but sufficiently pronounced to make them require, at all times, care, supervision and control for their own protection. Good schools and efficient teaching are capable of improving all mentally defective children above the level of idiocy. (*See also* CHAPTER XXX.)

FEET Painful, sweating and itching feet are annoying; crippled and deformed feet are incapacitating. When the doctor examines your feet he looks first for signs of pain or swelling; discoloration, as results from bruising or hemorrhage, points to some trouble. If the feet ache during the night or if pain begins early in the morning, the symptom is important. If swelling disappears after rest, the difficulty may be constitutional rather than related to the feet. People who stand long hours are most likely to be disturbed by painful feet, due to pressure on the arch of the foot.

Hygiene of the Feet The feet should be bathed at least once daily, preferably with soap, and afterward dusted with a simple powder. This helps to prevent ringworm, which thrives on moisture between the toes and on the feet. To aid circulation, the feet may be dipped alternately for a few minutes at a time in hot water and then in cold water. Among the troubles that can happen to a foot are: sprains, strains, dislocations, fractures, excessive sweating, corns, calluses, warts, chilblains, ringworm, bunions, hammertoes, painful heels, ingrown toenails, cracked toes, blisters, bruises, and disturbances of the circulation. These are discussed to some extent under the appropriate headings.

The shoe should have the shape of the foot and should fit the foot. The stockings should be right in size, so as to be free from wrinkles or pressures. Tight stockings tend to cause the toes to turn in, and may be a cause of ingrowing toenails.

Corns, like calluses, are due to rubbing; this may be rubbing by the shoe or by the stocking. Simple corns may be removed by cutting away with a sharp knife. For serious corns, particularly between the toes, surgical procedures may be necessary to remove the spur or bone that causes pressure. Soft corns usually occur on the inside of the little toe where the joint projects

against the inside of the fourth toe.

Bunions usually occur on the outer side of the large toe. Occasionally they occur on the middle of the foot, due to the modern practice of lacing shoes tightly. (*See also* CALLUSES; *and also* CHAPTER XXVIII.)

FENESTRATION An opening into any structure may be called by the Latin name *fenestra,* which means "window." The most frequent fenestration operation is the creation of a permanent mobile window into the internal ear. This is called the fenestration operation.

FEVER Elevation of the temperature of the human body above normal—namely, above 37° C. or 98.6° F. The temperature is taken with a medical thermometer, well shaken down, then placed in the mouth and kept there at least 3 minutes. Ordinary thermometers do not record above 110°; any temperature above that is likely to be fatal. A thermometer placed under the arm will record about a degree lower than one in the mouth, and a thermometer in the rectum will record about one degree higher. The temperatures of babies and small children should be taken preferably with a rectal thermometer which has a blunt tip. (Never go away and leave a child with a thermometer in place. The child may turn and break it and thus seriously injure himself.) A thermometer once used should be washed thoroughly with soap and not too hot water, then placed in alcohol for five minutes, dried, and returned to its case.

A doctor carefully studies and records changes in temperature because these changes may be so distinctive as to aid the diagnosis of the disease.

Many diseases begin with fever. Among diseases in which "fever" is part of the name of the disease are abortus fever (brucellosis or undulant fever), caused by infection with bacteria; black-water fever (hemoglobinuric fever), a disease like malaria that is associated with much bleeding; brain fever (meningitis); camp fever (typhus); childbed fever (infection after childbirth); enteric fever (typhoid); glandular fever (infectious mononucleosis); hay fever, a form of allergy; intermittent fever (malaria); Rocky Mountain spotted fever, a form of typhus, also called mountain fever; parrot fever (psittacosis); rabbit fever (tularemia); rat-bite fever, which includes two different diseases contracted from the bites of infected rats; cat-scratch fever, caused by germs that get into the body through scratching by cats; rheumatic fever, a condition affecting the heart (see *rheumatic fever*); scarlet fever, also known as scarlatina; Texas fever, an infectious disease of cattle; trench fever, caused by lice, like typhus fever; valley fever, an infection by coccidioidal mycoses, first discovered in California. (*See also* CHAPTER XXI.)

FEVER BLISTERS (*See* COLD SORES.)

FIBRILLATION A shivering tremor in a muscle. When the heart muscle fibrillates the symptom is serious, because it means that the heartbeat is not pushing the blood properly through the blood vessels.

FIBROMA A tumor composed of fiber tissue is called a fibroma. Fibromas are not malignant, as are cancers.

FIBROSITIS A rheumatic disease, of which the cause is not known. The patients do not do well when exposed to damp or cold weather, when fatigued, when submitted to overexertion or when suffering infection in other parts of the body. The pains of fibrositis are recurrent and tend to become chronic. People with fibrositis need to be protected from catching cold, from chilling, dampness or sudden changes in temperatures.

In the treatment of this condition, the salicylates such as aspirin frequently give great relief.

FILARIASIS A tropical disease caused by organisms named filaria produces swelling of the lymph glands, particularly in the groin. The filaria may block the lymph ducts and thus produce elephantiasis.

Another form of filariasis is the loa loa worm or eye worm which wanders across the front of the eye and leaves a serpentine track, damaging vision. The worm is carried by the fly called the mango fly. When such a worm is discovered, the doctor picks it out with a sharp hooked needle.

FINGERNAILS The toenails and the fingernails are composed of keratin. They grow faster in children than in adults. The fingernails grow faster than the toenails. The fingernail grows about 12/100ths of an inch a month. The nail of the middle finger grows more rapidly than the rest of the nails and the nail on the little finger grows slowest.

Since the development of manicuring and pedicuring, care of the fingernails and toenails is given much attention. The daily use of a handbrush to cleanse the skin under the nails is desirable, also the use of an orangewood stick for cleansing after washing. Weekly filing and trimming will keep the nails reasonably short. Any slight injury that breaks the skin near the fingernails will permit germs to get into the broken skin and set up a secondary infection. Infections around the fingernails are called felons. In severe cases, these felons or run-arounds, scientifically called paronychia, may require surgical attention.

Brittle fingernails are a constant annoyance. The exact cause is not known. A deficiency in the diet, perhaps of amino acids or of vitamins, may be responsible. Improper circulation to the nail plate may cause brittleness.

Cutting the toenails with a clipper is preferable to cutting with either a curved or straight scissors.

FISTULA An abnormal passage leading from the surface of the body into some cavity or organ beneath the surface. These are extremely frequent near the anus or rectum. They do, however, occur elsewhere in the body. They are sometimes treated by the use of caustic substances which seal up the passes. When they are more severe and cause symptoms, they are best treated by surgery which dissects the fistula and removes it.

FIXATION In psychiatry, when development stops, particularly emotional desire at an immature level, the condition is called a fixation. (*See also* CHAPTER XI.)

FLATFOOT *Pes planus,* a depression of the plantar arch of the foot. The condition may be present at birth or may be acquired as a result of loss of proper support by the muscles of the arch of the foot, sometimes caused by badly fitting shoes, by incorrect walking habits or by standing long hours in certain occupations. Frequently, flatfoot is associated with a turning-out of the foot in walking. The condition used to be considered incapacitating, preventing acceptance by the armed forces. Then it was found that men with so-called flat feet could frequently walk twelve or fifteen miles without tiring. The condition is not now considered a necessary cause of rejection for the army. (*See also* FEET; *and also* CHAPTER XXVIII.)

FLATULENCE When the bowel becomes distended with air or gas. The material, when passed from the bowel, is called flatus. Frequently, flatulence is caused by swallowing air during rapid eating. Occasionally, gas develops from bacteria.

FLEAS An insect comes to medical attention through biting people and producing inflammatory and itching areas which are a form of dermatitis. The flea is also a carrier of some diseases, such as plague. (*See also* CHAPTER XXIX.)

FLIES There are many varieties of flies, and some insects that are not properly flies are called flies. These include butterflies and dragonflies. Some insects of the same family are not known as flies, notably mosquitoes. Flies in general are dangerous because of their carrying certain filth diseases, which they pick up from manure and contaminated food. (*See also* CHAPTER XXIX.)

FOLLICULITIS Inflammation of the hair follicles frequently causes difficulty, an example being barber's itch. Inflammation of hair follicles on the head may result in baldness. (*See also* HAIR.)

FONTANEL The soft spot on a newborn baby's head. It represents a space where bones come together, eventually closed by the growth of bone.

FOOD POISONING The expression ptomaine poisoning used to be used for this condition because it was thought that germs acting on food produced poisons called ptomaine. This term is no longer used for food poisoning. Food may occasionally contain actual poisons like arsenic administered with malicious intent. The commonest form of food poisoning is that due to invasion of food by bacteria like the staphylococci or the salmonella organisms. The germs may produce poisons or may be poisonous in themselves. They may get into food from an infected wound, as from the finger of a cook or a baker. Food poisoning manifests itself by sudden abdominal pain, nausea, vomiting and diarrhea, any time from four to thirty hours after the food was eaten. Along with these symptoms come headache, cold sweat, shivering and occasionally, double vision. If death results, the cause is either shock or the great loss of water and salt associated with the vomiting and diarrhea. Typical of food poisoning is the sudden attack of half-a-dozen or more people who have eaten the same contaminated food. (*See also* CHAPTERS VII, XVIII.)

FOOD SENSITIVITY (*See* ALLERGY.)

FRACTURE The breaking of a bone. Many types of fractures are known, the classification depending on the bone involved and the way the fracture looks when examined by the X-ray. Certain fractures are associated with certain types of accidents. Chauffeur's fracture was a breaking of the small bones of the wrist or the arm due to sudden and violent reversing of the starting crank of an automobile engine. In a greenstick fracture, one side of the bone is broken and the other bent. This used to be called hickory-stick fracture. When the bone is splintered or crushed the condition is known as a comminuted fracture. When the fractured bone penetrates through the skin, the condition is called open or compound fracture.

FRECKLES Freckles are red spots of pigmentation in the skin, sometimes resulting fom exposure to sunlight. Other similar spots are the chloasmas, called liver spots. Pigmented areas may appear on the skin produced by powder marks, deposits of silver in the skin or unabsorbed material from bruises. For the prevention of ordinary freckles, ointments and oils may be purchased which protect the skin from the effects of the sun's rays. Freckles are sometimes removed by using substances on the skin which will peel off the superficial layers. A new drug discovered in Egypt, where it has long been used for the removal of pigment, is now sold under the name of Benoquin. All these methods are potentially dangerous and should be used only with proper advice.

FROSTBITE Damage to tissues resulting from exposure to extreme cold, particularly when there is a strong wind. Frostbite seldom occurs with a temperature above 20 degrees. Frostbite is first manifested by contraction of the blood vessels in the skin, so that it becomes pale. In severe frostbite, the blood does not come back to the skin. When it does seep back after the skin is warmed, the color is purplish or black. To prevent frostbite, postpone outdoor work when the temperature is below 8 degrees particularly when there is strong wind; wear clothing, shoes, socks and gloves that are well fitted and hold warmth. People who have to stay out of doors during cold weather should not stay out longer than two hours at a time and should have intervening rest periods of at least one half hour between work periods.

People with damaged circulation or with diabetes are more likely to frostbite than those in good condition. After freezing, the parts affected may be massaged gently for a few minutes to encourage circulation and

then wrapped in several layers of wool. (*See also* CHAPTER XIX.)

FURUNCLE (*See* BOILS.)

G

GALL A common name for bile which is stored in the gall bladder, a hollow pear-shaped sac on the under surface of the right lobe of the liver. The bile comes to it from the liver and passes from it to the intestines. Infection and inflammation of the gall bladder is called cholecystitis. The symptoms are usually severe pain and rigidity of the upper part of the abdomen on the right side, occasionally jaundice and coating of the tongue. The bowel is distended and becomes bloated quickly upon taking food. (*See also* CHOLECYSTITIS AND CHOLELITHIASIS; *and also* CHAPTER VII.)

GALLSTONES Hard masses formed in the gall bladder and bile passages. Nobody knows exactly what causes gallstones to form but this condition perhaps results from a blocking of the flow of the bile, caused by infections, and the surrounding of germs with calculus material. The gallstone is especially serious when it blocks the tube and causes the retention of bile in the gall bladder. Nowadays, a single severe attack of colic may be sufficient to suggest operation, which, while fairly serious, when performed by experts has an exceedingly low mortality rate, with recovery in the vast majority of cases from both the symptoms and the operation. (*See also* CHOLECYSTITIS AND CHOLE-LITHIASIS.)

GANGRENE Death of tissues due to stoppage of the blood supply. Gangrene may arise due to obstruction of the blood supply by inflammations of the blood vessels. Too-long an application of a tourniquet or constriction around a limb sometimes produces gangrene. Certain germs produce gangrene as a secondary effect. Diabetes is often accompanied in its late stages by gangrene. Very old people sometimes develop gangrene, particularly of the toes, because of interference with new blood supply. In most instances, gangrene will require amputation to save life.

GAS POISONING (*See* CARBON MONOXIDE POISONING; *and also* CHAPTERS XVIII, XX.)

GASTRIC The word "gastro" means stomach. Words which begin with gastro relate to conditions affecting the stomach. Gastritis is inflammation of the stomach; gastroenteritis, inflammation of the stomach and intestines; gastroectomy, the cutting-out or removal of all or part of the stomach. A gastroscope is a device for looking inside the stomach.

GASTRIC ULCER (*See* ULCER.)

GASTRITIS Inflammation of the walls of the stomach, due to infection; irritation by drugs; alcohol in excess; coarse foods; to the absence of certain vitamins in the diet; or,

sometimes, disorders of the blood.

Through a tube called a gastroscope, it is possible to see the lining of the stomach by reflected light, and to photograph it in color. This helps to make clear the nature of "gastritis." The symptoms of gastritis are, as with inflammations elsewhere in the body: pain, tenderness, nausea and vomiting. Usual attacks of gastritis are controlled by diminishing food and selecting easily digestible materials. Certain drugs overcome excess acid and irritation. Irritating foods such as alcohol, mustard, pepper, vinegar and spices and other irritants are avoided. A careful study of the gastritis points the way to its control. (*See also* CHAPTERS II, VII.)

GASTROPTOSIS Displacement of the stomach downward from its usual position, as shown by the X-ray, the condition is called gastroptosis.

GELATIN Gelatin is a colorless transparent substance, jellylike when moistened but hard when dried. Gelatin is mostly protein derived from animal tissues such as the skin, the ligaments and the bones. Gelatin is mostly used in desserts, artificially sweetened; pure gelatin does not have a sweet taste. Gelatin contains about twelve of the amino acids that constitute proteins. In cases of deficiencies of amino acids, feeding with gelatin may be helpful. Gelatin has had some use as a blood substitute.

GENETICS The science of heredity, and variations in heritage and growth. By this study, one determines the causes of resemblances and differences between parents and children, and between all living organisms. (*See also* CHAPTER IX.)

GERIATRICS The study of old age and its diseases. Geriatrics is derived from two Greek words meaning "old age" and "healing." The increasing number of aged people in the population has made necessary a specialty in medical practice for the care of the aged. (*See also* CHAPTER X.)

GERMICIDE A substance which kills germs, differing from antiseptic, which destroys any poisonous materials.

GIANTISM (*See* ACROMEGALY); PITUITARY GLAND; *and also* CHAPTER XVI.)

GINGIVITIS Any inflammation of the gums, including pyorrhea and trench mouth.

GLANDERS A highly contagious disease affecting chiefly horses, mules and donkeys but also communicable to dogs, goats, sheep and to human beings, but not to cattle. The chief symptoms are fever, inflammation of the mucous membranes, enlargement and hardening of the lymph glands and the formation of nodules which tend to break down into ulcers. In human beings, glanders is often fatal. It is popularly known as "farcy."

GLANDS The word glands has been used to describe the lymph nodes or lymph glands, but more particularly to describe certain organs which pour their secretions directly into the blood. Any organ that provides a secretion is a glandular organ. Glands which pour their material elsewhere than into the blood are those that provide material, such as the salivary glands which provide saliva, and the pancreas which provides digestive ferments. The glands which secrete internal secretions exclusively are the thymus, the pineal gland, the pituitary, the suprarenal glands and the sex glands.

The breasts are glandular, since they secrete milk. The stomach is glandular because it secretes hydrocholoric acid and pepsin. Overgrowth of the glands may result in all sorts of changes in the body, due to the secretion of too much of the material. Absence of the glands may also bring about changes resulting from deficiency of hormone substances. The glandular mechanism of the body is an interlocking chain; some glands affect other glands. In case of failure of certain glands, other glands may take up their function. In old age, the glands begin to break down and to degenerate, and to discontinue their activities. Nowadays, modern science has isolated the materials from the glands and can provide substitutes for the lacking secretions. (*See also* ADRENAL; GOITER; PINEAL; PITUITARY; THYMUS; *and also* CHAPTER XVI.)

GLAUCOMA A disease brought about by increase of pressure within the eyeball through interference with the circulation of fluid. It is responsible for 15 per cent of all cases of blindness. Associated with glaucoma may be the most severe headache. The doctor measures the tension of

325

the eye with a tonometer; he measures the extent of the disturbance of the field of vision with a perimeter. Various drugs are available for treating glaucoma. These lower the pressure in the eye and contract the pupil. A drug called Diamox, which causes elimination of fluid from the body, has been found to diminish tension in the eye. Frequently, it may be used in advance of any surgical procedures so that operation may be done under better conditions. (*See* EYE.)

GLEET Chronic discharge of muco purulent material from the sex organs. Chronic gonorrhea was formerly called gleet. Nowadays, effective treatment with penicillin and other antibiotic drugs has practically eliminated gleet.

GLIOMA A tumor of nerve cells.

GLOBULIN A general name for certain protein substances, the gamma globulin containing antisubstances against infections.

GLUCOSE Another word for dextrose.

GOITER Enlargement of the thyroid gland which lies in the front of the neck. The thyroid glands are important in handling iodine for the body. Practically all of the iodine which comes into the body in eggs, milk, bread, shellfish or salt is deposited in the thyroid gland.

Goiters are (1) simple enlargements of the gland; (2) excessive activity of the gland. The simple enlargement of the gland which may come on, particularly in girls,

around adolescence is due usually to a deficiency of iodine. Pregnant women need more iodine than at other times, to prevent the occurrence of changes in the thyroid in children.

When the thyroid gland enlarges and its activity becomes excessive, an excess amount of the secretion of the thyroid gland gets into the body. This secretion is called thyroxin. The condition is called exophthalmic goiter and is often associated with nerve strain. The eyeballs project, the heart beats rapidly and the basal metabolism rate is raised, showing that extensive chemical changes are going on in the body. With the nervousness, excitability and loss of weight come fatigue. Anyone with exophthalmic goiter needs careful attention by the doctor to determine the nature and extent of the condition. Various drugs have been developed to control exophthalmic goiter, including, for example, thiouracil and radioactive iodine. Treatment also may be application of X-ray or surgical removal of the gland.

Occasionally the thyroid gland becomes subject to tumors or cancers, which need prompt diagnosis by the doctor. (*See also* CHAPTER XVI.)

GONORRHEA A venereal disease with infection by a germ called the gonococcus. The usual method of infection is by sexual contact, although occasionally children are infected by the contact of their sex organs with the contaminated fingers of attendants, with towels, baths, or other materials. Babies used to have gonorrhea of the eyes, leading to blindness, at the time of birth but modern techniques for treating the eyes immediately following birth have practically controlled this type of infection. Nowadays, the use of sulfonamides and antibiotic drugs is not only curing gonorrhea but serving also to prevent its incidence, so that the disease may eventually disappear as have typhoid and diphtheria. (*See also* CHAPTER XXVII.)

GOUT A disturbance of the metabolism of uric acid in the body associated with a large amount of uric acid in the blood and an increased amount in the urine. Sudden attacks of acute pain in the joints occur; these may last from a few days to a few weeks, and recur at irregular intervals. The attack often begins with the great toe and involves only one joint, but later other joints may become affected. The joint involved is hot, red and tender and the skin around it becomes shiny from the stretching. Sometimes there are deposits of sodium urate called tophi in the skin over the cartilages of the ear, about the fingernails and in the cartilages of the joints. Gout usually comes on around thirty-five years of age but may not occur until people are advanced in years. Excessive intake of purines or protein substances and of alcohol does not cause gout but may be associated with an attack.

A drug called colchicine is the most specific drug used against gout. Drugs of the salicylic acid type are helpful. New drugs much used are benemid, butazolidin and Anturan[R]. Much comfort is given to people with gout by rest, by warmth applied to the affected parts, and by protection from contact with the bedclothing by cradles. People with gout also should take diets which are low in fats, rather rich in sugars and proteins, and free from most purine substances. Purine substances include: livers, sweetbreads, anchovies, beef kidneys, brains, meat extracts and heavy gravies. On the other hand, milk, eggs, cheese and most vegetables are relatively low in purine substances.

GRAND MAL (*See* EPILEPSY.)

GRANULOCYTOPENIA A condition in which certain important cells called leukocytes are diminished or absent in the blood. The condition is also called agranulocytosis. This condition is often associated with sensitivity to certain types of drugs. It is a severe condition, since the defending cells of the body are absent. Treatment under such circumstances, with penicillin to control infection, may save the life. (*See also* CHAPTER IV.)

GYNECOLOGY The specialty of medicine which is concerned with the diseases of women and with their surgery. A gynecologist is a specialist in conditions affecting women.

GYNECOMASTIA Any enlargement of the breasts of men which causes them to resemble the breasts of women. The condition in men is usually associated with a glandular disturbance—a deficiency of male sex gland material or an excess of female sex gland material.

327

H

HABITUATION A tolerance to the effects of drugs or poisons or addiction to them so that there is a craving when the drug is withdrawn. (*See also* ADDICTION; DRUG; *and also* CHAPTER XVIII.)

HAIR Hair grows from follicles, growing to its full length in about eight weeks. Then comes a resting period for the follicles. Many tests related to shaving have shown that shaving hair does not affect it except to cut it off.

The hair growth is not increased by applying oils or alcohol or quinine or other stimulants. Ultraviolet will not produce any increase in the growth of hair, nor will tanning; neither will they stop the growth of hair, unless carried to excess sufficient to destroy cells. X-ray will cause the hair to fall out, and X-ray can burn the underlying skin.

Baldness Alopecia is the scientific term for baldness. Most baldness is hereditary, not only the baldness but actually the pattern of the baldness. Thus far a cure for baldness has not been discovered. Apparently, growth of hair is affected by hormones, but exactly how to control this is not known.

Care of the Hair Rapid falling of the hair may follow sickness. This is temporary, and the hair will grow out again in a few months. Cutting the hair shorter or shaving the head will not make it grow faster. Apparently, the use of a stiff brush and occasional massage of the scalp with fingers is helpful to some people, particularly if carried on in a routine and regular manner.

Hygiene of the Hair The hair should be washed often enough to keep it clean. For most hair any ordinarily good soap will do, but special shampoos are available. Experts say the use of an egg in the shampoo does not help, any more than throwing an egg into an electric fan. After the hair has been washed with soap and water, it should be rinsed thoroughly, so that the excess soap is removed, and dried rather slowly without too much heat.

Nothing is gained by singeing the hair, except to make a bad smell and to improve the finances of the barber.

Gray hair appears to come with age to most people. Attempts have been made to relate the grayness of hair to hormones, but thus far consistent results have not been secured.

Superfluous Hair The scientific name for superfluous hair is hypertrichosis, meaning excessive hair. Men ordinarily have hair on their chests and around the sex organs and on the face. Excessive hair on the breasts of women or on their faces gives them anguish. Such excess growth is apparently related to glandular activities but thus far does not seem to be consistently controllable. Studies are being made in the use of estrogenic hormones taken internally and applied locally, and in some cases there seemed to be success. In women, excess growth of hair is more likely to occur after the menopause. The certain method for the removal of excess hair is the use of the electric needle. Use of the X-ray for this purpose is dangerous.

HALITOSIS The word halitosis has been popularized as the generally used term for bad breath. Bad breath may arise from decay of the teeth, from infection, from insufficient cleaning of the mouth and the teeth, but no mouth wash yet known can prevent the bad odor arising in this way. Good dentistry helps. Infections in the tonsils may cause bad breath, in which case gargles will wash the surface, but will not get down to the infected material. Occasionally the lungs may develop materials which give a bad odor. The eating of garlic will release a bad odor.

Chlorophyll has been advocated as a means of controlling such odors but the evidence that it will do so is not satisfactory. A bad odor can sometimes be covered up by a good odor. (*See also* CHAPTER XXXIV.)

HAMMERTOE Bending of a toe, usually the second, from wearing shoes that are too short. Often this is not controllable except by surgery. (*See also* CHAPTER XXVIII.)

HARELIP (*See* CLEFT PALATE.)

HAY FEVER Hay fever is the form of allergy produced by ragweed or related pollens, as of the trees and flowers. Hay fever caused by grass pollen is called rose fever. The symptoms are: coryza, sneezing, mucus from the nose, headache and intense itching of the eyes and upper air passages. Nowadays, hay fever is helped by antihistamine drugs. Allergists determine the cause and prevent contact, and may undertake desensitization. (*See also* ALLERGY; *and also* CHAPTER XII.)

HEADACHE Among all the pains that send people hurrying to the doctor, headache is among the most frequent. The American Association for the Study of Headache has classified major headaches into three types: one related to circulation of the blood, another to tension of muscles, and the third to infections, tumors and inflammation. The exact causes of headaches from the biochemical point of view link them to a substance called serotonin developed by the tissues, and to another substance called tyramine found in some foods. Beyond all this are the psychogenic or stress headaches related to mental causes like depression.

Migraine is a special kind of headache often occurring in families. With this headache there are visual sensations of seeing bright circles of light. The migraine headache is not a sharp pain, but throbs and pulsates. People with migraine get nausea. More women have migraine than do men. For the most severe types of headache there are various specific remedies that can be prescribed by the doctor, but cannot be purchased otherwise, chief among these are drugs of the ergotamine type. There are many other drugs for treating depression and relief of tension which also must be prescribed by the physician. For the great mass of common headaches, most people try aspirin or other pain-relieving drugs. These attacks may make the patient ill for more than three or four days, but usually headaches disappear in a few hours. (*See also* CHAPTERS II, XXXI.)

HEAD BANGING AND HEAD ROLLING Occasionally, normal healthy infants when put to bed roll their head from side to side or bang it up and down, even to the point of creating bruises. The symptom may be frightening, but in general it is not serious and disappears as the child grows older. The exact cause of this habit is not known but apparently it yields some sort of satisfaction to the infant. Children develop strange habits, and more harm is done by attempting to control the habits by extraordinary punishments than by trying to substitute for the habits pleasurable activities.

HEARING, HARDNESS OF (*See* DEAFNESS; OTOSCLEROSIS; EAR; *and also* CHAPTER XXVI.)

HEART Organ whose function is to keep up the circulation of the blood. At birth the heart beats about 130 times a minute, gradually diminishing to 100 at 6 years, 90 at 10 years, 85 at 15 years, and, among adults, anywhere from 60 to 80. Sixty to 65 beats per minute is exceedingly slow but has been noted, particularly in long-distance runners. The heart beats more than two billion times during a lifetime and pumps millions of gallons of fluid. The heart lies inside a sac, called the pericardium, a little to the left of the breastbone, at about the fifth rib. It is essentially a muscle about as big as a fist. It beats from before birth until death and seldom rests,

even by diminishing its rate. It is an involuntary muscle that responds to excitement, effort, and other activities by beating fast.

You can give it rest by lying down so as to slow the beat a little and decrease its force.

Coronary Arteries The heart gets its own nourishment from small blood vessels that pass into its muscle tissue from the large blood vessels that carry the blood away from the heart. Blocking of these coronary arteries is called coronary thrombosis; the symptoms that follow such blocking are known as coronary disease. In hardening of the arteries, blocking of the coronary blood vessels is more frequent than otherwise. Associated with temporary spasms of these vessels or temporary lack of blood supply to the heart is angina pectoris.

Heart Block The heartbeat is controlled by electric currents which activate the beat. Any interruption along the path causes heart block. Particular places where interruption occurs are called bundle branch block or atrioventricular block.

Heart Failure Failure of the heart to carry on its work is serious because the whole body depends on the blood. Failure may be due to inability of the muscle to pump, inability of the pump to force out enough blood at one time, or failure of the pump to force the blood all the way around and back again. If any of these failures occur, fluid collects in the feet and in the abdomen; the brain gets insufficient nourishment; occasionally the heart muscle will enlarge in an attempt to do what it cannot. Signs of heart failure are shortness of breath, and a blue tinge to the skin resulting from lack of oxygen in the blood.

Heart Disease Heart disease is not a single illness but may be one of several, such as that resulting from rheumatic fever (*which see*), one of the foremost foes of health in children, which is related frequently to streptococcus infections of the throat. People of advanced years sometimes suffer breakdown of the heart; death may be prevented by seeing to it that the victim avoids stress and strain.

Coronary Thrombosis Coronary thrombosis is the forming of a clot or clots in the coronary arteries. The moment an attack occurs, the victim should be put immediately at complete rest in bed. Then, by careful study involving the use of the electrocardiograph, the doctor will determine the nature and scope of the condition and take the necessary measures to relieve pain and, if possible, bring about improvement. Any attack of acute indigestion in a person past forty-five years may actually be the beginning of coronary thrombosis and should not be regarded lightly.

In general, the following ten heart commandments will help to prolong life:

1. Do not subject the heart to sudden strenuous or prolonged physical exertion.
2. Eat regularly, slowly, and temperately.
3. If excessively overweight, seek sound advice on how to reduce.
4. Avoid physical activity for at least 30 minutes after eating,

particularly after a heavy meal.
5. Avoid emotional stress and strain, since worry is an important factor in relation to heart strain.
6. Keep the body as free of infection as possible.
7. Maintain regular bowel activity.
8. Try to get sufficient sleep in a room abundantly supplied with air.
9. Try to observe a proper balance between work, play, relaxation, and rest.
10. After forty-five years of age have an examination regularly. It may reveal defects of which you are unaware and thus save life.

When the heart is damaged by disease so that the connections between the upper and lower portions of the heart are interrupted, these portions will beat independently of each other. The condition is called heart block. Any interference with the rhythmical, steady beat of the heart demands careful investigation. (*See also* CHAPTER VI.)

HEARTBURN A burning sensation over the chest or beneath the breastbone is sometimes related to spasm of the esophagus, sometimes associated with a gall-bladder inflammation. Many cases are related to regurgitation of gastric juice into the esophagus. The conditon can be regulated by the doctor, who listens to the heart to determine that it is "heartburn" and prescribes a proper course to correct this condition.

331

HEAT PROSTRATION Exposure to high temperatures often will be followed by moist, cold skin, poor circulation, elevation of the body temperature, restlessness and anxiety, and may be so severe as to initiate shock. Prompt recognition and treatment are important. "Heat stroke" is avoided by making sure that the body has enough salt, since loss of salt from perspiration may aid in causing heat stroke. (*See also* SUN STROKE; *and also* CHAPTER XIX.)

HELMINTHIASIS A scientific name for the presence of parasitic worms in the body.

HEMATEMESIS Vomiting of blood, a serious sign, since it may indicate the hemorrhage of tuberculosis, a hemorrhage of the stomach, a hemorrhage from a varicose vein of the esophagus, or a hemorrhage from an ulcer or a cancer. This serious symptom requires that the person be immediately put at rest, and get as quickly as possible a diagnosis of what is wrong. Blood transfusion may be needed to save life. (*See also* CHAPTERS III, VII.)

HEMATURIA The appearance of blood in the urine, often associated with diseases of the kidneys. Frequently the cause of blood in the urine cannot be determined. The blood may come from any part of the passage down which the urine goes from the kidney through the ureters into the bladder and out through the urethra. Bleeding may be from the kidneys, or from a stone that has damaged the walls of any of these structures mentioned; bleeding may occur as a result of blood

disorders in which the capillaries rupture easily and the blood does not coagulate. Careful examinations are necessary to determine the cause. (*See also* CHAPTER VIII.)

HEMOGLOBIN The red pigment of the red blood corpuscles that carries oxygen. Normal, as measured by the various types of color scales, is called 100 per cent, or the equivalent of fifteen to sixteen grams of hemoglobin per 100 cc. of blood. (*See also* CHAPTER IV.)

HEMOPHILIA A blood disorder in which the blood fails to clot. It may result in death. Such a condition occurs, apparently, through absence of an important constituent in the blood and has affected the royal families of Spain and of Russia. It is limited to the men of the family but transmitted by the women. The chief symptom is the bleeding, which follows even a minor injury and persists almost indefinitely. Packs of gauze, the stitching of wounds and various other methods have been tried to control this condition. Transfusion of blood has been used. Quite recently, what is apparently the missing substance has been found by the laboratories of Harvard University and is available for use in such cases.

HEMORRHAGE Bleeding may occur in any person due to a wound or to the cutting of a blood vessel. Usually a clot forms. For the formation of a clot, calcium is necessary and also certain materials derived from the blood itself. In some people various of these necessary substances may be absent. When a doctor finds that a person bleeds too often and too easily, he examines the blood to test the clotting-time, the number of blood platelets, the presence of fibrin and the other substances necessary for the proper clotting. Whenever bleeding occurs, regardless of cause, the "hemorrhage" must be stopped. One of the simplest ways is to put on a pack of sterile gauze and to bandage tightly. If a large artery is cut, a tourniquet may be necessary to stop the flow. Bleeding from the pocket of a tooth after the pulling of a tooth may be controlled by packing with sterile gauze, applying heat and applying substances which clot the blood. In serious bleeding, get a doctor or dentist immediately. For persistent nosebleeds, called "epistaxis," put the person flat, preferably with the face down. Apply cold to the nose, or pack with sterile gauze. If nosebleeds occur frequently, a careful examination should be made of the blood pressure and of the blood vessels in the nose, and of the blood itself.

HEMORRHOIDS Varicose veins at the lower end of the bowel, commonly called piles. At least one-third of all grown people have hemorrhoids.

Anything that interferes with the proper flow of the blood in the blood vessels may be associated with hemorrhoids. A sedentary life, overweight, pregnancy, constipation, or the excessive use of cathartics all have been associated with this condition. Obviously, such conditions are treated directly. Hemorrhoids are painful when the blood in the dilated vein becomes clotted. Secondary infection with fungi produces severe itching. Sometimes hemorrhoids push through at the time when the bowels have an action. These are called "protruding hemorrhoids." If the hemorrhoids are scratched and bleed, they are called "bleeding hemorrhoids." Numerous ointments, suppositories and other preparations have been developed to relieve the symptoms of hemorrhoids. In more serious cases, electric coagulation is attempted, or they may be removed by surgery.

HEPATITIS (*See* JAUNDICE.)

HERNIA Hernia is the scientific name for a rupture. Nowadays, people know that there are spots in the walls of the body through which the tissues below may push or protrude, and they know that these occur most often in the groin but also in the midline of the abdomen or elsewhere in the body. When the tissues underneath the body force their way through an opening in the body wall, a lump will appear. If this is surrounded by tight tissues, it may lose its blood supply and become gangrenous. Sometimes ruptures are present at birth; sometimes they follow attempts to lift heavy objects; occasionally athletes get them from strain in competition.

Formerly, people tried to control ruptures by wearing trusses and supports and many of them still follow this uncomfortable procedure rather than to have the simple surgical operation that brings about permanent cure. The treatment of every rupture, naturally, depends upon the place where it is located. A method called the injection method has been tried, with a view to putting in substances which will create fibrous tissue and thus block the rupture. In the surgical method, the stitching is placed in such a way as to bring about permanent improvement. The surgical method is exact and the risk is slight. Today, with modern anesthetics and antibiotic drugs to prevent infections and blood transfusions to prevent shock, the patients usually get well in a very short time and are returned to an active, useful and more pleasant life.

HERPES Cold sores or fever blisters. (*See also* COLD SORES.)

HERPES ZOSTER (*See* SHINGLES.)

HICCUPS Hiccups are due to a spasm or constriction of the diaphragm. Anything that disturbs co-ordination in the breathing mechanism can cause hiccups. A sudden distention of the stomach will disturb the action of the diaphragm and bring on hiccups. An irritation of the brain such as occurs in encephalitis may be responsible. Hiccups may also be associated with nervousness, worry, anxiety, shock or accident.

Popular treatments for hiccups, in addition to coughing, sneezing, or swallowing ice, vinegar, or cold water, include pulling on the tongue; pressing the upper lip with the finger; breathing into a paper bag so that the breath is reinhaled and, finally, new drugs like chlorpromazine and reserpine, which seem to have a definite effect in modifying the stimuli that come from the brain to the diaphragm. Doctors sometimes spray ethychloride as a refrigerant on the front of the abdomen, make slight

pressure on the eyeballs or press on the ribs near the diaphragm, as simple measures which may be successful. (*See also* DIAPHRAGM.)

HIVES Urticaria; blisters, wheals, or breaking-out of the skin, usually associated with allergy. Such eruptions develop after insect bites. The common name for hives is nettle rash. Hives appear after eating certain foods; sometimes they come in crops, representing successive attacks of sensitivity.

Symptoms of hives are alleviated by stopping certain foods, cleaning the intestinal tract and using of the skin lotions like menthol in calamine or other anti-itching preparations included with antihistamines. Garments that produce much warmth to the skin and perspiration should be avoided in the presence of hives, since they, apparently, tend to increase the extent of the eruption. (*See also* ALLERGY; *and also* CHAPTERS XII, XXIII.)

HOARSENESS Inflammation and irritation of the vocal cords. Singers who use the voice too frequently for long periods of time sometimes develop small nodules on the cords and thus develop hoarseness. Excessive eating, drinking, smoking in business conferences may increase hoarseness. Tuberculosis and cancer of the throat are also serious conditions which may affect the throat. Any hoarseness that lasts more than a short time and does not yield to simple remedies should require an immediate investigation of the larynx by a competent specialist in throat conditions. He will have the apparatus and the facilities which enable him to look directly at the spot to see what is wrong. (*See also* LARYNGITIS; *and also* CHAPTER XXVI.)

HODGKIN'S DISEASE A disease of the lymph glands in the throat, characterized by swelling of the lymph glands, the spleen, and the tonsils. This condition is sometimes believed to be a form of cancer. It occurs twice as often in men as in women. The condition usually begins with a painless enlargement of one side of the neck but then spreads to the other side, and may gradually involve all the glands. A specific method for treating this condition is not known. The X-ray and radium are used and, internally, some of the newer drugs like the nitrogen mustards.

HOMOSEXUALITY When people are attracted sexually toward those of the same sex, rather than to those of the opposite sex, the condition is called homosexuality. Female homosexuality is sometimes called lesbianism.

HORMONES The glandular substances which pass from the glands of internal secretion into the blood. Among the common hormones are estrogens, the female sex hormones; testosterone or androgens, the male sex hormones; thyroxin, the hormone from the thyroid gland; pituitrin, the hormone from the pituitary gland; Cortisone and adrenalin from the adrenal glands. (*See also* GLANDS; *and also* CHAPTER XVI.)

HYMEN The membrane at the entrance to the female sex organs is called the hymen; the presence of this tissue is often considered synonymous with virginity, although it may be absent in women who have not had sexual contact. Its absence is not to be construed as certain evidence of loss of chastity.

HYPERHIDROSIS Scientifically, excessive sweating is called by this long name. (*See also* PERSPIRATION.)

HYPERTENSION (*See* BLOOD PRESSURE, HIGH; *and also* CHAPTER V.)

HYPERTHYROIDISM (*See* GOITER; *and also* CHAPTER XVI.)

HYPOCHONDRIASIS Enjoyment of ill health. Hypochondriacs seem to get pleasure out of being ill and having other people wait on them. Of course, few people are completely healthy. Different people have different thresholds of irritation. Minor pains and aches disturb some people much more than they do others. To the hypochondriac, every cough is a threat of consumption. Actually, a cough is just a sign that there is irritation somewhere in the breathing tract. Hypochondriacs sometimes fix upon some one organ of the body, relating everything to the stomach, the liver, the intestines, or even to a fear of mental disturbance. A hypochondriac who fixes his attention on the gastrointestinal tract can develop such symptoms as loss of appetite, nausea, belching, fullness in the stomach and distress after meals.

Obviously, the symptoms associated with hypochondriasis can also be the actual symptoms of a variety of diseases. Thus every person should be given the benefit of the doubt, and have careful study to determine whether anything is definitely wrong that can be corrected. Actually, hypochondriasis itself may need the help of a psychiatrist, to treat the mind as well as the body. (*See also* CHAPTER XXX.)

HYPOTENSION (*See* BLOOD PRESSURE, LOW; *and also* CHAPTER V.)

HYSTERECTOMY Total or partial removal of the uterus.

HYSTERIA A psychoneurotic disorder characterized by much emotionalism. Hysteria may imitate a variety of diseases. Usually, hysteria disturbs activities of daily life. Queer actions take place, related to eating, sleeping, working, remembering, listening or talking. Most important in hysteria is to be certain of the diagnosis. Failing to detect a real condition and calling it hysteria is serious. Charlatans sometimes develop great reputations by exploiting hysteria and bringing about miraculous "cures" through hocus-pocus. (*See also* CHAPTER XXX.)

I

IATROGENIC DISEASE A "disease" induced by a physician—i.e., mental disturbance in a patient caused by something the doctor said or by a diagnosis made too bluntly or a drug prescribed which induces undesirable symptoms.

ICHTHYOL Proprietary name for a coal-tar product which was formerly much used in conditions affecting the skin.

ICHTHYOSIS When a baby is born with a skin that is dry, rough and scaly like that of a fish, the condition is called fishskin disease or ichthyosis. The cause is not known, but there is some evidence that it may be related to deficiencies in the diet of the mother. Hence, nutrition in pregnancy is always of great importance.

ICTERUS (*See* JAUNDICE.)

IDIOSYNCRASY Any special or peculiar characteristic by which a person differs from other people, or any peculiarity of constitution that makes a person react differently from most people to drugs or treatment. (*See also* ALLERGY; *and also* CHAPTER XII.)

ILEITIS Inflammation of the ileum. Food enters the body through the mouth, passes downward through the stomach into the intestines. The first portion of the small intestines is called the duodenum, next the jejunum and then the ileum. The ileum connects with the cecum from which juts off the appendix. The ileum may become blocked so that food does not pass through by masses of indigestible residue, by collections of roundworms, by tumors, by having one part folding into another called *intussusception*. The walls may be infected by germs or viruses or become inflamed with swelling, redness due to congestion and pain. Such inflammation is called *ileitis*. The doctor diagnoses the conditions from his examinations including use of the X-ray, feeling the area, and listening for the movement of the tissues. According to the extent and severity of the condition the treatment may be palliative or radical which includes surgery. Surgery may involve removal of portions of the bowel, or bypassing the damaged portion through short circuiting which connects the bowel above the damaged portion to the bowel below it.

IMMUNIZATION The act or process of protecting against disease. A child is born with substances in his blood derived from the mother which enable him to resist certain infections. These gradually disappear from the blood, so that after from six to nine months, the child needs extra protection against common infectious diseases.

At about nine months of age, children used to be vaccinated against smallpox; by the twelfth month, they should be protected against diphtheria with the toxoid; inoculations are also available against lockjaw, or tetanus. Newest among the inoculations is the one against infantile paralysis. This is given now in three injections: the first two, two weeks apart; the third, ten months later. Also the Sabin vaccine which is taken by mouth. Sometimes inoculation against diphtheria, whooping cough, lockjaw and poliomyelitis is given in one injection. For protection against measles gamma globulin may be given, which also protects against infectious hepatitis and, to some extent, against infantile paralysis. An antimeasles vaccine is now available. Substances are available for protection against typhoid and

paratyphoid and against typhus, yellow fever, cholera and dysentery. These inoculations are used particularly when persons are going to areas where they will be especially exposed. (*See also* CHAPTER XXII.)

IMPETIGO A serious infection of the skin which brings on blisters, often filled with pus. Impetigo is often transferred from one person to another by the fingernails or the hands, which carry streptococci and staphylococci or other pus-forming germs. Women occasionally get the disease from children. In men, the most frequent source of infection is the barbershop. For the prevention of this infection, the possibility of contamination must be avoided. Use a separate washcloth and towel; wash the hands frequently before touching the skin; exclude children from contact with other children who are infected. Formerly, impetigo was treated with various antiseptics. Nowadays, pus infections are controlled with sulfonamides and antibiotics like penicillin, terramycin and others, so that impetigo is more easily controllable. (*See also* CHAPTER XXIII.)

INDIGESTION Incomplete or difficult digestion. Symptoms related to stomach disturbances should not be dismissed as indigestion or dyspepsia, due to "something I ate." Most people with so-called indigestion have nervous indigestion, accompanied by palpitations, cold hands and feet, sweaty hands, headache, fatigue and similar symptoms. They complain of fullness after eating. They eat too frequently and too fast, often swallowing air. These people feel better with massage and with diets which are easily digestible. (*See also* CHAPTER VII.)

INFANTILE PARALYSIS Poliomyelitis, an infection by a family of viruses that gets into the body and eventually reaches the anterior cells of the spinal cord which it destroys, bringing on paralysis. The virus, one of the smallest known, is now known to be one of several different types. The condition may vary, from an attack that seems like a slight cold with a little stiffness of the neck to complete paralysis of the arms and legs and even of the breathing apparatus. In the preparalytic stage, there is fever, sore throat, a cough or a cold, along with headache, nausea or vomiting. Important and alarming symptoms include trembling of the hands or other parts of the body and pain or stiffness in the neck and back. A trained physician quickly detects the difference between infantile paralysis and the ordinary cold or the beginning of an infectious disease of a mild type.

The spinal fluid may show changes in the number of cells, and the doctor may want to put the needle into the spine to get some of this fluid for examination.

Vaccines called the "Salk vaccine" and the "Sabin vaccine" have been discovered, and a test involving millions of children has shown that these have protective value against infantile paralysis. The use of splints, frames and plaster casts in early cases is gradually giving way to the application of hot packs, which bring about the relief of pain and spasm which are typical of the early stages of infantile paralysis. During the acute early stage, the child should be subjected to a minimum of handling.

Difficulty with breathing may be controllable by some one of the special respiratory devices which are now available. After the acute illness has subsided, the patient may be treated by physical therapists and by orthopedic surgeons to bring about the maximum recovery possible. Underwater exercises, because they enable the development of muscles, are most useful. These muscles may take the place of those paralyzed. Braces and supports are used to encourage restoration to full activity. (*See also* CHAPTER XXII.)

INFANTILISM If certain glands fail to function properly at the time of birth, a condition called infantilism develops which includes mental retardation, underdevelopment of the sex organs, and sometimes diminished height.

INFARCT Occlusion of an artery which cuts off the blood supply so that the tissue affected cannot live. Most important is myocardia infarct, referring to blocking of circulation in the blood vessels of the heart. Most important symptoms are chest pain, fall of blood pressure, and often shock.

INFLUENZA The distinction between influenza and the common cold is difficult even for experts. Influenza commonly occurs in epidemics and has been definitely related to viruses known as influenza viruses. Conditions similar to influenza are caused by other viruses. Influenza occurs in epidemics, whereas the common cold goes on all the time. A person may have an influenza virus mixed with ordinary germs. In the ordinary attack of influenza there is a sudden fever, with severe protraction, pains in the back and legs, redness of the eyes and inflammation of the throat. Usually the person comes down with the disease from one to three days after exposure. After influenza a period of depression and weakness follows which, for most people, is more serious than the disease itself. For people who seem to have little resistance against influenza, vaccination with the viruses produces increased resistance. The person with influenza or the common cold or a similar condition should take plenty of fluids, eat a light diet, and stay in bed until the depression and weakness are gone. Antibiotic drugs are useful in keeping away invading germs which may cause streptococcus infections or pneumonia. Influenza vaccines are used to protect against some viruses. (*See also* CHAPTER XXII.)

INSOMNIA Failure to sleep. The exact cause of the regular onset of sleep is not known. Contributing factors to insomnia may include noises, light, internal disturbances, difficulties with breathing, anxiety, and physical discomforts of all kinds. Innumerable drugs are available which depress the activity of the brain, reduce sensitivity, and thus induce sleep. These drugs are known as hypnotics. Exceedingly strong drugs are known as narcotics. People get into the habit of taking such drugs, and then discover that they cannot sleep without them. They may take

more and more of the drugs, and accidental deaths have occurred. Reasonable warmth of the body and the presence of fresh air is helpful toward sleep. A heavy meal should not be taken within four hours of the time of going to bed, but a light snack just before going to bed stops hunger pains and aids sleep. The reading of a relaxing book to reduce tension also aids sleep.

INTERMITTENT CLAUDICATION (*See* BUERGER'S DISEASE; SPASM.)

INTERTRIGO (*See* CHAFING.)

INTESTINES The intestines, commonly called the bowels, are divided into the small and large intestines. They extend from the stomach to the lower opening or anus. The small intestine is about twenty feet long; the large intestine about five feet long. The small intestine includes the duodenum, the jejunum, and the ileum. The large intestine includes the cecum (with the appendix), the ascending, transverse, and descending colon (including the sigmoid) and the rectum. The walls of the intestine are covered by mucous membrane which includes glands.

IODINE A germicide much used in the form of a tincture to prevent infections. If the alcohol evaporates, the iodine becomes extremely concentrated and may burn the skin. Surgeons use iodine to disinfect the skin. Iodine is used in various skin diseases to destroy germs. Taken internally, strong iodine is corrosive. Minimal doses of iodine are taken,

339

perhaps best as iodized salt, to prevent simple goiter.

IRITIS Infection attacking the colored portion (iris) of the eye. With this infection the iris becomes swollen, dull, and discolored. The pupil gets small, gray, and sluggish. Iritis may be secondary to infections elsewhere in the body by such germs as those of the streptococcus group or by the organism that causes syphilis. Diabetes may cause the development of iritis, in which case, of course, treatment of the diabetes is most important. (*See also* EYE; *and also* CHAPTER XXV.)

IRON An element used in medicine chiefly for its effect in stimulating the formation of red blood cells with plenty of hemoglobin. Iron-deficiency anemias are discussed under ANEMIA. (*See also* CHAPTER XIV.)

ITCHING Itching has been defined as "unpleasant sensation in the skin provoking the desire to scratch." Scientifically, itching is a combination of the sense of touch and pain. People can itch while they are asleep or unconscious. Some people itch more readily than others, simply because their threshold of feeling in the skin is lower than usual. Old people itch more often and more easily than young people. Itching may be associated with contact with various chemicals, with fungi, with insect bites, with changes in temperature. Winter itch is about the same as bath itch, both apparently associated with drying the skin. Winter itch disappears in warm weather because perspiration helps to keep the skin moist and soft. Many sub-stances are known which relieve itching, such as menthol and camphor, also ointments containing tar and other substances so toxic that they are prescribed only by doctors.

ITCH MITE (*See* SCABIES.)

J

JAUNDICE Yellowness of the skin and of the whites of the eyes due to circulation of bile in the blood; also called icterus. When red corpuscles break down in the blood, the residue is eliminated through the liver as bile. The bile goes from the liver to the gall bladder, where it is stored and occasionally discharged into the intestines. Blocking in this system may cause the bile to get into the blood, producing jaundice.

When the liver becomes infected, as in hepatitis, the condition is called "catarrhal jaundice." Hepatitis is caused by a virus. Jaundice is a symptom, and not a disease in itself. Usually it is a symptom of damage to the liver or the bile system. The cause should be determined, because jaundice, unless suitably controlled, may result in death. (*See also* CHAPTER VII.)

JOINT DISTURBANCES (*See* ARTHRITIS; BACKACHE; GOUT; *and also* CHAPTER XIII.)

JUGULAR VEINS The veins at the front of the throat.

JUNGLE ROT Soldiers in the tropics, frequently affected with ring-worm because of the moisture on the skin due to heat, called the condition jungle rot. (*See also* RINGWORM; *and also* CHAPTER XXIII.)

K

KALA-AZAR A tropical disease accompanied by fever, progressive anemia, enlargement of the spleen and liver, and filling of the tissues with fluid. This disease is seen along the shores of the Mediterranean, in West Africa, in India, China and Brazil. The disease is transmitted to people by the bite of the sand fly. Some American soldiers developed the condition in our wars. It has been called dumdum fever, black fever and Mediterranean fever. (*See also* CHAPTERS XXI, XXII.)

KELOID When scars overgrow in recovery from wounds, the condition is called keloid. People thus suscep-tible may get such overgrown scars even from a pin prick, a broken pim-ple or a flea bite. The exact cause has never been determined. They may grow anywhere on the body. Usually they are painless, although fixation on the scars may cause women to feel itching or burning or pricking sensations in the keloids.

Apparently they can be suitably removed by surgery. Recently a sub-stance has been discovered, called hyaluronidase, which apparently acts to break down the cells and thus stop keloids. Careful plastic surgery,

accompanied by the use of this sub-stance, in which the scar is cut away and the tissues sewed together again, is helpful in many instances in re-moving keloids without new ones being formed. Radium and X-ray have been used on small keloids with success.

KIDNEYS On either side of the spine, toward the back of the abdo-men, are the two organs called the kidneys. The kidney is shaped like a bean. Each kidney weighs about a quarter of a pound. The kidney has two parts: a central portion and an outside portion. These parts work together, as the blood passes through them, to produce the urine and to eliminate waste material from the body. All the blood in the body passes repeatedly through the kid-neys. Fortunately, each person has two kidneys; these are vital organs, and if one is damaged, the other carries on the work. An infection of the kidneys is called pyelitis. The kidneys become infected by germs brought from elsewhere in the body. Nowadays many useful drugs are available for stopping infection in the kidneys, including the sulfon-amides, the antibiotics, and mandelic acid. The drug to be used depends on the nature of the infection. The kidneys may be so seriously dam-aged that they become inflamed and fail to do their work. This condition is called nephritis. A damaged kid-ney gives off albumin. If a kidney vessel becomes blocked, the cavity swells, producing a cystic kidney. Doctors can obtain material coming from each kidney separately, and thus determine what is wrong and how the condition is best attacked.

(*See also* NEPHRITIS; *and also* CHAPTER VIII.)

KNOCK-KNEE A condition in which the legs are not straight but come together at the knees, scientifically called genu valgum. In all deformities of shape and position, orthopedic surgeons can help by braces or by surgical procedures.

KRAEUROSIS A condition of the skin which is progressive, with hardening and shriveling. This condition sometimes affects the genital organs of both men and women.

KYPHOSIS Hunchback or curvature of the spine, usually situated in the middle of the spine and involving one or many of the bones of the spine. A similar condition is brought about by progressive arthritis. The condition produces not only a convex shape in a portion of the spine but also round shouders.

L

LABIA A Latin term meaning "lips."

LABOR A common term referring to the mechanism of childbirth.

LACRIMATION The pouring of tears from the eye.

LAMENESS Limping or weakness and loss of function of the leg, with the production of an abnormal gait.

Lameness may result from many causes, including arthritis, damage to the tissues, hemorrhage into the muscles (called charley horse) or difficulties with the bones. Lameness is itself simply a catchall term for a great variety of conditions which interfere with locomotion.

LARYNGITIS Inflammation of the vocal cords may follow overuse of the voice. Irritation by chemical substances or infection may also be causes.

In serious inflammation of the larynx, go to bed and keep quiet. Nothing helps the vocal cords more than rest. Speak only in whispers. Applications of warmth or cold to the throat may bring some comfort. Inhalation of steam, into which aromatic oils can be added, seems to aid recovery. The larynx is the organ of speech. Loss of the vocal cords due to serious diseases which require surgical procedures is now met by the application of several new devices, which are called "artificial voice boxes" and which can aid speech. (*See also* HOARSENESS; *and also* CHAPTER XXVI.)

LAXATIVE Any substance that aids in elimination from the bowel. (*See also* CATHARTICS AND LAXATIVES; *also* CHAPTERS VII, XXXI.)

LEFT-HANDEDNESS Using the left hand in preference to the right. People are left-handed or right-handed according to the structure of the brain. Attempts have been made to correlate "left-handedness" with vision, speech, hearing, etc., and with mental activities, but apparently the left-handed are as mentally sound as the right-handed. One side dominates. Attempts to change domination may lead to mental problems, like stuttering or difficulties with speech.

LEPROSY An infectious disease characterized by the gradual development of areas of tissue without feeling which eventually dies and becomes gangrenous, mutilating the body. Leprosy is a transmissible disease which has been known for thousands of years. However, it is not nearly so fearsome as its reputation would indicate. In the United States, patients with transmissible leprosy are confined in a leprosarium. There are only some hundreds of these persons in the United States. Estimates indicate that there are about an equal number not confined. In some parts of the world, thousands of people with leprosy mingle freely in the population. Leprosy is better known as Hansen's disease, named for an investigator who discovered the organism. The suggestion has been made that it be called hansenosis, so as to get rid of the evil repute of the word leprosy. Modern treatment with chaulmoogra oil and diasone and other sulfa derivatives is often effective.

LEUKEMIA One of the most fatal of all diseases of the blood, called a cancer of the blood. The normal human being has about 7,500 white blood cells in every cubic millimeter of blood. In leukemia the number increases, getting as high as 1,000,000 white blood cells for every cubic millimeter. These white blood cells crowd out the red blood cells and the platelets, producing

anemia and bleeding. In the modern treatment of leukemia, radioactive phosphorus has been used, also nitrogen mustards and other products which inhibit the creation of the excess white blood cells. (*See also* CANCER; *and also* CHAPTER XXIV.)

LEUKOCYTES The technical name for white blood cells. There are many different kinds. In some diseases they are tremendously increased, as in leukemia. In granulocytopenia, on the other hand, they may disappear from the blood. Either such circumstance may be most serious and lead to death. (*See also* CHAPTER IV.)

LEUKOPLAKIA A condition in which white patches develop on the tongue, the cheeks, and the gums. The condition is believed to be related to smoking and has been called smoker's tongue and smoker's patches. The exact cause is not known however.

LEUKORRHEA Excessive formation of mucus and secretion from the cells of the female sex organs. The word comes from two Greek words meaning a white flow; in slang, the condition is called the whites. Perhaps repeated use of irritating douches may be responsible. If harmful germs are absent, the condition is annoying and uncomfortable but not serious.

LIBIDO A term used, chiefly by psychoanalysts, to refer to sexual desire and to the energy developed by primitive impulses.

LICHEN Lesions of the skin which

consist of solid papules with exaggerated markings on the skin. Most common is lichen planus, a common inflammatory skin disease. Itching may be slight or severe. The condition may be acute and widespread, or it may be chronic and localized. Some are convinced that its cause is a nervous one.

LINIMENT A liquid intended for application to the skin by friction. Liniments are made with turpentine, ammonia, belladonna, calamine, chloroform, soft soap or other ingredients. They are often used in rheumatic pains to produce increased circulation and a sense of tingling and warmth which seems to be helpful.

LIPOMA Tumors consisting mostly of fat. Lipomas may become mixed with other tumors. They are not especially malignant.

LIPS Inflammation of the lips may occur from irritation or infection. Sensitivity to chemical ingredients of lipsticks may produce eruptions. Cold sores and fever sores may appear on the lips. Deficiency of certain vitamins, particularly riboflavin, which is a part of vitamin B, may be followed by cracking at the corners of the mouth and the appearance of blisters. Such infections as carbuncles and boils may occur around the lips, where they are especially serious because of the large blood supply which may carry the infection elsewhere. Most serious of conditions affecting the lips is cancer. Chronic irritation from holding a warm pipestem, or from other irritation to the lips, may result in cancer, which is usually treated by radium, X-ray or surgery. (*See* CLEFT PALATE.)

LIVER The largest gland or organ in the body. It weighs approximately four to five pounds. It lies in the upper right part of the abdomen, immediately under the diaphragm. The liver has several lobes, and a rich blood supply. It is the great chemical storehouse of the body. It develops the bile, handles the breakdown of protein products, stores glycogen and fat, maintains the composition of the blood, and helps the body get rid of poisonous substances.

Most serious of the conditions affecting the liver are: tumors, cirrhosis or hardening, atrophy or wasting, and infections by a variety of bacteria or parasites, causing inflammation or hepatitis. Vitamin deficiency may definitely harm the liver and interfere with the carrying out of its function. Fortunately the liver, like other vital organs, is a hardy tissue and tends to repair itself. (*See also* CHAPTER VII.)

LIVER EXTRACTS In the treatment of pernicious anemia the use of liver extracts has, in general, been supplemented by folic acid and vitamin B_{12}. However, many people believe that whole liver still contains substances which have not been isolated, and certainly vitamin B_{12} protects the nervous system beyond the extent of what is secured from folic acid. (*See also* ANEMIA, PERNICIOUS; *and also* CHAPTER XIV.)

LIVER SPOTS (*See* CHLOASMA.)

LOCKJAW (*See* TETANUS.)

LOCOMOTOR ATAXIA This was the old name for a condition of the nervous system now called tabes and recognized as a form of infection of the brain by syphilis.

LORDOSIS Forward curvature of the spine.

LOUSE A parasitic insect. Wherever great numbers of people are crowded together infestation by lice is a possibility. Head lice are a frequent annoyance among children in school. To kill head lice, mix kerosene and sweet oil, and rub well into the scalp. Then cover the head with a piece of muslin for at least two hours, or better, overnight. Be careful to keep the head away from contact with any lighted flame. When the muslin cover is removed, wash the hair and scalp with soap and hot water, then rinse well with clear water. Repeat the procedure as often as live vermin are found in the hair. For the removal of nits, wet the hair thoroughly with hot vinegar and comb it with a fine-toothed comb; repeat until all the nits are gone. Always dry the hair thoroughly before going out.

Other substances for removal of "lice" are known. However, these demand control by experts and should not be used except under such conditions.

For removal of lice from clothing and disinfectization, live steam is used. (*See also* CHAPTER XXIX.)

LUNGS The organs of respiration which change the blood coming through their veins by adding oxygen from the air that is inhaled. There are two lungs—the right which has three lobes, and the left which has two lobes. The lungs are in the chest or thoracic cavity and they are surrounded by a membrane called the pleura. (*See also* BREATHING; PNEUMONIA; TUBERCULOSIS; *and also* CHAPTERS III, IV.)

LUPUS A chronic tuberculosis disease of the skin, associated with the formation of nodules.

LUPUS ERYTHEMATOSUS A chronic or acute disease of the skin with red scaling patches of various sizes. The condition occurs on the exposed areas of the face, scalp and hands. This form of lupus is not caused by the germ of tuberculosis. The condition is now recognized as a special disorder of the connective tissue system related to such conditions as xeroderma, periarteritis nodosa, and other disorders. Usually young girls are affected.

LUPUS VULGARIS True tuberculosis of the skin. This condition develops slowly and produces scars and serious changes in the skin. (*See also* TUBERCULOSIS.)

LYMPH Most of the tissues of the body are connected through little channels which collect materials from the spaces between the cells. These are called lymphatic vessels, and they contain a transparent, slightly yellow fluid called "lymph."

LYSOL A solution of cresol is sold under the proprietary name of *Lysol*. This is an antiseptic solution which is caustic and is poisonous in high concentrates. The solution should be kept away from children, because on occasion children have taken the fluid into the mouth and burned the mouth and throat.

M

MADURA FOOT Infestation of the foot by organisms known as mycetes which can get into the tissues through an opening in the skin, and set up inflammation. Also known as mycetoma. Especially serious among American troops in the tropics. (*See also* CHAPTER XXVIII.)

MAGNESIA Various salts of magnesia are used as purgatives. Magnesium citrate is most popular. This is usually bought by the bottle and taken in the morning on arising, in amounts prescribed by the doctor.

MAIDENHEAD (*See* HYMEN.)

MALARIA An infectious disease caused by a parasite known as the "plasmodium" and transmitted by infected mosquitoes of the Anopheles family; several forms of malaria are known. At least four different plasmodia have been associated with human malaria. These plasmodia get into the red blood cells and ultimately destroy them. As a part of the process, malarial chills or paroxysms occur, giving rise to the different forms of malaria—the types that are irregular, the types that come regularly every two, three, or four days. A typical malarial paroxysm begins with a feeling of coldness, then of heat and finally of sweating. New drugs have been discovered which are extremely effective against ma-

laria. Most of them are related to quinine. Malaria is probably the most widespread disease in the world. It can be controlled through control of the mosquitoes that spread it. Such control involves the cleaning up of swamps, removal of excess rain water, spraying of areas with oils or insecticides that destroy the mosquito in various stages. People who are constantly exposed to malaria in tropical areas take either quinine or the new drugs every day one hour before sunset. They screen their beds at night and keep the air moving to get rid of the mosquitoes. During the day suitable clothing is worn to prevent access of the mosquito to the skin. (*See also* CHAPTER XXIX.)

MALINGERER A person who fakes illness or disability to escape military duty or to collect insurance.

MAMMARY GLAND The scientific name for the breast.

MARASMUS Malnutrition with gradual wastings of the tissues, caused by an insufficient, imperfect food supply or failure to absorb a good food supply. (*See also* CHAPTER XIV.)

MASOCHISM Derivation of sexual pleasure from pain, flogging, and humiliation. Named after the novelist, Sacher-Masoch, who described such a case.

MASSAGE Rubbing, kneading or stroking of the superficial portions of the body, with the hand or by various devices to improve circulation and promote well-being; also to break up adhesions in the body. Following massage, often there comes relief of pain, decrease in swelling, and increase of motion in much of the body that has not moved easily.

MASTITIS Inflammation of the breast, from injuries and infections by various germs. If abscesses form, they are eliminated by surgery. Ordinary infections of the breast in either men or animals are now controllable through use of sulfonamides and antibiotic drugs.

MASTOIDITIS Infection in the mastoid, bone cells behind the ear. Often mastoiditis is brought about by infection from blowing the nose with the nostrils closed, forcing the infected material back into the internal ear and the mastoid. Mastoiditis includes a swelling behind the ear, with the point painful on pressure, usually preceded by a severe earache. Infection of the mastoid has in the past frequently followed such diseases as measles, scarlet fever and diphtheria. Formerly hundreds or thousands of operations used to be done on the mastoids. Now, however, the early use of sulfonamide drugs and antibiotics in streptococcal infections of the nose and throat has cut down the number of such operations to exceedingly few. (*See also* EAR; OTITIS; *and also* CHAPTER XXVI.)

MEASLES A virus disease, with running of the nose and sore throat, resistance of the eyes to light, and an eruption of the skin which is characteristic. In the mouth, white spots appear called "koplik spots." Usually the eruption fades in three or four days, and the skin peels in a mild way. Once perhaps the most frequent of all childhood diseases, measles is now to a considerable extent controlled by inoculation with gamma globulin or measles virus vaccine for prevention. The use of antibiotic drugs has eliminated the dangerous complications of measles. (*See also* CHAPTER XXII.)

MEASLES, GERMAN Rubella; an infectious disease usually appearing in children of grade school and high school age, seldom in children under five years of age. The condition is highly contagious, spreading rapidly from one person to another. The eruption appears on the chest as pale pink spots which spread rapidly and finally become bright scarlet. In this condition, the lymph glands at the back of the neck become swollen. Occasionally German measles is mistaken for scarlet fever or ordinary measles. The condition is seldom serious. Patients put to bed recover rapidly, with the fall of temperature and the disappearance of the rash.

German measles has come to be considered more serious nowadays, because a connection has been developed between infection with the virus of German measles during pregnancy and serious damage to the body of the unborn child. A high incidence of disturbances of vision, hearing and of the heart has been found in babies whose mothers have had German measles during pregnancy. (*See also* CHAPTER XXII.)

MELANCHOLIA In some forms of mental disorder, the most prominent symptoms are extreme depression, with fear, brooding and painful delusions. Such patients are usually exceedingly quiet, and show no desire to move about. The symptoms frequently come on during the menopause or "change of life" in women and at about the same age in men. Such people find life disturbing, and become exceedingly anxious about their financial condition, problems in the family and fancied slights. Women suffer more often than do men. The use of glandular preparations to take the place of the diminished secretions of the glands has been found helpful in some instances, and good psychiatric attention, food, rest and good hygiene seem to help greatly. (*See also* CHAPTER XXX.)

MELANOSIS Pigment in the body derived from the blood. This deposit may occur in various portions of the body and produce what is called melanosis. In the skin, deposits of melanin are observed in sunburn, around the nipples during pregnancy, and in various infections of the skin. Particularly serious are melanotic cancers in the skin; highly pigmented growths producing what is called "melanoma" (tumor of the skin) are especially dangerous and should have prompt attention.

MÉNIÈRE'S DISEASE A common condition which includes difficulty with hearing, ringing in the ears, and sudden attacks of dizziness. The exact cause is not known. Suspected causes include allergy, viruses, insufficient activity of the adrenal glands and physical changes in the internal ear. Treatment includes avoidance of allergens, low-salt diet, and in the most severe cases surgical decompression in the internal ear.

MENINGES The coverings of the

brain and spinal cord. Infection and inflammation of these coverings produces meningitis. Tumors affecting the meninges are meningiomas.

MENINGITIS Infection and inflammation of the meninges. Many forms of meningitis are known, depending on the infecting germ, the portion of the meninges that is involved and the pathological condition that develops. Most common is cerebrospinal meningitis which occurs in epidemic form, and which is due to a special germ that attacks the meninges. The symptoms arise from the changes that the germs and their poisons produce in the tissues of the nervous system. Meningitis begins, as do most infectious diseases, with sore throat, dullness, fever, chills, rapid pulse, and general soreness of the body. A delicate pinpoint-sized red rash may be found on the chest, or even large spots over the body. This condition spreads rapidly, when it begins in areas where people are overcrowded. The discovery of a serum against meningitis resulted in cutting down the death rate greatly. More recently, use of sulfonamides and antibiotics has been found more effective than serum and is the method of control commonly employed. Bear in mind that meningitis may be caused, however, by other germs, such as the germs of tuberculosis, of pneumonia, the various streptococci, and even rarely seen germs. The method of treatment is definitely related to the causative organism. For the tuberculous germs, streptomycin is more effective than some of the other antibiotic drugs. (*See also* CHAPTER XXII.)

MENOPAUSE The climacteric or climax, change of life. Between the ages of forty-five and fifty the average woman undergoes gradual changes in the sex glands that bring on certain symptoms. These symptoms are definitely related to the breaking down of the glands. Most common is the appearance of what are called hot flashes, during which the entire body becomes warm and there is excessive perspiration, followed by chilliness. Changes in the circulation bring on palpitation, headache and dizziness; frequently are associated with irritability and also with sleeplessness. Fortunately, new discoveries have developed substitutes for the glandular materials which are effective in stopping the most serious symptoms. These are mostly estrogenic hormones, and synthetic forms are known, called stilbesterol. These drugs, when suitably prescribed by the doctor, have been of the greatest importance in freeing women from the fears associated with the menopause and in overcoming the disagreeable symptoms.

MENSTRUATION Periodic bleeding from the uterus. The period represents the development of an egg cell by the ovaries and the passing of this egg cell into the uterus. The uterus gets ready for the egg cell by a congestion, and the bleeding is the sign that there has not been a pregnancy and that the congestion is disappearing from the uterus. In fact, one poetic doctor said that menstruation is the weeping of the uterus at its failure to become pregnant. Girls in the United States mature between twelve and sixteen years of age, although some are earlier and some later. In other countries girls may mature much sooner—this apparently being true in the hot countries. Failure to menstruate may be associated with a variety of symptoms. If the appearances of maturity are unusually delayed, a young girl should be taken to the doctor for a careful and complete examination to find out the cause.

When pregnancy occurs, menstruation stops until after the child is born.

Formerly, many girls were incapacitated during menstruation because of pain and, customarily, sedatives and pain-relieving drugs were used. The newer attitude toward this normal function has freed women from this terror, and dysmenorrhea is not as frequent as formerly. The relationship between the mind and menstruation is more clearly established and a condition known as premenstrual tension has been described, for which special treatment is also available. Ordinarily a young woman need not change her habits greatly during this period. Most doctors believe that strenuous exercise should be avoided, tub baths may not be desirable, but many women do not permit menstruation to interfere with any of their ordinary habits. (*See also* DYSMENORRHEA; *and also* CHAPTER XVI.)

METABOLISM When food stuffs are taken into the body, they are broken down into various constituents, which are then picked up by the blood, and new materials are developed to be used by the body. This whole process is called metabolism.

The basal metabolism is the minimum amount of energy expenditure necessary to maintain the activity of the cells of the body when it has had complete rest in a warm atmosphere; the metabolism is measured about twelve to eighteen hours after any food has been taken. This is the basal metabolic rate. The basal metabolic rate is raised during activities. It may be raised by excessive action of the thyroid gland. The basal metabolic rate is lowered during sleep and rest and under the influence of various drugs. (*See also* CHAPTER XIV.)

METRITIS Metro usually refers to the uterus. Metritis or endometritis is an inflammation of the lining of the uterus. Metrorrhagia is a hemorrhage from the uterus.

METRONIDAZOLE A new drug, also called Flagyl^R, found specific against Trichomoniasis infection of the genital tissues.

MIGRAINE (*See* HEADACHE; *also* CHAPTERS II, XII.)

MISCARRIAGE (*See* ABORTION.)

MISCEGENATION Marriage of two people of different races.

MITRAL VALVE The valve on the left side of the heart between the upper and lower chambers. (*See also* HEART; *and also* CHAPTER VI.)

MOLES Growth of the skin, usually colored and with hair; also called nevus. Also masses formed in the uterus by membranes or by discontinued growth of a fetus may

be known as a mole. Proliferation and cystic degeneration of masses from the forming membrane may be called hydatidiform mole.

MONILIASIS Infection with a fungus of a group that is scientifically called *Candida*. Various portions of the body may be involved, such as the skin, the nails, the bronchial tubes, the lungs, or the genital organs. Recently, doctors have found that the taking of antibiotics in excess may destroy the ordinary germs for which the germs causing moniliasis then substitute.

MONONUCLEOSIS When leukocytes with a single cell develop in increased numbers in the blood. One form of this condition, believed to be caused by a virus, is called infectious mononucleosis. This begins with fever, sore throat, swelling of the lymph glands, particularly in back of the neck, and the characteristic increase in the mononuclear cells of the blood. Epidemics have occurred, particularly among students and in barracks. In a recent outbreak, evidence was assembled indicating that the disease was spread particularly by the practice of petting or necking, with the exchange of saliva from person to person.

MOTION SICKNESS (*see* AIR SICKNESS.)

MOUNTAIN SICKNESS A condition occurring particularly at altitudes over 15,000 feet, apparently due to the diminished atmospheric pressure. The symptoms include: rapid pulse, headache, dizziness, loss of appetite, blueness, shortness of breath, muscular weakness. The control of this condition is, obviously, to get the person down to a lower altitude. (*See also* AIR SICKNESS.)

MOUTH, DISEASES OF (*See* PYORRHEA; TONGUE.)

MUCUS A thick, glary liquid secreted by mucous glands. The substance consists of water, mucin, inorganic salts and cells held in a suspension.

MULTIPLE SCLEROSIS A disease of the spinal cord in which there is degeneration and scarring resulting in paralysis. The cause is unknown. The condition is slowly progressive. Treatment includes drugs which have the ability to encourage circulation of blood. In this condition the myelin sheaths of the nerves are destroyed. Apparently a person may be sensitized to his own myelin. Injections of Cortisone directly into the spinal fluid have been reportedly helpful. (*See also* SCLEROSIS.)

MUMPS An acute infectious disease caused by a virus and characterized by swelling of the parotid glands and also by occasional damage to other glands. About two to three weeks after exposure, the disease begins, with fever, pain below the ear, and swelling of the parotid gland. This usually subsides in about a week without suppuration. Mumps is especially serious in time of war, when men are crowded together in barracks. Usually the disease affects children between the ages of five and fifteen. Most often, it occurs in early winter and spring. The danger of the condition is in the spread of mumps to other glands, particularly the sex glands. A vaccine has been developed against mumps; otherwise, the treatment is usually the provision of a good diet with plenty of fluids, rest, drugs, if necessary, to relieve the pain and lower temperature. (*See also* CHAPTER XXII.)

MUSCLE CRAMPS An involuntary severe contraction of muscle fibers. At least half the people, if not all of them, occasionally develop cramps in the muscles of the legs, which come on during exercise or at night when they turn or stretch. These cramps come on more frequently in the presence of fatigue or lack of sufficient blood supply and, occasionally, with deficiencies of vitamins and of calcium. Many suggestions have been made for relieving these cramps including, for instance, breathing into a paper sack, which acts as a stimulus to taking more oxygen. Calcium has been used. Quinine has been suggested as a specific, and in severe cases the new drug chlorpromazine has been tried. In the vast majority of cases, such cramps are hardly of sufficient significance to demand much more than an encouragement to keep the legs warm and to use enough exercise to encourage the circulation.

Somewhat similar is a condition described in Sweden called restless legs. The person concerned seems to be unable to keep the legs quiet upon lying down, and is constantly moving them.

MUSCULAR DYSTROPHY Most

351

serious of muscular diseases are the muscular dystrophies in which the muscles waste away and lose their strength. Causes are not definitely known, nor is there a specific method of treatment. In a typical case, a child who seems to be normal at birth will begin at the age of four or five to be unable to use the legs properly, and to tumble about. The back muscles become weak, so that the child cannot sit erect. Soon he finds difficulty in getting up from the floor. The wasting of the muscles may be complete, or there may be progressive weakness. As certain muscles become weak, stronger muscles pull, and this produces distortion of the body.

MUSCLE INJURIES Muscles may be injured by any of the accidents that injure other tissues. When the fibers are torn, they bleed. Bleeding into a muscle produces a painful condition known as charley horse.

Treatment depends on the nature and scope of the injury. Rest and the application of heat, in most instances, takes care of ordinary minor hemorrhages into the muscles. Severe damage usually requires surgical procedures.

MUSTARD PLASTERS An old home remedy, used as a counterirritant to draw blood to the area where the mustard plaster is applied. These can be so strong that they will blister the skin. The mustard plaster seems to be falling into complete disuse. It should never be left on for more than fifteen to thirty minutes.

MYASTHENIA This term is used to indicate weakness of the muscles. (*See also* MUSCLE DISEASES.)

MYCOSIS Infection caused by fungi.

MYELITIS Inflammation of the spinal cord, as in *polio*myelitis, or inflammation of the bone marrow as in *osteo*myelitis.

MYELOMA Tumor of the bone marrow. It may be malignant or cancerous, and demand prompt diagnosis and surgical procedures for removal. (*See also* CANCER; *and also* CHAPTER XXIV.)

MYIASIS Invasion of the eye or the ear or the intestines by the larvae of flies. (*See also* CHAPTER XXIX.)

MYOPIA Nearsightedness, an extremely frequent disability of the eye. (*See also* EYE; *and also* CHAPTER XXV.)

MYXEDEMA A disorder due to deficient secretion of the thyroid gland caused by a failure of the gland to perform suitably at birth, or growth of a simple goiter due to a lack of iodine, infection, or damage to the gland. The chief symptoms are a sallow, puffy appearance, especially of the face and hands, a low metabolic rate, increased sensitivity to cold, dryness of the skin, absence of perspiration, dryness of the hair, brittle nails, decreased interest in living, a thick tongue with coarse speech, and many changes in the blood. Myxedema, which is associated with cretinism, is completely controlled by the taking of thyroid extract or thyroxin. (*See also* GLANDS; *and also* CHAPTER XVI.)

N

NAIL BITING A common habit of children and adolescents; onychophagia is the highly fancy name given to this. Some even bite the fingernails down to the quick. The habit is difficult to break and may even persist into adult years. As little girls grow up, they are broken of the habit more easily than boys, because of manicuring, the use of nail lacquers, and other cosmetic uses.

NARCISSISM A term used by psychiatrists to indicate self-love or fixation of the libido upon one's own body. Named for the beautiful Greek boy who fell in love with his own reflection.

NARCOLEPSY An uncontrollable tendency to acts of deep sleep, which are usually of short duration. Observed in various diseases and also simply as a condition in itself. Sometimes the muscles of the body would seem to lose their strength, so that the person falls to the ground without loss of consciousness. The person with "narcolepsy" has a sleepy look upon his face and is disinclined to move around much. Few people die of this condition, unless as the result of an accident. Ephedrine sulfate helps to prevent these attacks of sleep. More recently, benzedrine or amphetamine has been found useful in controlling narcolepsy, and also psychic energizing drugs.

NARCOTIC ADDICTION (*See* ADDICTION.)

NAVEL, DISEASES OF The navel (umbilicus) is the scar left when the umbilical cord is cut. After the cord is cut the excess tissue shrinks, leaving the scar. In the newborn child, the care of the navel is important to prevent infection. The navel is covered with a sterile dressing and watched carefully until it heals. If hemorrhage occurs, prompt attention is necessary to stop serious bleeding. The navel contains creases and folds, and therefore demands regular washing, preferably with soap and water. Any condition that affects the skin may also affect the navel, including attacks by germs or even insect bites.

NEPHRECTOMY Surgical removal of the kidney. (*See also* CHAPTER VIII.)

NEPHRITIS Inflammation of the kidney. Several forms are known, depending on the portion of the kidney attacked or the cause of the infection. Interstitial nephritis attacks the tissue between the cells of the kidney and, when it becomes chronic, is associated with a rise in the blood pressure and other serious changes in the body. The nephritis may attack the tubules of the kidney or the glomeruli, which are the portions that develop the urine. In an acute infection of the kidney, the tissues swell and enough poisoning of the body may occur to cause convulsions or unconsciousness.

Chronic inflammation of the kidney or chronic interstitial nephritis is known as Bright's disease.

353

The conditions likely to cause suspicion of infection of the kidneys include headache, mental depression and fatigue; the skin develops a pale or pasty appearance, with swelling or puffiness under the eyes, on the backs of the hands and around the feet; the blood pressure rises; accumulation of fluid in the body may become enormous. The diagnosis is made through examination of the urine, which will show a large amount of albumin and also cells from the kidneys, sometimes in the form of actual moldings in the shape of the tubules. These are called casts. In the presence of acute inflammation of the kidney, immediate rest in bed is desirable, with a simple and nutritious diet. Everything should be done to protect the kidneys against an overburdening of material. There has been a popular belief that meat in any form is harmful in Bright's disease but protein is so necessary for the building and repair of body tissue that an adequate amount of body protein must be supplied. During a severe attack of disturbances of the kidney every tissue of the body must be watched, and particularly the blood.

Stone in the kidney may be called nephrolithiasis. (*See also* KIDNEYS; *and also* CHAPTER VIII.)

NERVOUSNESS When people get excited too easily, when they are disturbed or when they have tremors and weakness, the condition may be called nervousness. This is just a catchall term, and exact diagnosis gives the condition a more definite name. (*See also* CHAPTERS XI, XXX, XXXIII.)

NEURALGIA Pain in the nerve. It may be severe and definitely along the course of a nerve, or it may vary in its extent and scope in many ways. The facial nerve has three branches, and pain may occur in any or all of them. This is called trigeminal neuralgia and when limited to the part along the cheek is usually known as *tic douloureux*. Pain over the eye is called supraorbital neuralgia and affects the nerve of the same name. Sciatica is neuralgia of the sciatic nerve.

The pains of neuralgia are sharp, stabbing, and come in paroxysms which may last just a short time but recur. Sometimes the nerve is so sensitive that merely blowing on the skin will produce a paroxysm of pain.

Pain associated with the nerves of the teeth is called dental neuralgia.

Many ways of controlling pain in nerves have been detected. Alcohol has been injected directly into nerve areas. Inhalations of various drugs that produce insensitivity to pain have been tried. Surgical operations are done, to cut or remove nerves. Vitamins are helpful in some cases and, conceivably, neuralgias are related to deficiencies of vitamins. Among the vitamins most frequently helpful are thiamin and vitamin B_{12}. (*See also* CHAPTER XXXIV.)

NEURASTHENIA Symptoms formerly ascribed to exhaustion of the nerves, including fatigability, lack of energy, and various indiscriminate aches and pains, were formerly thought to be a special disease of the nerves. Nowadays the term psychasthenia is preferred, since in most instances this represents a condition associated with mental rather than physical effects. (*See also* CHAPTER XXX.)

NEURITIS Inflammation of nerves and changes that are either degenerative or inflammatory are accompanied by pain, hypersensitivity, loss of sensation, paralysis, and the disappearance of the reflexes which doctors test to determine the nature of the nerve involved.

Neuritis may arise from various toxins or poisons like lead or alcohol, from diseases like diphtheria or malaria, or from rheumatic conditions. If more than one nerve is affected, the condition may be called multiple neuritis or polyneuritis. Treatment depends on determining the cause and removing it. For relief, many pain-relieving drugs and sedative drugs are used. If infection is detected, antibiotic drugs may be tried.

NEUROSIS Mental disturbances of a mild character. Sometimes called anxiety neurosis or psychoneurosis. In anxiety neurosis the chief symptoms are emotional instability, irritability, apprehension, and great fatigue. This form of neurosis is associated with emotional problems. Other manifestations include palpitations, nausea, a rapid heartbeat, occasionally diarrhea, and tremors. Other forms of neuroses are those due to fright, to obsession, or associated with various occupations. (*See also* NEURASTHENIA.)

NEVUS Birthmark or angioma of the skin. A circumscribed area of pigmentation of the skin, usually with large blood vessels, may appear shortly after birth or at the time of birth. These angiomas are described according to their appearance and whether or not they are covered with hair. Examples are port-wine nevus, spider nevus, warty nevus, and others. These nevi are now controllable by X-ray or radium and also by surgical treatment. Sometimes they are removed with carbon dioxide snow or by electric coagulation.

NIGHT CONDITIONS Many conditions of disturbance of living are related to the night. Nightmare is a terrifying dream that usually awakens the sleeper with a sense of oppression and distress. A night cry is a shrill cry uttered by a child during sleep, which is sometimes related to the beginnings of definite disorders; on the other hand, far more often it is simply the reflection of a dream. Pain at night in the hips or knees may occur as a symptom of hip disease but also, like muscle cramps at night, may be without great significance. Frequently night palsy develops. This is a numbness of the extremities occurring during the night or upon waking in the morning, and which is related to the circulation of the blood. Lying long in one position may produce it, or lying on an arm such as happens in what doctors call "honeymoon paralysis." Night sweats frequently accompany fevers, and especially the fever of tuberculosis. Some people see better at night than others; they have night vision, which seems to be related to the supply of vitamin A. Nightwalking is called somnambulism, and is obviously quite definitely related to dreams which cause the person to get up and move about. Night terrors (pavor nocturnus) are descriptive of conditions which occur in children, perhaps because of bad psychological conditioning of adults. If it were not for adults, babies would never be afraid. They become frightened because older people frighten them with stories of the bogeyman. Older people teach them to fear policemen and doctors and burglars, and no doubt television and radio have helped this process. Babies have a fear of loud, sudden noises and they fear falling. When parents are overanxious and excessively affectionate, their attitudes are reflected in the child's thoughts and dreams. A common source of the development of night terrors is the threat that the child's hand or his sex organs will be cut off, because the parent or nursemaid has become displeased at something the child has done.

NOISE Unnecessary noise is a health hazard, and even necessary noise may need to be controlled by the wearing of earplugs or other devices to lessen its impact. Experiments have proved that the constant impinging of sound on the nerves may be damaging to health. Hardness of hearing, dizziness and headaches have developed in persons who work in boilermaking plants or in other occupations in which the noise may be tremendous and without much cessation or rest.

NOSE Prominent organ in the center of the face composed of small bones and cartilages and the soft tissues which surround two cavities; the nose itself is surrounded by the sinuses. Minor infections may occur in the hair follicles or in the roots of the hairs in the nose. Such infections are manifested by redness, swelling, discomfort, and pain which increases steadily. Infections in the nose are particularly serious because they may spread into the blood vessels. The right way to take care of the nose is to remove carefully by proper use of the handkerchief such material as can be reached easily; what cannot be reached can be washed out. (*See also* CHAPTER XXVI.)

NOSEBLEEDS (*See* EPISTAXIS; HEMORRHAGE.)

NOSE, FOREIGN BODIES IN Children and particularly infants put into their mouths anything they can pick up, and occasionally push things into the nose. Buttons, beans, pieces of chalk or erasers have been taken out of noses, and are especially dangerous if they are inhaled and go on down into the windpipe. They should never be pushed around with knitting needles or toothpicks or other devices. Doctors have special instruments for extracting such materials. The X-ray picture will show exactly where the foreign material is, and permit the doctor to grasp and extract it without harm to the delicate tissues. (*See also* CHAPTER XXVI.)

NUTRITION (*See* AMINO ACIDS; CARBOHYDRATE; VITAMINS; WEIGHT, OVER- AND UNDER-; *and also* CHAPTERS XIV, XV.)

NYCTALOPIA Night-blindness, inability to see at night, due to deficiency of vitamin A. (*See also* CHAPTER XV.)

NYMPHOMANIA Excessive desire for sexual activity in a woman.

NYSTAGMUS Oscillatory horizontal movements of the eyeballs. Miners' nystagmus occurs particularly in men who work in cramped quarters with insufficient illumination. The oscillation which occurs only when the patient's head is placed at an abnormal plane is positional nystagmus. Finally there is rhythmic nystagmus, in which the eyes slowly wander a few degrees in one direction and then adjust back. This is seen in passengers in moving vehicles who watch the landscape and also in viewers at tennis championships.

O

OBESITY (*See* WEIGHT, OVER- AND UNDER-; *also see* CHAPTER XIV.)

OLD AGE (*See* SENESCENCE; *and also* CHAPTER X.)

OLFACTORY The sense of smell. Disturbances of the sense of smell may include anosmia, which is loss of the sense of smell. In some disturbances of the brain, tests are made of the ability to smell various odors, which may indicate the portion of the brain involved.

OMENTUM The organs of the abdomen are covered with a membrane called the peritoneum. That portion which connects the abdominal organs with the stomach is called the omentum.

ONYCHIA Inflammation of the matrix of the fingernails. This may occur from infections of various kinds, particularly infection by ringworm.

ONYCHOPHAGIA (*See* NAIL BITING.)

OPHTHALMIA Inflammation of the eye, especially when the conjunctiva is involved. This term is modified by other words, to indicate the form of inflammation. *Ophthalmia neonatorum* is a purulent infection of the eyeball, usually by gonorrhea, which occurs at the time of birth. Egyptian ophthalmia is another name for trachoma. Sympathetic ophthalmia is the inflammation of an eye which follows a serious infection or inflammation of the other eye. Then there is paralysis of the eye, termed ophthalmoplegia; the ophthalmoscope which is used to examine the eye; and ophthalmology, which is the name of the specialty. A specialist who devotes himself to diseases affecting the eye is an ophthalmologist. (*See also* EYE; TRACHOMA; *and also* CHAPTER XXV.)

ORCHITIS Inflammation of the testicle. This may result from any kind of an infection, particularly gonorrhea. The symptoms are pain, swelling, and a feeling of weight. Treatment depends on the nature of the disturbance. Surgery may be required.

ORGASM The culmination or climax of the sexual act is usually, in the male, ejaculation of fluid, associated with intense excitement. In women, there is similar sensation, without the elimination of fluid but with gradual decongestion and relaxation. Difficulties with this process are more frequently psychic than physical.

ORTHODONTICS The branch of dentistry which straightens teeth and makes the bite normal. Formerly called orthodontia.

ORTHOPEDIC The branch of surgery concerned with the correction of deformities of the joints and spine.

ORTHOPSYCHIATRY A subdivision of psychiatry, concerned with the prevention and treatment of disorders of behavior, particularly in adolescents.

ORTHOPNEA A condition in which it is necessary for the person to sit up to breathe easily.

OSTEOMYELITIS Infection of the bones involving the bone marrow. In most cases it is due to pus-forming germs like the staphylococcus and the streptococcus, but other germs may be involved. The long bones of the body are the most frequently affected, but any bone can be involved. Osteomyelitis of the jawbone is among the most serious of its forms.

Osteomyelitis is painful and is associated with fever, rapid pulse, and all the usual signs of infection. The use of the X-ray helps to establish the location of the damage. Because bones are associated with the production of blood, infections from bone marrow may be carried throughout the body, and especially to other areas of bone marrow.

Once the presence of osteomyelitis is determined, modern medicine requires the use of the antibiotic drugs to destroy the infection; opening of the bone may be necessary to release the infected material which is under pressure and to give opportunity for direct application of antibiotic drugs to such areas. (*See also* CHAPTER XVII.)

OTITIS An inflammation of the ear, which can be called internal or external otitis, or otitis of the middle portion of the ear (otitis media) according to the part of the ear involved. Infections of the ear come most frequently from extension, by way of the nose or from the outside, and occasionally through the blood. The symptoms of otitis include severe pain, which is relieved when the eardrum is opened. This is especially important, because failure to relieve the pressure of the infected material may extend it to the mastoid cells producing mastoiditis. (*See also* EAR; MASTOIDITIS; *and also* CHAPTER XXVI.)

OTOSCLEROSIS Progressive deafness, associated with hardening of the small bones of the internal ear so that they fail to function. The exact cause of this condition is not known. Most authorities consider it a chronic inflammatory disease.

Otosclerosis occurs more often in women than in men. Sometimes the first complaint is a ringing in the ears, with gradual progressive loss of hearing. Sufficient hearing may remain to permit the person to follow ordinary conversation. In other cases the deafness is so severe that it becomes necessary to learn lip reading or to wear a hearing aid. The nature of the hearing aid should be determined by actual trial.

Some authorities have thought that otosclerosis was related to vitamin deficiencies, but this has not been proved. When the doctor examines the patient with otosclerosis, he makes certain that all of the accessory factors involved in hearing are properly functioning. The Eustachian tubes are cleaned, by blowing through them. The diet is investigated. Sedative drugs may be tried to control the ringing in the ears.

Recently, surgical operations have been developed to make a window from the outside into the internal ear. This has proved of vast benefit in many cases. Another new operation is called mobilization of the stapes which loosens up the ossicles or small bones inside the eardrum. (*See also* EAR; DEAFNESS; *and also* CHAPTER XXVI.)

OUTLET The lower opening of the pelvic canal is called by obstetricians the outlet. This is measured before childbirth, to determine whether or not the child can be born safely.

OVARY A female sex gland. There are two ovaries, one on each side, in the lower portion of the abdomen.

The ovary provides the female egg cell which passes each month down the Fallopian tube to the uterus. The ovary also develops glandular substances important for establishing the female body structure and the functions peculiar to women.

The ovary may become twisted on the tissues which support it, which will affect its blood supply and bring on pain and swelling. Blocking of the ovarian ducts may cause the formation of ovarian cysts as large collections of fluid. Pain may arise, and it will become necessary to open the abdomen and to get rid of such cysts.

Ovaries may become infected by any of the germs that are carried in the blood or that pass through the ovary by extension from other organs and tissues. Infections are responsible for more than 90 per cent of disturbances of the ovary. If pus forms in the Fallopian tubes, it may extend over to the ovary. Pain, swelling, high fever and similar symptoms demand attention. Again, adequate use of antibiotic drugs in many instances brings about complete relief.

Tumors of all kinds can affect the ovary, including cancer.

The doctor cannot determine from any examination that he can carry on from the outside of the body the exact nature of such tumors. In the examination of the ovary he may insert a finger into the rectum; he may press on the abdomen from the outside; he may take X-ray pictures; in cases of extreme doubt, when diagnosis is important, the abdomen may be opened in an exploratory operation, to find out exactly what is wrong. (*See also* GLANDS; *and also* CHAPTER XVI.)

OXYGEN Used for many purposes in medicine, practically all of which relate to relieving difficulties of breathing. The iron lung and the chest respirators are used when there is paralysis of the breathing apparatus in infantile paralysis. In pneumonia when the lung is incapacitated by congestion, oxygen may be given through tubes or in oxygen tents. Oxygen is used after carbon monoxide poisoning to provide air for breathing. The shortage of air which occurs with diseases of the heart may be treated by oxygen, but if the difficulty is primarily due to slowing of the circulation the oxygen is only a temporary relief. (*See* also CHAPTER IV.)

OZENA An extraordinary, unfortunate disease resulting from drying of the mucous membranes of the nose, with crusting and infection. (Ozena is derived from a Greek word meaning "stench.") In this disease gradual degeneration of the membrane that lines the nose occurs; discharge collects and drys, causing foul-smelling crusts. Vitamin deficiencies may be related to the development of this condition. A recent point of view is that continued infection of the nose in infancy gradually produces atrophy and death of the mucous membrane. Physicians treat such conditions by suitable washes of the nose, by packing the nose with gauze containing antiseptic materials, by feeding of diets that are adequate in salts and vitamins.

P

PACIFIER Any article, such as a rubber nipple or a little bag filled with sugar, that is placed in the mouths of irritable children to pacify them. For a while doctors forbade their use, believing that they deformed the mouth or created dependence on the device. More recently, particularly in England, pacifiers have returned to good standing, and are being developed of suitable materials to encourage teething.

PAIN The human skin is sensitive to touch, heat and cold, and also to pain. In the skin are little nerve endings which respond with pain when touched with the point of a pin. Pain also occurs wherever there are nerves of sensation. Tests are developed for measuring the intensity of pain, but have not yet been so definitely accepted as to constitute standards. There may be pain from excessive heat applied to the skin; there is also pain from pressure on the skin. In order to test pain-relieving drugs, tests have been developed, using the pricking of a pin, burning of light rays, pressure or pinching; but these tests are only relative.

Pain is diminished in surgical operations by using anesthesia, by blocking nerves, by cutting nerves and by the use of pain-relieving drugs. Pain on the surface must be distinguished from pain in the bones, blood vessels or organs of the body. The neurologists have traced the pathways of pain, from the point of origin to the brain. Psychiatrists recognize psychogenic pain which is wholly mental. Psychogenic pains are vague, irregular in appearance, inclined to be exaggerated, and often accompanied by signs of excellent health otherwise. Psychiatric pains may be treated by psychiatry rather than by drugs. Finally, there are the indeterminate pains which people develop when they want to collect from insurance companies after accidents. (*See also* CHAPTER II.)

PAINTER'S COLIC (*See* POISONING; *and also* CHAPTER XVIII.)

PALATE The roof of the mouth. (*See also* CLEFT PALATE.)

PALPITATION A fluttering or throbbing, especially of the heart, or any motion of the heart of which the person is aware. Ordinarily, we are not aware of the actions of the heart. Palpitations are often psychosomatic phenomena. (*See also* HEART; *and also* CHAPTER VI.)

PALSY Paralysis. Most frequent is shaking palsy. (*See also* BELL'S PALSY; PARALYSIS AGITANS; *and also* CHAPTER III.)

PANCREAS A large gland situated in the abdomen near the stomach, liver and gall bladder, which secretes digestive ferments and makes insulin for the metabolism of sugar by the body.

Inflammations of the gall bladder often extend to the pancreas, and this makes them especially serious. Sometimes the pancreas is infected by germs brought from elsewhere in the body by way of the blood.

Infection of the pancreas may be associated with severe pain and difficulties of digestion. The determination of pancreatic infection in its relationship to the gall bladder is a difficult diagnosis.

Other conditions that affect the pancreas include cysts, stones and tumors. Excessive tissue in the pancreas results in excessive insulin, and this may produce a condition called hyperinsulinism. People with excessive amounts of insulin in the blood may have symptoms which have caused them to be diagnosed as alcoholics. Most serious is cancer of the pancreas, because it is a vital organ and its removal is hazardous to life. (*See also* GLANDS; *and also* CHAPTER XVI.)

PARALYSIS (*See* CEREBRUM; ENCEPHALITIS; INFANTILE PARALYSIS; PARAPLEGIA; *and also* CHAPTER III.)

PARALYSIS AGITANS Involuntary, tremulous motions of the body, with lessened muscular power, is typical of paralysis agitans or the shaking palsy. Because this condition was discovered by James Parkinson, it is called Parkinson's disease and the tremors Parkinsonism. There are several different types of Parkinsonism; some follow brain inflammation, some are without any known cause, and others are related to hardening of the arteries in the brain.

As this condition develops, the face develops a masklike appearance, and there is a tendency to bend the trunk forward and to pass from a walking to a running pace to keep from falling over. Paralysis agitans comes on late in life as a distinct condition, but occurs in younger people following infections of the brain. The rate of progress of the condition varies. In many instances it may be confined to one limb, or even a finger, for months before other portions of the body are affected. Strong emotional stimuli may bring about sudden temporary stopping of the shaking.

The most important drug now used in the treatment of Parkinson's disease is L-Dopa (an abbreviation of a long chemical name). L-Dopa can be given by mouth after the physician has determined just how much of the drug is necessary to control the symptoms. The effects of the drug, which must be prescribed by a physician, vary. Sometimes side effects occur which must also be controlled. Parkinson's disease is no longer considered to be uncontrollable or necessarily progressive. (*See also* ENCEPHALITIS; *and also* CHAPTER III.)

PARAPLEGIA Paralysis of the lower limbs. It may result from a variety of causes, including various poisonings, and damage to the spinal cord such as results from industrial or war injuries. (*See also* CHAPTER III.)

PAREGORIC A camphorated tincture of opium which is used to stop pain and also diarrhea.

PARESIS A slight paralysis.

PARESTHESIA A sensation of tingling, crawling or burning of the skin, without any obvious cause, which occurs in neuritis involving the nerves near the surface of the body and also in certain disturbances of the spinal cord.

PARKINSON'S DISEASE (*See* PARALYSIS AGITANS.)

362

PAROTITIS Inflammation of the parotid glands, as in mumps. Inflammation of the lymph glands that lie over the parotid glands may also be called parotitis.

PARTURITION The process of giving birth to a child. (*See also* PREGNANCY.)

PATCH TEST In making a patch test, a small patch of adhesive, with gauze containing a substance to which a person may be sensitive, is applied to the skin. If redness and inflammation appear, the test is positive. (*See also* ALLERGY; DESENSITIZATION; *and also* CHAPTER XII.)

PEDIATRICIAN A specialist in the treatment of children's diseases.

PELLAGRA A condition characterized by spinal pain and digestive disturbances, redness, dryness and peeling of the skin, nervous symptoms like spasm, and even mental disturbances. Known for centuries, particularly in Italy, southern France, Spain, and the southern part of the United States. For a long time it was associated with the eating of spoiled maize or corn. Research proved that pellagra is more likely related to a deficiency of certain essential substances in the diet. Most important is nicotinic acid (also known as niacin) which is part of the vitamin-B complex. Feeding with yeast, liver extract, fresh milk, eggs and lean meats brings about recovery in people with pellagra. Often they have been living on pork fat, corn bread, soda biscuits and corn syrup. (*See also* VITAMINS; *and also* CHAPTER XV.)

PELVIMETRY Before childbirth, the obstetrician measures the dimensions and capacity of the female pelvis—the basin-shaped ring of bones at the bottom of the trunk, joining the legs below and the spine above.

PEMPHIGUS A skin disease in which large blisters form, which break and leave pigmented spots. Itching and burning occurs with the blisters. Many varieties of pemphigus are known, and also other skin diseases which are like pemphigus.

PENICILLIN The powder extracted from a mold called *penicillium notatum*. First of a long list of antibiotics, this product is immensely effective in treating infections by germs of many varieties. Other antibiotics widely used include: bacitracin, aureomycin, terramycin, chloramphenicol or chloromycetin, tetracycline, erythrocycline, and at least two hundred more that are now undergoing active experimentation.

PENIS The male sex organ; it becomes erectile and is used in sexual intercourse. At its center is the urethra, which carries the urine from the bladder to the outside. Surgical procedures are used to correct structural disorders. Circumcision removes the foreskin, which sometimes is painful or infected. Hypospadia is a splitting of portions of the organ, so that its opening is at the bottom or on the inner side instead of at the front.

PERLECHE When angles of the mouths of children, and sometimes adults, develop inflammatory conditions with the formation of cracks, the condition is called perleche. It may result from infection. Most often it is associated with a deficiency of vitamins, particularly vitamin B_2, called riboflavin, and vitamin B_6, called pyridoxine. (*See also* CHAPTER XV.)

PERICARDITIS Inflammation of the pericardium, the sac enveloping the heart. Symptoms include pain, rapid pulse, often severe coughing. The doctor hears sounds with his stethoscope that indicate to him infection of the pericardium. Many varieties are known, depending on the nature of the germs infecting. If fluid or pus forms inside the pericardium between it and the heart, the doctor may insert a needle to take off the excess material and permit the heart to beat properly. (*See also* HEART; *and also* CHAPTER VI.)

PERINEUM The space between the genital organs and the anus or lower opening of the bowel. This may be torn in childbirth, or attacked by infections, particularly by ringworm, which also attack the groin. These infections produce severe itching and sometimes blistering. Perineal disturbances are uncomfortable, and should have prompt treatment.

PERITONITIS The peritoneum is the name of the membrane that lines the abdominal cavity. It may push through the wall of the abdomen, in the case of a rupture. Cysts occur in folds of the peritoneum. Part of the peritoneum is called the mesentery and cysts in the mesentery are called mesenteric cysts.

363

Most serious of the conditions that affect the peritoneum is peritonitis. The tissue becomes infected and inflamed, particularly after injuries to the abdomen, rupture of appendix, or abscess in the appendix. Occasionally the peritoneum becomes infected from an ulcer of the stomach or duodenum, from an infection in the gall bladder or, in fact, from infection in almost any abdominal organ. Absorption of the toxic materials threatens life. Signs of peritonitis include fever, rigidity of the abdominal wall, and tenderness when the wall is touched. When there is severe abdominal pain, accompanied by tenderness of the whole abdominal wall, vomiting and fever, the doctor suspects peritonitis. In some instances, surgical operation may be necessary.

Since the germs that affect the peritoneum are usually the types that yield to sulfa drugs and penicillin, the record of peritonitis has become much less alarming since these drugs have come into use. (*See also* OMENTUM.)

PERSPIRATION The sweat glands cause water to reach the surface of the skin, and by its evaporation the temperature of the body is controlled. Perspiration, or sweat, is about 98 per cent water. The odor of sweat varies, according to the part of the body from which it is secreted. Perspiration under the arms is likely to be odorous, because of the invasion of bacteria. Perspiration is increased by the drinking of warm drinks, by fright and anxiety, and by a number of drugs which stimulate the flow of water from the skin. Perspiration is decreased by cold, and

by drugs which can stop perspiration. Many drugs are associated with dryness of the throat and skin.

Among the diseases that affect the sweat glands is hyperhidrosis, which is excessive sweating. This may sometimes be a symptom of a serious general condition.

People who perspire frequently should have underwear that does not retain moisture. They should not wear too much clothing. They may use dusting powders which help to limit perspiration. An offensive odor to the sweat generally is called bromidrosis. Colored perspiration is called chromidrosis.

PERTUSSIS (*See* WHOOPING COUGH; *and also* CHAPTER XXII.)

PERVERSION Any deviation from the normal or average in sexual conduct is called perversion.

PESSARY Appliances have been developed which are placed in the vagina in order to hold up the uterus. Similar devices are sometimes used to stop the opening of the uterus and prevent conception.

PHARYNGITIS Between the mouth and the opening of the esophagus which leads to the stomach is an area called the pharynx. Here are the tonsils, and much lymphoid tissue. This area may become infected and inflamed. The condition is pharyngitis. The pharynx is likely to become inflamed when other neighboring tissues are inflamed. In the center of the pharynx there hangs a little piece of tissue called the uvula. Occasionally, this becomes swollen.

In septic sore throat, usually a

streptococcus infection of the pharynx and throat, one is gravely ill, and the breath develops a foul odor. The infection may spread elsewhere, even entering the blood, and cause serious symptoms. Occasionally the septic sore throat occurs in epidemics.

Vincent's angina is a form of infection of the throat, caused by organisms. These are especially susceptible to several different remedies and may be thus controlled. *See also* VINCENT'S ANGINA; *and also* CHAPTER XXVI.)

PHENOLPHTHALEIN A neutral drug that acts on the bowel as a purgative. The drug is almost wholly eliminated from the human body after being taken in, and seldom causes any incidental effects. Rarely, a person may be sensitive to phenolphthalein, which sensitivity manifests itself by red spots developing in the skin. (*See also* CATHARTICS *and* LAXATIVES.)

PHLEBITIS Inflammation of the veins. Clots may be formed when veins are inflamed and, when carried elsewhere in the body, do great harm. Slowing of the circulation of the blood may cause clots in the veins. This happens particularly after surgical operations or childbirth. Hence, doctors now get patients up out of bed earlier and have them move about, to prevent clotting. Swelling of the legs and feet may require elastic bandages; elevation of the foot of the bed tends to aid in elimination of the congestion.

Inflammation of blood vessels, with the formation of clots in the veins, is called thrombophlebitis.

About 1 per cent of cases in childbirth, and about 2 per cent of people who have had severe operations develop thrombophlebitis as a secondary complication.

Thrombophlebitis may cause severe pain. Taking the pressure off is one of the most important methods for reducing pain and aiding healing in thrombophlebitis.

PHTHISIS The name means a progressive wasting and emaciation. This used to be the name for pulmonary consumption or tuberculosis.

PICA Children often crave unnatural articles of food. They attempt to eat sticks, plaster, dirt, or other similar materials. The condition is called pica.

PILES (*See* HEMORRHOIDS.)

PINEAL GLAND A little gland which lies within the skull below the brain, and tends to disappear as the child grows. The gland is tiny—about the size of a pea. When infected or enlarged from any cause, it may close the canal by which the cerebral-spinal fluid circulates from the brain into the spinal cord. Closing of this canal develops a high pressure of fluid in the brain, and may do serious harm. The exact effect of the pineal gland and its exact purpose in life is not positively determined.

PITUITARY GLAND A small reddish-gray organ lying in the skull, below the brain. It has several parts, and a variety of hormones have been obtained from these parts. The hormones produced by the front of the

365

pituitary regulate the growth of all body tissues; control the development and function of the thyroid, the adrenal glands, the sex glands, possibly the parathyroid glands, and also induce the flow of milk. Portions of the posterior lobe affect the blood pressure, the contraction of smooth muscles in the body, and the function of the kidneys. Other portions of the gland seem to be related to the growth of cells generally, to the formation of pigment, to the growth of hair, and to maintaining the general functions of the body against stress. From the pituitary a hormone called ACTH, the adrenocorticotropic hormone, has been developed, which is used in what are called collagen disorders and against any of the disorders which result from stress. (*See also* CHAPTER XVI.)

PLAGUE A contagious, epidemic disease. The two most common forms of plague are bubonic and pneumonic plague, both serious conditions. Plague is carried by lice derived from rats. Modern medicine has developed methods of vaccination against plague and techniques to control it. Seldom does either pneumonic or bubonic plague appear in modern civilized countries.

PLEURISY Infection of the pleura, the lining of the cavity of the chest. It may be infected by any one of a variety of germs, resulting in pleurisy. If the wall has become thickened or roughened, there are sounds that can be heard by the doctor. If pus forms, it must be removed with a needle. Pleurisy is exceedingly painful, and must be controlled by

stopping movement of the ribs, using adhesive straps, and controlling the infection by the use of antibiotic drugs. (*See also* CHAPTER XXII.)

PLEURODYNIA A sharp pain in the muscles between the ribs, the sign of an infectious condition which may occur in epidemic form, with fever. This condition has been called Bornholm's disease, after the Danish island where it was first observed; also devil's grip. The condition is now related to infection with a virus which is called the Coxsackie virus, as it was identified in the Coxsackie area of New York State. The condition is not serious, but its virus is occasionally confused with the virus of infantile paralysis. (*See also* CHAPTER XXII.)

PLEXUS At any point in the body where groups of nerves come together as a network, or where blood vessels come together, or lymphatic glands come together. There are many such plexuses. When such an area becomes damaged by a variety of accidents and infections, it is known, for example, as brachial plexus injury, if it is located in the area under the armpit; or a renal plexus injury, if it is located in the area near the kidneys, etc.

PNEUMA The word comes from the Greek word meaning breath. This prefix, before any other term, refers most often to conditions related to breathing or the lungs.

PNEUMOCOCCUS A germ which affects the lungs.

PNEUMOGRAPH An instrument to record the breathing.

PNEUMONIA Inflammation of the lung. The usual cause of pneumonia is the pneumonia germ, which exists in many varieties. Pneumonia can, however, be caused by the streptococcus or other germs, or by viruses. Pneumonia was once the most feared of diseases, but sulfonamides and antibiotics now control it. The condition can be diagnosed by use of the X-ray, since it produces a congestion and solidification of the lungs which shows in the X-ray pictures. In a typical case, pneumonia follows a cold or some infectious disease. There is a chill. A sharp stabbing pain is felt in the side; the pain is made worse by breathing. Then comes coughing, with bloody or brownish expectoration, and fever. Headache, nausea and vomiting occur, and sleep is difficult because of the general misery and pain. Prostration and weakness occur often. The outpouring of blood and serum into the lung cause it to solidify, so that there is insufficient breathing space and difficulty in the circulation of blood through the lungs back to the heart. As a result fingernails and skin turn blue, indicating shortage of oxygen. The patient will recover suddenly by what used to be called crisis, or gradually by lysis. With the development of the antibiotic drugs, particularly such drugs as sulfadiazine and penicillin, the pneumonia now is brought quickly under control. What used to be a six weeks' illness has been shortened to one week in most instances. The greatest danger of pneumonia is to the young and to the very old. The condition is more dangerous to women than to men. The sustaining of the pa-tient's heart action is obviously of the greatest importance, in order to maintain body strength until the disease is broken up and the patient begins to convalesce. Unlike other infectious diseases, pneumonia may occur more than once in the same person, and as a result certain types of people seem to be frequently its victims. (*See also* CHAPTER XXII.)

PNEUMONIC PLAGUE (*See* PLAGUE.)

POISONING Poisons have serious effects on the human body, and there are many of them. Any drugs, such as acetanilid, alcohol, anilines, atropine, belladonna, boric acid, chloral or other drugs, may produce poisoning. Also poisoning may result from gases, like ether, chloroform, carbon monoxide, acetyline or sulphur dioxide. Poisoning results from food which has been contaminated by germs. Poisoning may result from sensitivity to substances like ivy. For each poison, there is a specific method of controlling it, called an antidote. In general, the first step is to get the poison out of the body. Before the doctor arrives, give whites of eggs, milk, or strong tea, which are antagonistic to many poisons. Vomiting may be provoked by tickling the back of the throat or by giving warm water with salt. With a stomach tube, to be swallowed, a person who knows how to use the tube can wash out the stomach. The simplest procedure is said to be a heaping teaspoonful of salt in a cup of lukewarm water—stir until the salt is dissolved, and have the poisoned person drink the mixture, repeating every three or four minutes

367

until vomiting occurs. (*See also* FOOD POISONING; *and also* CHAPTER XVIII.)

POLIOMYELITIS (*See* INFANTILE PARALYSIS; *and also* CHAPTER XXII.)

POLLUTION Air pollution is a significant factor in disability and disease. The pollutants include carbon monoxide, nitrogen compounds, hydrocarbons, lead, and particles called particulate matter. The major source of pollution is industry and internal combustion engines, also residential heating and smoke from incinerators. Soft coal and high-sulfur oil when burned are sources of pollution. People subjected to much pollution have high rates of respiratory illness.

POLYCYTHEMIA When the red blood cells are increased far above normal of five million to six million in each cubic millimeter of blood, the condition is called polycythemia. In this condition, the red blood cells may reach as many as fifteen million to a cubic millimeter of blood. Polycythemia is accompanied by such symptoms as dizziness, fainting, a feeling of fullness in the head, nosebleed, and sometimes disturbances of vision, and ringing in the ears. The condition usually affects older people rather than young ones. Careful examination of the blood with a microscope will show the presence of the disease. Among new methods of treatment is application of radium or X-ray to the long bones which manufacture red blood cells. Certain drugs have been developed which definitely reduce the excess red blood cells. Most important of recently used drugs is the radioac-

tive isotope of phosphorus or iodine, which has a specific effect on polycythemia. (*See also* CHAPTER IV.)

POLYNEURITIS The inflammation of a number of the nerves of the body.

POLYPS When nodules in the nose or the intestines or the bladder become filled with fluid and hang by connections to the wall, the condition is called polyps. These are removable by surgical procedures or, in the nose, by the use of electric desiccation.

POSTURE The human body is a machine which moves on two feet, standing erect. Since man was originally an animal that walked on four legs, he has a tendency to develop bad posture, with rounded shoulders, stooped shoulders, sunken chest, twisted back, protruding abdomen or lame hips. Constantly there is stress in the body on the various portions that adapt to the new position. Good posture means that the body is held in a correct position when standing, sitting or lying down and also in motion. When standing, the human being must stand tall, the abdomen drawn in, the shoulders squared and high, the chin straight back, the weight properly distributed on the feet, the curve of the back within normal limits. In a correct sitting position, the body is erect, the head poised to bring the center of gravity in the line joining the bones of the hip. This position must be practiced, to become routine. Constant assumption of a bent posture or a drooping position, while at work or at rest, results in a stretching and a relaxing of the ligaments, with a tendency toward permanent sagging; the back gets rounded and the chin shoved forward. (*See also* BACKACHE.)

POULTICE A poultice is a soft, semiliquid mass made from any particular substance which is mixed with water. This is applied to the skin to supply heat and moisture or to produce stimulation. Bread-and-milk poultices used to be used for this purpose. Mustard plasters are occasionally used. The clay poultice is sold under the trademark Antiphlogistine.

POX Any eruption with blisters or pustules, such as chicken pox (varicella), cowpox (vaccinia), smallpox, swine pox. The term pox used to be used as synonymous with syphilis.

PREGNANCY The time from conception until birth; the average pregnancy is 280 days. Every organ and tissue of the body of the mother is affected by pregnancy. The time when a woman is most likely to become pregnant is the period between the sixth and eleventh days after the first day of menstruation.

Signs of Pregnancy The breasts begin to enlarge as early as the second month, and with a first baby, even, sometimes, as early as the second or third week. Among the most definite signs of pregnancy are cessation of menstruation, morning nausea, and vomiting which begins usually during the second month and rarely lasts beyond the fourth month. Another symptom is increased emotionalism, with peevishness, fretfulness and irritability. Cravings for strange foods may appear. Fluttering (called "quickening") is experienced between the sixteenth and eighteenth week. The usual changes in the shape and size of the body are well known. X-ray will show the presence of the child and, later, its position. The doctor can hear the heartbeat of the child between the eighteenth and twentieth weeks and sometimes even earlier. Laboratory tests like the Aschheim-Zondek test, made on rabbits and on frogs, are accurate determinations of the presence of pregnancy.

Prenatal Care The modern doctor is careful about prenatal care in pregnancy. Just as soon as a woman believes she is to become a mother, she should consult her doctor. He will make a complete physical examination, laboratory studies of the secretions and excretions of the body, and a record of the past history of the patient. He will study the blood, the blood pressure, the work of the kidneys. He will make accurate measurements of the organs concerned in childbirth, and thus anticipate any difficulties that may arise. Examinations continue at intervals of a month, and later even at intervals of two weeks or oftener, depending on the development of various symptoms.

Diet The prospective mother may gain about 15 per cent in weight during the nine months previous to the birth of the child. A gain of anything more than 20 pounds is a sign for additional studies of the diet and health of the prospective mother. The prospective mother must have enough vitamins, calcium and phosphorous to provide for the needs of the child. Milk and milk products provide most of the calcium. Diets ordinarily are low in iron, and iron is absolutely necessary for the building of the red blood cells. Among mineral salts, iodine is of great importance. The prospective child makes demands upon the body of the mother, and iodine is needed for the prevention of simple goiter.

The Birth of the Baby Before the baby comes, the mother should assemble the materials required at childbirth, depending on whether she is going to the hospital or having the baby at home. Today, in the United States, more than 85 per cent of all babies are born in hospitals. In most cases the time required for childbirth for a first baby will be between sixteen and eighteen hours, and for later babies, between eight and ten hours. But many women have them faster, others slower. A common belief holds that more babies are born at night than in the daytime. Actually, there is no such variation.

The body of the woman, in most instances, returns to normal in six to eight weeks after childbirth. During this period, rest and diet are important. About the fourth day, in most cases, the mother may begin light exercises, sit up in bed and increase her activity. The tendency nowadays is to get the mother up much earlier than formerly.

PRESBYOPIA When people get old, their eyes change. Slight changes occur after the age of forty. The changes in the eye are due to loss of elasticity of the lenses, and sometimes to changes in muscles. In presbyopia people see well at a distance. One of the chief symptoms is tiredness on reading, culminating sometimes in headaches at the end of the

day. Older women find it difficult to thread needles or to work on fine patterns. Changes in the hearing also occur with old age, inclining toward hardness of hearing. This is called presbycusis. (*See also* EYE; SENESCENCE; *and also* CHAPTERS X, XXV.)

PRICKLY HEAT A condition of the skin with little blisters and spots, accompanied by a pricking or tingling sensation, occurring usually in hot weather and in the tropics. Also called heat rash and scientifically miliaria.

PROCTOLOGY A specialty of medicine concerned with the anatomy, functions and diseases of the rectum; from the Greek word for this organ. Many words are associated, such as proctoscope, the device for looking into the rectum; proctostenosis, a narrowing of the rectum; proctotomy, cutting into the rectum.

PROJECTION Ordinarily, anything that extends forward. In psychopathology, a process of the mind whereby a person overcomes his feelings of inadequacy or guilt by transferring the responsibility to some other person or object. This is especially frequent in paranoia, a form of mental disturbance. (*See also* CHAPTER XXX.)

PROSTATE The organ which surrounds the neck of the male bladder. It consists of several lobes. In advancing years, the organ becomes enlarged, and may interfere with the emptying of the bladder. Swellings occur in connection with any infections or inflammations. Among the greatest advances made by medicine in recent years is the improvement of methods for removing the prostate in cases of simple enlargement. Formerly this required a long surgical procedure. Nowadays, by the use of an electric dissection, the procedure is made safe and may be completed in a short time, without significant mortality.

PRURITIS (*See* ITCHING.)

PSEUDO A prefix indicating that something actually is not, but may resemble, a particular condition. Examples are pseudopregnancy, also called phantom pregnancy and pseudosyesis; pseudojaundice; pseudohermaphroditism; pseudomalady.

PSITTACOSIS An acute disease caused by a virus and producing symptoms in human beings like those of pneumonia. Usually transmitted to human beings by contact with sick birds like parrots, parakeets and lovebirds. (*See also* CHAPTER XXII.)

PSORIASIS A chronic inflammatory skin disease characterized by the development of red patches covered with silvery white scales. This occurs particularly on the scalp and on the extensor surfaces of the limbs. Several varieties have been described. The exact cause is not known. A variety of treatments, including changes in diet, the use of hormones and local applications, are used with some success in diminishing the symptoms. (*See also* CHAPTER XXIII.)

PSYCHO This prefix indicates mental conditions and processes. Examples are psychiatrist, one who spe-

cializes in conditions affecting the mind; psychoanalysis, a method developed by Freud for investigating and treating conditions affecting the mind; psychology, the science that studies the functions of the mind; psychometry, a method of measuring mental processes; psychoneurosis, a large group of conditions which are based not on physical but on mental causes; psychopath, a mentally irresponsible person; psychosis, a mental disorder; psychosomatic, pertaining to conditions which affect the mind and the body, with body effects frequently dependent on the mind.

PTOMAINE An alleged cause of food poisoning. (*See also* FOOD POISONING.)

PULSE A regular throbbing in the arteries caused by contractions of the heart. A finger applied to an artery anywhere near the surface permits counting of the pulse rate. The pulse rate of adults varies from 67 to 72; of infants, between 100 and 120. The fastest pulse rates recorded are over 300 beats per minute. This condition is called tachycardia. A slow pulse is known as bradycardia. (*See also* CHAPTERS I, VI.)

PURPURA Hemorrhages occurring in the skin, the mucous membranes or elsewhere without definite cause or due to slight injury. A special form is *ideopathic thrombocytopenic* purpura due to decreased numbers of platelets in the blood. The condition may follow infections or allergic manifestations. The blood platelets are markedly diminished in number. Fragility of the capillary blood vessels is related. Recent discoveries have shown that ACTH and Cortisone are frequently helpful in overcoming this condition. Removal of the spleen is successful, in a considerable number of cases, in causing discontinuance of the bleeding.

PYELITIS Inflammation of the kidneys. This condition is detected by examination of the urine, by taking X-ray pictures of the kidneys, called pyelograms, after injecting various substances which make them visible with the X-ray. Pyelonephritis is another term for infection of the kidney. Treatment involves accurate diagnosis of the exact nature of the condition, the use of drugs such as sulfonamides, antibiotics and mandelic acid. When control by drugs is impossible, surgical procedures are used. (*See also* KIDNEYS; *and also* CHAPTER VIII.)

PYEMIA Any infection with germs that produces pus which gets into the blood.

PYLORUS The valve which releases food from the stomach into the intestines. Ulcers may occur at the pylorus; spasm in the pylorus occurs in babies, and sometimes requires surgical operation.

PYORRHEA Purulent inflammation of the gums and outer covering of the roots of the teeth. The teeth become loose, and pus can be seen coming from the gums. Pyorrhea is preventable by good dental attention and routine cleanliness. Once pyorrhea has occurred a high quality of dental care is needed, with the use

of specific remedies against infection and careful study of the general health.

Q

QUARANTINE Infectious diseases used to be quarantinable. People were limited as to movements, and had to remain home if there was a case of any infectious disease in the family. "Quarantine" is still used in smallpox, but seldom is it seriously established for other diseases. Of course the sick person may be isolated, which means kept alone and from contact with others, during the time of the infection. Whenever a child has an infectious disease make certain that secondary complications have healed before he is permitted to mingle with other children. (*See also* CHAPTER XXII.)

QUICKENING The first feeling, on the part of a pregnant woman, of movements of the prospective child. This occurs between the fourth and fifth month of pregnancy.

QUININE Used specifically in malaria with great efficiency. Quinine is also employed to lower fever, to prevent pain, as a bitter tonic in convalescence, and to stimulate contraction of the uterus. Because of the side effects of quinine and because, possibly, better products could be developed, thousands of quinine derivatives were studied during the war, and new substances have been developed which are substituted with good effect. Quinine is also occasionally used for fibrillation of the heart and for muscle cramps, in the form of quinadine, which is a substance developed from quinine. (*See also* MALARIA.)

QUINSY An acute inflammation of the tonsils and the tissue around the tonsils, usually with abscesses. A better name is peritonsillar abscess. (*See also* CHAPTER XXVI.)

R

RABIES An acute infectious disease transmitted from animals to man and from animals to other animals by a virus. Most frequently, the wolf, the cat and the dog are affected, but also cattle, foxes and other wild animals may be affected. This virus attacks the nervous system and is found in the saliva. Because serious dryness of the throat occurs in this condition, it is sometimes called hydrophobia.

Vaccines have been developed which protect against rabies. Use of such vaccine is called Pasteur treatment. In treating a dog bite, cauterization is used to destroy the virus completely. Animals are not killed after biting, but are watched for a period of time to make certain that they do not have rabies. If the animal dies, examination is made for the presence of negri bodies, which are diagnostic of rabies.

RADIATION The use of rays of various kinds for the diagnosing and treatment of disease. Radiography is used to describe the use of the X-ray; it is also called roentgenography from Roentgen, who discovered the method. Radioactivity is the power of certain substances to give off certain kinds of rays. A radiologist is a physician who specializes in the use of rays in the diagnosing and treatment of disease. Radium is a highly radioactive substance which is used like the X-ray. (*See also* CHAPTER XIX.)

RALE Any abnormal sound arising in the lungs or air passages heard with the stethoscope on listening over the chest. Doctors have classified many different types of rales.

RASH To the public, any eruption on the skin is a rash. The term is more commonly used for the acute inflammation. Such rashes as diaper rash, drug rash, heat rash, metal rash are exceedingly common.

RAT BITE FEVER (*See* FEVER; *and also* CHAPTER XXII.)

RAUWOLFIA A plant, long known in India, which has recently been carefully studied and found to be of special value in producing relaxation in both mind and body, lowering blood pressure, and for other purposes. The active principle from the drug is known under a variety of names. Since the total name of the drug is *rauwolfia serpentina,* some of the names depend on the word rauwolfia and some on the word serpentina. Examples are rauwolfine and serpasil.

373

RECTUM The portion of the bowel between the sigmoid colon and the anus. The prefix recto is used with a variety of words in relation to conditions which affect the rectum and processes related to diagnosing and treating conditions affecting the rectum.

REFLEX The word reflex describes reaction movements reflected from a stimulus elsewhere in the body; a reflex is an involuntary action. Most widely known reflexes are the knee jerk (absent in many diseases of the brain and spinal cord); the oculocardia reflex (slowing of the rhythm of the heart following depression of the eyeballs); laughter brought on by tickling; vomiting when the throat is tickled with a feather; swallowing anything put on the back of the tongue; a baby jumping when it hears a loud sound (startle reflex).

REFRACTION Testing of the eyes to determine the state of the vision. (*See also* EYE; *and also* CHAPTER XXV.)

RELAPSE After convalescence has begun, the disease sometimes becomes active again, and the symptoms recur. This is called relapse.

RENAL Any condition pertaining to the kidney. (*See also* CHAPTER VIII.)

RESISTANCE A person may be resistant to a disease because he has the antisubstances in his blood. The resistance may be measured by taking samples of the blood and testing them against the organisms or the toxins of the disease. In psychoanalysis, resistance is the reluctance of the person being studied to give up his usual patterns of thinking, feeling and acting and to take on other methods or to adapt himself to other ways. (*See also* CHAPTER XXII.)

RESPIRATION The act of breathing with the lungs—taking in air and expelling it. Taking in air is inspiration, letting out air is expiration. Forcing the person to breathe is called artificial respiration. A respirator is a device for producing breathing and includes what is commonly called an iron lung. Other types of respirator cover only the chest. A new technique in process of experimentation involves using make-and-break electric current to stimulate the nerves that control the diaphragm and thus to produce respiration.

RESPIRATORY TRACT (*See* ALLERGY; BREATHING; COLDS; HAY FEVER; INFLUENZA; PNEUMONIA; RHINITIS; *and also* CHAPTERS III, XII, XXII.)

RESUSCITATION Artificial respiration. Following unconsciousness from any cause such as submersion in water, or electric shock, resuscitation is practiced to restore ordinary breathing. The average person breathes from sixteen to twenty times a minute. Many different techniques have been known and practiced, including the so-called Schaeffer prone method, and the Eve method, which involves rocking the patient on a board, alternately lowering and raising the head. Respiration mixtures of oxygen with carbon dioxide are used to stimulate breathing and to provide the necessary oxygen. People who are getting artificial respiration may need stimulation to the circulation of the blood, which is sometimes helped by rubbing and massage; also body warmth must be maintained.

Now most widely recommended is mouth-to-mouth breathing. Several simple tubular devices have been developed which hold down the tongue of the unconscious person while air is breathed into his lungs. (*See also* CHAPTER XXXIV.)

RETINA Vision is brought about when light rays pass through the eye to the nervous tissue back of the eye, called the retina. Detachment of the retina is a loosening of this structure, resulting in blindness. An operative procedure is now used for treating such cases, causing the retina to become again attached.

An inflammation of the retina is called retinitis; it may be due to infection, hemorrhage, or injury. (*See also* EYE.)

Rh FACTOR Examinations of the blood have indicated that there are, in addition to the usual agglutinating substances, factors now known as Rh positive and Rh negative which are associated with reactions in the blood. About 15 per cent of people are Rh negative. When such people are injected with positive antiserums in blood transfusion, other substances, called agglutinins, are developed, so that subsequent transfusions will cause severe reaction. In babies, at the time of birth, these factors act to produce a serious disease that breaks up the blood vessels and may cause death. The disease is called "erythroblastosis."

A product named Rhogam[R] is used by physicians to desensitize the Rh factor and to prevent severe reactions. Intramuscular injection of one dose of Rhogam will prevent the mother's blood from producing antisubstances which become permanent. By genetic studies the physician can predict which infants may be affected. One in eight marriages brings together an Rh negative woman with an Rh positive man. About one in 200 pregnancies produces an affected child. The mother's blood produces antibodies between incompatible blood passing from the fetus to the maternal blood circulation. In some instances babies born with severe Rh disease have been treated by having all of the infant's damaged blood removed and replacing it with fresh blood from the blood bank. The fresh blood must be of the same type as that of the mother. (*See also* BLOOD TYPES; *and also* CHAPTER IX.)

RHEUM The prefix rheum—is used for a number of conditions, coming from a Greek word which means "flow." Rheumatoid means, "resembling rheumatism." Rheumatism is a general term that indicates diseases of muscles, tendons, joints, bones and nerves, resulting in discomfort and disability. A variety of conditions are called rheumatism, including, for example, rheumatoid arthritis, degenerative joint diseases, inflammations of the spine, bursitis, fibrositis, myositis, neuritis, lumbago, sciatica and gout.

RHEUMATIC FEVER A severe disease characterized by painful arthritis which moves from joint to joint and which is likely in most in-

375

stances to damage the heart. Sometimes the heart only is affected, and joint damage does not occur. The cause of this condition is not definitely known. However doctors are now convinced that it is related to streptococcal infection in the throat, with some hereditary susceptibility to the condition. The disease attacks children, girls more frequently than boys. Although it is stopped, by various methods of treatment, there is a tendency to recurrence.

Much has been learned about rheumatic fever in recent years. Most important is the fact that the treatment of any sore throat immediately with sulfonamide drugs or antibiotic drugs will stop the streptococcal infection which leads to rheumatic fever, and the incidence of this disease is steadily decreasing. When an acute attack occurs, the inflammation may be controlled by ACTH or Cortisone. The patient is, of course, put at rest, and frequently salicylic-acid drugs are given which, when given in sufficient dosage, are also effective in allaying the inflammation. Children with rheumatic fever do better in warm climates than in cold. The period between attacks should be devoted to building up the child's health generally. Parents and teachers should be discouraged from making chronic invalids of children with rheumatic fever.

Of the greatest importance is the prevention of coughs, colds, sore throats and similar conditions. Nowadays, many of the children with rheumatic fever are given special attention in institutions like Irvington House, Irvington-on-the-Hudson, New York; La Rabida Sanitarium,

Chicago; St. Francis Sanitarium, New York, or the Cardiac Hospital in Miami, Florida. Here physicians who understand the condition and good nursing services are available. Many cases are helped and enabled to survive by care in such institutions. (*See also* ARTHRITIS; HEART; *and also* CHAPTERS VI, XIII.)

RHINITIS Any inflammation of the mucous membranes that lie in the nose. This takes serious forms. (*See also* ALLERGY; NOSE; OZENA; *and also* CHAPTER XXVI.)

RHINOPHYMA Changes in the blood vessels that cause the nose to become swollen with big nodules. The condition is treated by plastic surgery of the nose.

RIBS The human being has twenty-four ribs, which form the cage for the chest. They may become bruised or broken. This condition demands treatment in which the ribs are held in place by adhesive tape or other methods until healing occurs. The X-ray picture will reveal the location of the fractures. These are common fractures in motor accidents. Sometimes an extra rib which grows at the top of the chest will cause disturbance by pressure on the tissues. This is called a cervical rib. The ribs at the bottom which are not connected at the front are called floating ribs.

RICKETS When lime salts are not deposited in sufficient amounts in growing cartilage in newly formed bone, the bones are soft, and bend. The condition is called rickets. Once it was little understood; now it is known that it is due to a deficiency of ultraviolet rays and of vitamin D. Since children have been given cod liver oil, halibut liver oil, and similar substances, adequate amounts of calcium, and outdoor exercise in the sun's rays, rickets has practically disappeared. (*See also* CHAPTER XV.)

RINGWORM A fungus infection which may affect any portion of the body. On the feet it produces what is called athlete's foot; in the groin, it produces redness, swelling and often complete disability. Many drugs are now known which can destroy ringworm. Obviously, the greatest cleanliness is necessary to prevent its spread. One of the difficulties in treating ringworm is the fact that people try to treat it themselves and, as a result, suffer from overtreatment, with damage to the skin.

In the prevention of ringworm, dryness is of great importance, because it grows most profusely in warm, moist places. (*See also* CHAPTER XXIII.)

ROCKY MOUNTAIN SPOTTED FEVER (*See* FEVER; *and also* CHAPTER XXII.)

RUBELLA Another name for German measles. (*See also* GERMAN MEASLES.)

RUPTURE (*See* HERNIA.)

S

SACROILIAC (*See* BACKACHE.)

SACRUM A triangular bone formed by five vertebrae at the lower end of the spine. Many backaches are due to disturbances of the joint between the sacrum at the back and the bones of the pelvis in front. (*See also* BACKACHE.)

SADISM Derivation of sexual pleasure from cruelty to others. The word comes from the name of the Marquis de Sade, who wrote a book describing such practices.

SALIVA The fluid secreted by the salivary glands. These glands are under the jaw, in front of the ear, and under the tongue. Saliva contains a starch-digestive ferment which keeps the mouth moist and softens foods. Sometimes stones get in the little tubes leading from the glands. These salivary calculi may have to be removed surgically. (*See also* GLANDS.)

SALPINGITIS Infection of the Fallopian tubes. The infecting agent may be one of a variety of organisms. Gonorrhea used to be the infection most frequent. Salpingitis may be responsible for sterility. (*See also* FALLOPIAN TUBES.)

SARCOMA Tumors like cancer, but consisting of connective tissue.

377

They may involve cartilage of bone or fibrous tissue. They are characterized by the kind of tissue involved—thus *fibro*sarcoma, *chondro*sarcoma, *osteo*sarcoma, or *lipo*sarcoma. The doctor determines the type by examination of a portion of the tissue under the microscope. (*See also* BIOPSY; CANCER; *and also* CHAPTER XXIV.)

SCABIES   Inflammation of the skin with intense itching, occurring chiefly at night. The disorder is caused by the itch mites; the female insect, burrowing beneath the skin to lay eggs, causes the irritation. This condition is sometimes called Cuban itch and seven-year itch. Animals may acquire it, thus there are scabies of canaries, cats, horses and other animals. (*See also* ITCH; *and also* CHAPTER XXIX.)

SCARLET FEVER   An acute contagious disease beginning, usually, from several hours to a week after a person has been exposed to it. Like other infectious diseases, scarlet fever begins with vomiting or chills, followed by high fever, rapid pulse, sore throat, swelling of the glands in the neck and a scarlet-red eruption which appears on the skin. The tongue is heavily coated at first, and red at the tip and edges. Later, the papillae of the tongue become red and swollen, giving the tongue the appearance that is called strawberry tongue. Scarlet fever seems especially to damage the kidneys and one of the most important steps is to make sure that everything possible is done to protect the vital organs.

The discovery of the sulfonamide drugs and the antibiotics is chiefly responsible for the tremendous control that has developed over scarlet fever. The condition is now kept mild, and the secondary complications related to the nose, throat, ears and kidneys are quite rare. Scarlet fever is a member of the group of diseases that are caused by streptococci, which, fortunately are especially susceptible to the antibiotic drugs. (*See also* CHAPTER XXII.)

SCIATICA   The long nerve known as the sciatic nerve passes from the lower part of the spinal column out of the spinal canal through some openings between the bones, then down the back of the thigh and onward to the leg. This nerve, the longest in the body, may become inflamed from a number of causes, and when it does it causes the neuritis called sciatica. In examination for the presence of sciatica, the doctor looks for curvature of the spine or any pressure that might result from bones in wrong positions. He studies the legs for signs of spasms of the muscles. A simple test is to raise the leg in a straight position while lying flat on the back. This puts a strain on the large hamstring muscles, which in turn refer the strain to the nerve. Studies are made with the X-ray of the condition of the sacroiliac joint. Of utmost importance in sciatica are rest, relief from tension, and support to the inflamed tissues. Heat is helpful in relieving pain. Infections are controlled by the usual methods. Surgical procedures include work on the bones and muscles or on the nerve itself. (*See also* CHAPTER XXXIV.)

SCLERODERMA   A condition in

which the skin becomes hardened and yellow, changing its consistency and its color. Women are far more commonly affected than men—most often between twenty and forty years of age. The management of scleroderma includes a warm environment (approximately 78° continuously), adequate nutrition with small amounts of food eaten six times per day, and sleeping with the head of the bed elevated to prevent regurgitation of acid into the esophagus.

SCLEROSIS Hardening which may involve tissues of the eye, the spine, the breast and other portions of the body.

SCOLIOSIS (*See* SPINAL CURVATURE.)

SCURVY (*See* VITAMIN; *and also* CHAPTER XV.)

SEASICKNESS Relationships have been established between the eye, the ear, and the sensation of motion responsible for nausea. Seasickness, of course, is also related to airsickness and car sickness. Among measures found helpful are the wearing of a tight belt, taking champagne before sailing, stuffing the ears with cotton or wool to keep out noises, bandaging the eyes to overcome visual disturbances, eating fruits or alkaline foods, taking baking soda, and a dozen superstitious methods. In fact, one man says, "If you are smoking, don't stop smoking," and the other says, "If you are smoking, stop smoking."

Since seasickness is definitely related to the circular canals in the internal ear, the drugs known as Dramamine, Bonamine, and Merazine have proved highly helpful in diminishing the sensations, and many people now sail with great pleasure, who formerly spent most of their time in bed. Have plenty of sleep before going on the boat, relax, and do everything in moderation. (*See also* AIRSICKNESS; *and also* CHAPTER XXXIV.)

SEBACEOUS CYST (*See* WEN.)

SEBORRHEA A condition characterized by much perspiration and activity of the oil-forming glands. People with unusually greasy skin do better with diets rich in proteins but restricted as to sugars, fluids, fats and salts. A diet high in vitamins, particularly leafy green vegetables and fresh fruits, seems to be helpful. There may be relationships to the glands, particularly the sex glands. Dandruff on the scalp is a form of seborrhea. Dandruff can be removed by washing the hair at least once a week, bathing the body regularly at least once a day, and avoiding the wearing of clothing that produces heat, such as heavy, hot hats. When there are pimples on the face, with a greasy complexion and enlarged pores, when there is scaling and inflammation of the skin behind the ears and in the groin, seborrhea becomes a serious condition.

SENESCENCE The gradual aging of the body. In senility this aging process is complicated by a variety of conditions. Old age is seldom uncomplicated. The cells of the body break down and lose their power of repair. Tissues become fibrous or calcified. Normal old age comes on

379

gradually and is usually well established by age sixty-five, but there are exceptions. The condition of the blood vessels is very important, probably the most important single factor in aging. Hardening of the arteries is likely to be associated with more rapid degenerative changes. The muscular tissues of the bowels wear out, and difficulties of digestion are seen. The diseases most likely to occur in old age are enlargement of the prostate, which is said to occur in at least half of all men over the age of 70; cancer, a disease particularly of advanced years; and arthritic changes in the bones and joints. (*See also* CHAPTER X.)

SEPTICEMIA Invasion of the blood by the toxins of germs or by germs themselves.

SEPTIC SORE THROAT A condition that begins with a chill, a high fever, difficulty in swallowing and stiffness of the head and neck, caused by a streptococcus. As the infection extends downward, the voice becomes hoarse, coughing occurs and there may even be shortness of breath. Septic sore throat is not in itself fatal, but invasion of the blood by the germs, attack on the heart and on vital organs may cause death. The person with a septic sore throat should go to bed immediately and have the physician who is called determine the nature and extent of the condition. With the use of the sulfonamides and the antibiotics septic sore throat can be quickly brought under control. (*See also* CHAPTERS XXI, XXII.)

SHINGLES The term comes from a Greek word meaning "belt," since the blisters which are typical of shingles follow the course of the nerve around the body like a belt. Another term is herpes zoster. Crops of blisters appear, and with them come sensations of burning and sometimes pain. Young people get over shingles quickly, but older people suffer longer and probably more severely. In persistent cases of shingles specialists now use X-ray and ultraviolet ray. Certain antibiotics, particularly aureomycin, seem to be able to control the viruses, under some circumstances.

SHOCK A condition in which blood pours into the large vessels in the abdomen or when there is extensive dilation of the blood vessels on the surface of the body. Coupled with this change is severe perspiration; the skin seems warm. A person in shock should be placed with the head low, so that blood may get to the brain. He should be kept comfortably warm. Severe pain can be relieved by suitable drugs which the doctor can inject. Sometimes blood transfusion is necessary in shock to restore the quantity of blood. People with secondary shock are pale, weak, or exhausted. Shock may follow a severe burn, a severe pain, a severe mental condition (such as fright), or it may result from sudden loss of blood.

SINUSES The cavities in the bones of the head around the nose. When infectious germs gain access to the sinuses and infect the membranes that line their walls, the openings are blocked and congestion occurs, with severe pain, particularly headache. An ordinary cold will clear up in three to five days, but infected sinuses may last for weeks and weeks. The infection can be attacked principally through the blood, although the modern techniques of the nose-and-throat specialist may aid in draining the sinuses. The X-ray is used in study; also light cast through the sinus, to show the extent of the involvement. Sinus infections are sometimes related to nutritional deficiency. People with infections of the sinuses should avoid swimming, diving and strenuous outdoor exercise. They do better in climates that are hot and dry. (*See also* CHAPTER XXVI.)

SKIN The covering of the body. The outer layers called the epidermis or cuticle and the lower layers known as the corium or derma. The skin is made of fibrous elastic tissue, sometimes containing muscles which can actually cause hairs to stand on end. In the lower layers are the blood vessels, some fat, the sweat glands, the oil glands, and the roots of the hair. The skin also contains the ends of nerves which give the sense of touch, pain, and changes in temperature.

SLEEP (*See* INSOMNIA.)

SMALLPOX A contagious, infectious disease, often fatal. It begins with severe fever, followed in a few days by an eruption which appears all over the body. The red spots become pustules; and then crusts form. If the crusts do not heal well, pock marks are produced. Smallpox ap-

pears from twelve to twenty-one days after the person has been exposed. There are various divisions of smallpox according to the part of the body involved and the nature of the eruption (whether hemorrhagic or single). The condition is prevented by smallpox vaccination, which often used to be required before entrance to school, before a new occupation, or travel abroad. Serious epidemics of smallpox are practically never seen now, since the introduction of smallpox vaccination. (*See also* CHAPTERS XXI, XXII.)

SNEEZING A violent expulsion of air from the nose following irritation of the mucous membranes of the nose. The nerves send their messages through their facial nerves to the brain, which responds. The sneeze begins with the taking of a deep breath. When you sneeze, most of the droplets that are expelled come from the mouth, but also many come from the nose. The material is carried forward horizontally. The size of the drops varies greatly, and their number may reach 19,000 or 20,000 with a single strong sneeze.

In times of respiratory epidemics, face masks of gauze may be worn to hold back the germs and prevent their dissemination.

SNORING The actual noises made in snoring are due to passage of air at places in the nose and throat where there may be partial obstruction. The tongue may fall back in sleep, partially closing the openings through which air passes. When lying on the back, the muscles controlling the soft palate may fail to hold it. Inflammatory reactions

381

cause mucus to collect in the nose or in the passages behind the nose. If the nose is blocked and the lips are held close together, a whistling sound occurs as the air passes out. The most that can be done to prevent snoring is to make sure that obstructions in the nose and throat are cleared.

SOMNAMBULISM Sleepwalking. Obviously, this is associated with restless sleep and dreaming.

SPASM Any sudden contraction of a muscle that occurs without any desire or wish on the part of the person concerned. Spasm of the muscles of the calf of the leg is called intermittent claudication or intermittent limping. Spasms also occur in chorea, or "St. Vitus' dance," which is a rheumatic disorder. Drugs have been developed which are capable of controlling spasm.

SPEECH The ability to express thought by spoken words is peculiarly a phenomenon of human beings although some birds and animals may imitate speech. The voice is produced by the vocal cords in the larynx, modified by the actions of the tongue, the palate, the teeth, and by the presence of the sinuses and the nose. Disorders of speech include stuttering, stammering, slurring, slow and rapid speech, repetitive speech, and inarticulate sounds.

SPINA BIFIDA In one out of every 1,000 childbirths the spinal column fails to grow together as it should, creating a condition called spina bifida. In a way, this is like

cleft palate or harelip. The condition is especially bad if the spinal fluid drains, or if there is an infection which may damage the spinal cord and produce paralysis. A child with this condition should be taken to the doctor immediately, as it is possible to correct such malformations by surgical operation.

SPINAL CURVATURE Curving of the spine too much backward or forward, too much to one side or the other; also called scoliosis. The curves are given other names as well, depending on their direction. Posture is important in preventing curvature of the spine. However, most cases result from infection of the bones of the spine, occasionally with tuberculosis. Spinal curvature requires the attention of an orthopedic surgeon, who helps the condition by the use of braces, supports, plaster casts, and surgical procedures.

SPINAL FRACTURE A broken back, among the most serious of all injuries. Immediately after an accident affecting the back, the X-ray should be used to detect any break in the bones of the spine. Most such injuries occur when people fall from a height, when they are struck by motorcars, when they are thrown from a horse, when they dive into shallow pools, or when they are subjected to sudden pressure resulting from lifting or straining. When there is a break directly into the spinal cord with hemorrhage into the cord or tearing of the cord, paralyses occur, and every such case should be in a hospital where the best that modern surgery and medicine can provide is available. A neurologist should be consulted, as well as a surgeon.

SPLEEN A large pulpy organ on the left side of the abdomen. All of its functions are not clear, but definitely it is associated with blood formation and destruction of red blood cells, perhaps also with maintaining blood volume and, conceivably, with some of the reactions of the blood to various infections and other conditions. The spleen may be damaged in accidents, even broken, resulting in severe hemorrhages. Under such circumstances, an operation must be performed immediately. There are other organs and tissues in the body apparently capable of undertaking the duties of the spleen, so that it may be removed, as is done frequently in thrombocytopenic purpura.

SPRAINS Stretching of a ligament so that it tears, sometimes bleeds internally. Sprains or strains of the ankles and the wrists are frequent. Every serious sprain should be subjected to an X-ray picture. Ordinarily, a simple sprain is treated by rest, elevation of the leg and ankle and the application of an ice bag. In more serious conditions, physical therapy is used; sometimes the orthopedic surgeon will wish to apply tape to hold the joint firmly, or even a cast. The value of heat is greatest in the final stages when repair has begun, since it encourages circulation of the blood and absorption of the excess fluid.

SPRUE A disease with symptoms like those of pellagra and pernicious anemia, associated with the growth of a yeastlike fungus like monilia. The word sprue comes from a Dutch word meaning an inflammation of the mouth. For two thousand years this condition has been known. Sprue is believed to be primarily a disease of nutritional deficiency which, like pellagra, will improve with good diet rich in proteins and vitamins. (*See also* VITAMINS; *and also* CHAPTERS XIV, XV.)

SQUINT (*See* CROSS-EYE; EYE; *and also* CHAPTER XXV.)

STERILITY The condition of being unable to produce a child. In any such instance a careful investigation must be made of the physical condition of both the husband and the wife, since either may be entirely or partially responsible for the condition. The first step in examining the woman is to determine if the passage from the ovary to the uterus is clear. The male sperm may be examined under the microscope to be sure that enough active sperm is secreted to produce conception. (*See also* CHAPTER XVI.)

STOMACH A large sac which lies across the abdominal cavity below the diaphragm, immediately following the esophagus or swallowing tube. The lower end of the stomach or pylorus connects with the duodenum, the first portion of the small intestine. The stomach is lined by mucous membrane which contains the gastric glands and these provide gastric juice containing hydrochloric acid and pepsin and mucus. The walls of the stomach contain muscle which provides the stomach with the ability to mix the food and move it along the gastrointestinal tract.

STOMACH ULCERS (*See* ULCER; *also* CHAPTER VII.)

STOMATITIS Inflammation of the mouth, often infectious, such as trench mouth or Vincent's angina, sometimes from biting or chewing the cheek or irritation from a rough tooth. Occasionally resembling canker sores which are of unknown cause. Often relieved by applying mild alkaline or peroxide (half strength) mouth washes. Occasionally the blisters are like herpes and related to either viruses or allergy.

STRABISMUS (*See* CROSS-EYE; EYE; *and also* CHAPTER XXV.)

STROKE A common term for hemorrhage into the brain. Also called apoplexy.

STUTTERING AND STAMMERING Difficulties of speech associated with physical and mental factors. Examination should determine whether swollen adenoids, abnormal length of the uvula, abnormal size of the tongue or improper development of the mouth are present. Psychologists and psychiatrists study behavior changes that may be due to lack of confidence and the fear of appearing ridiculous. Children who have a dominant left eye and left hand sometimes develop speech difficulties when forced to change to right eye or right hand dominance.

STYES Scientifically called hordeolum. Styes are infections of the hair follicles on the eyelid, resembling pimples or boils. Antibiotic drugs are helpful. (*See also* EYE; *and also* CHAPTER XXV.)

SUNBURN A red condition of the skin caused by the sun; the technical name is *erythema solari*. A similar condition can be caused by ultraviolet rays. The inflammation varies from a slight flush to severe burning with blistering and loss of skin. Lotions are now available which can be put on the skin, and which will prevent sunburn by interfering with the passing of ultraviolet rays. A severely burned person may be dizzy, have headache, fever and vomiting, and other symptoms of a constitutional disturbance. Certain skins are more delicate than others. Blonds with thin skin react much more quickly than brunettes with thick skin. The skin of an infant is more delicate than that of an older person, and burns more easily. Upon being exposed to the sun, it is well to begin with just a few minutes and work up gradually to the time when the skin is sufficiently tanned that longer exposures may be indulged.

SUNSTROKE (*See* HEAT PROSTRATION; *and also* CHAPTER XIX.)

SWEAT (*See* PERSPIRATION.)

SYMPATHETIC NERVOUS SYSTEM The nervous system controlling functions of the body that go on without any conscious activity by the brain. The nerves of this system go to all important organs and tissues of the body, to the sweat glands of the skin and to the salivary glands. For this reason, emotions may be reflected in perspiration, dryness of the mouth or similar symptoms. The blood supply to any part of the body can be increased by interrupting the sympathetic nerves that go to the blood vessels. Another operation on the sympathetic nervous system is used as a relief for high blood pressure, increasing the flow of blood into the abdominal area and the legs. Interruption or treatment applied to the sympathetic nervous system is used in conditions of the heart like angina pectoris or in severe pain involving the uterus. Sometimes such operations are done in cases of cancer, to relieve unbearable pain. (*See also* CHAPTER V.)

SYNDROME A number of symptoms occurring together regularly. For example, there is Cushing's syndrome, due to certain tumors which cause an excess of secretion by the cortex of the adrenal gland; Froehlich's syndrome, in which there is increase in fat and weakness of the nerves and muscles; Korsakoff's syndrome in which there is multiple inflammation of nerves with loss of memory; apparently caused by excessive use of alcohol, with severe deficiency of certain vitamins. The condition called Ménière's disease is also known as Ménière's syndrome.

SYNOVITIS Infection and inflammation of the synovial membranes, the membranes which line the joints.

SYPHILIS A communicable venereal disease which usually begins with a sore on the sex organs called a chancre. Syphilis is sometimes called the pox, sometimes lues. The cause is an organism known as the *treponema pallidum* which, seen under the microscope, has a corkscrew appearance. Syphilis is usually acquired in sexual contact, but may be acquired also through other contamination. So wide is the variety of symptoms syphilis can produce that it is said to be able to imitate every other disease. It may involve any organ of the body. A child may be infected at birth with syphilis. Fortunately this condition, formerly hardly controllable, is now promptly diagnosed with certainty by the Wassermann, Kahn or similar tests, and treatment with penicillin or terramycin can bring the disease under complete control within a week. As a result of these new treatments, the disease is decreasing in its frequency and can, with proper control, be completely eliminated. (*See also* CHAPTER XXVII.)

T

TABES (*See* LOCOMOTOR ATAXIA.)

TACHYCARDIA An overrapid heartbeat. When this occurs at intervals, it is usually called paroxysmal tachycardia.

TACHYPHAGIA Rapid eating. The United States is full of rapid eaters. Not only do they eat rapidly, but frequently they swallow air while eating and thereafter belch, and suffer with bloating.

TALIPES A deformity of the foot.

When a child is born with this condition, it should have prompt treatment to correct the condition. When the weight of the foot is on the toe, the condition is called *talipes equinus,* because it resembles the foot of a horse. When twisted to the side, the condition is *talipes valgus.* (*See also* CLUBFOOT.)

TATTOOING Tattooing invariably becomes popular in time of war, and one sees great numbers of former soldiers and sailors bearing all sorts of designs which have been made by pricking the skin and inserting dye substances.

TAY-SACHS DISEASE Children affected with Tay-Sachs disease develop symptoms of deterioration at six to nine months of age with progressive loss of muscle strength. Coordination becomes poor. After the first year of life, blindness and other defects occur, followed usually by death between two and four years of age.

Especially interesting about Tay-Sachs disease is the frequency among Ashkenazi Jews in whom the carrier frequency is 1 in 30 for this classification and 1 in 300 for non-Jewish people. Approximately 52 new cases of this disease occur yearly in the United States, of which 40 are in the Jewish group.

With the development of the use of amniocentesis before birth, a method of control has developed which may point the way to the ultimate elimination of this disorder. The diagnosis is confirmed in fetuses by chemical and ultrastructural analyses of all of the fetal tissues. Parents who possibly anticipate the birth of a child with Tay-Sachs or any other ganglioside-storage disease may be informed that the chance is 1 in 4 that the prospective child may have the condition, that the condition may be determined in the fetus, if present, by amniocentesis and examination of the amniotic fluid. A family which carries a ganglioside-storage disease or any instance in which such a condition has appeared in a child may now prevent its occurrence in subsequent pregnancies. In 75 per cent of pregnancies the fetus will be free of the disease. (*See also* CHAPTER IX.)

TEETH Each tooth consists of dentine which surrounds a pulpy cavity in which are the nerves and the blood vessels. The crown of the tooth is covered by enamel. The root may be a single projection, a double one or a triple one. The roots are covered by bone called cementum. The ordinary classifications include the incisors, the canine, the premolar (or bicuspid), the molar, and third molar (called wisdom teeth). The upper canine is known as the eye tooth. The milk teeth of childhood are replaced by the permanent teeth of which there are 32—8 incisors, 4 canine, 8 premolars, and 12 molars.

TENDONITIS Inflammation of the tendons which pass from the bones to the muscles.

TENIA (*See* WORMS.)

TESTICLE The common name for one of the pair of male sex glands. Inflammation of these glands is discussed under the medical name, *orchitis. (See also* CHAPTER XVI.)

TETANUS Lockjaw, a condition caused by a germ which creates one of the most powerful poisons known. Tetanus may begin about seven days after a wound which permits the germs to get into the tissues. Tetanus is associated with irritability, headache, chills and fever; then comes the stiffness of the muscles of the jaw and neck, which gives the disease its name. Fortunately, a specific vaccine is available for the prevention of tetanus, and when there is possibility that the wound has been contaminated with these germs, the vaccination should be used. Also available are antitetanus antitoxins.

THROMBOANGIITIS OBLITERANS (*See* BUERGER'S DISEASE.)

THROMBOPHLEBITIS (*See* PHLEBITIS.)

THROMBOSIS The formation of a clot in a blood vessel. (*See also* GANGRENE; HEART.)

THRUSH An infection by various fungi which attack tissues of the mouth. Seen most often in children.

THYMUS A gland which lies in the chest in front of the windpipe, between the lungs and above the heart. This gland is believed to be associated with growth, since it is gradually absorbed and disappears after the first eight or nine months of life. If it fails to become smaller and continues to send substances into the body, changes may occur that affect health. Research now

shows that the thymus is associated with the development by the body of antibodies to infectious agents. (*See also* GLANDS; *and also* CHAPTER XVI.)

THYROID (*See* GLANDS; GOITER; *and also* CHAPTER XVI.)

TIC Any spasmodic movement or twitching, particularly of the face. Habit sometimes develops movements of this kind, which are then called habit spasms. Inflammations of the facial nerve may produce painful spasms called *tic douloureux*. (*See also* CHOREA.)

TOBACCO Vast numbers of persons smoke—they are estimated at more than 60,000,000 in the United States—and as a result, physicians are interested in the effects of tobacco on health. Apparently, smoking is a pleasurable process which aids relaxation. The effects of tobacco are primarily the effects of the nicotine and, obviously, much depends on the dosage, since nicotine can slow the circulation of the blood. Smoking of filtered cigarettes cuts down the total dosage of nicotine. Tobacco is forbidden in Buerger's disease.

Secondary effects are on the digestion, the throat and the lungs. Other effects relate to the tar in tobacco. The argument has been made from statistics that tobacco tar is the cause of the gradual increase of cancer of the lung that has occurred in the past thirty years. Similarly, cancer of the lung is credited to industrial wastes, exhaust gases which contain tar, and other irritants of the lung.

TONGUE A tongue that is dry, dark and furred indicates an unhealthful condition. A tongue that is moist and clean is of the normal appearance. The healthy tongue can be moved quickly or slowly in all directions. In people who have overactivity of the thyroid gland, the tongue moves quickly. Those who have underactivity of the thyroid, have a sluggish tongue. People who are weak or exhausted and those in a stupor or a coma cannot project the tongue far. Sometimes a nervous condition causes the tongue to tremble. Paralysis may affect one side of the tongue only, so that the healthy side will push the tongue toward the paralyzed side. People may suffer with a burning of the tongue, which seems in many instances to be a psychosomatic condition. Teeth made of dissimilar metals may create electrical currents, which have been associated with burning of the tongue. Burning of the tongue occurs in pellagra and in various vitamin deficiencies. Elevations of the papillae of the tongue develop in a condition called geographic tongue. In pernicious anemia, the tongue assumes a most unhealthful appearance, which is overcome by taking vitamin B_{12}.

TONSILS One pair of lymphoid masses in the throat. Infectious germs that get into the throat are picked up by the tonsils; the tonsils swell, and with this comes pain, soreness, difficulty in swallowing, swelling of the glands in the throat, fever, a rapid pulse and general illness. This condition is called tonsillitis. If tonsils in children are repeatedly inflamed, it is best, in a quiescent interval, to have the tonsils removed. It is not desirable to remove tonsils in times of epidemics, particularly of infantile paralysis, since this may leave open areas through which viruses invade. An enlarged tonsil is not necessarily an infected tonsil. Tonsils have been made smaller by exposure to X-ray and other methods have been tried. The medical profession generally is inclined to believe in a good surgical removal, best performed in a hospital, with anesthesia. (*See also* CHAPTER XXVI.)

TORTICOLLIS Twisting of the neck so that the head leans or is tilted toward one shoulder or the other; also called wry neck, twisted neck. The cause may be just a bad habit, but in most instances the condition is associated with paralysis of certain nerves, with excess action of certain muscles. Occasionally, other nervous conditions will result in wry neck. Infection of the lymph glands may cause the head to be held toward one side or the other. In the most difficult cases, surgical operations are used to produce straightening. By the use of suitable braces or casts, the head is held in proper position until recovery has occurred. Regular exercises and massage help the postoperative result.

TRACHEA The windpipe. It may become infected as may any other part of the body, and infection is to be treated according to the germ involved, with various sulfonamides and antibiotic drugs. Inhalations of warm steam will relieve a trachitis (inflammation of the trachea). In a tracheotomy, a hole is made in the windpipe in order to permit breathing. This is done nowadays in cases of bulbar infantile paralysis, which interferes with respiration.

TRACHOMA The most widespread eye disease of the world is the inflammation caused by a virus called trachoma. This condition is most common in Egypt, Palestine and India. The disease can be transmitted by secretions from the infected eye on the hands, towels, handkerchiefs, pillows, or even by sneezing.

In trachoma the eyes become inflamed and red, blisters and crusts form, and scarring follows. Everything possible must be done to prevent such an infection. Modern treatment involving the use of sulfonamide drugs and antibiotics is successful, particularly if the condition is seen sufficiently early to stop it before it has reached the point of destroying the tissue. (*See also* EYE; *and also* CHAPTER XXV.)

TRANQUILIZING DRUGS Tranquilizing drugs have come prominently into medicine. They include extracts of *rauwolfia serpentia* such as reserpine and serpasil, chlorpromazine (also known as Thorazine and Larjactil), Promazine (which is the same drug called the chlorine radical), Miltown or Equanil (which is a meprobamate), Frenquel (which is derived from a drug called Meratran), and several others still in process of investigation. These drugs have the effect of quieting activity of the brain at various levels. (*See also* CHAPTER XXX.)

TRENCH MOUTH (*See* VINCENT'S ANGINA.)

TRICHINOSIS A disease caused by eating pork infected with an organism called trichina. When this pork is eaten without proper cooking, the symptoms of trichinosis develop. A temperature of 137 degrees Fahrenheit for a sufficient time will destroy the organisms of trichinosis. The disease begins with headaches, chills and a general feeling of illness. The eyes become swollen and painful, the throat sore, and the muscles sore. Fever appears. Examination of the blood reveals an increase in the number of white blood cells. When a piece of muscle is taken, the organisms will be found encysted in the muscle. The way to avoid trichinosis is to make sure that all pork products are properly inspected, properly stored and properly cooked. The feeding of swine on garbage helps to spread the disease. Sterilization of garbage by electrical or other methods will help to prevent it.

TUBERCULOSIS An infectious disease caused by the tubercle bacillus. This disease was for centuries considered the most serious of all, and was called "captain of the men of death." Nobody knows how many millions of human beings have been destroyed by tuberculosis. Fortunately, new discoveries have made possible an attack on tuberculosis which is efficient, and today many states in the United States have death rates as low as 5 per 100,000, compared with a death rate in 1900 of over 300 per 100,000 population. Tuberculosis is a germ disease

389

which spreads to those who are well from those who are sick and are giving out the germs in their sputum. The X-ray is used to determine the presence of tuberculosis. The tuberculin test, in which a small amount of material called tuberculin is applied to the skin, is also a test of the presence of tuberculosis.

Tuberculosis of the bones and lymph glands used to be frequent, being spread through tuberculosis of cattle. Now that tuberculosis of cattle has been gradually eliminated, these forms of tuberculosis are rarely seen.

In the modern prevention of tuberculosis, a vaccine called "BCG" is being used. More than 40,000,000 children throughout the world have already been inoculated with this vaccine, and it seems to have the power to control infection, although not absolutely 100 per cent protection is secured.

Sanitariums are still used for the severe open cases. For early cases or for cases without the germs in the sputum, ambulatory methods are used. Patients come to dispensaries, where they may receive streptomycin, paraminosalicylic acid, isoniazid or a new antibiotic called cycloserine. Extensive use of these methods in the treatment of veterans with tuberculosis has proved that they are efficient. Many sanitariums widely known throughout the world have now closed their doors, because of an insufficient number of patients.

In the treatment of severe tuberculosis, artificial pneumothorax is used. This is a method by which air is injected into the chest cavity, to cause the lung to collapse and be at rest. While at rest the lung will heal; it is later allowed to re-expand. Lungs can also be put at rest by cutting the nerve (the phrenic nerve) which goes to the diaphragm. Another method, wholly surgical, is thoracoplasty, in which ribs are removed and the lung is put at rest permanently so that healing can take place. Also, infected lobes may now be removed surgically.

TULAREMIA An infectious disease caused by an organism called *pasteurella tularensis,* which is transmitted to men by handling infected rabbits or squirrels, or other small animals. The condition can also be transmitted by insect bites.

This condition gets its name from Tulare County, California, where wild game was found to be dying by the thousands from this condition. Since wild rabbits are the chief animals infected, the condition has been called rabbit fever. Men who hunt rabbits should be warned of the danger of bringing home any rabbit which can be knocked over with a stick. Healthy rabbits can run. People who handle rabbits for any purpose after they are dead ought to wear rubber gloves, and should wash their hands with antiseptic solutions. Never let a scratch, cut, or sore come in contact with the flesh of the rabbits or with a dish or pan in which rabbit meat has been kept. Wrapping paper which has contained the bodies of dead rabbits should be burned. A cut or a sore developing after handling rabbit meat must be suspected of this infection. (*See also* CHAPTER XXII.)

TUMORS Tumors are new growths of tissue. They may be benign or malignant. (*See also* CANCER; *and also* CHAPTER XXIV.)

TYPHOID FEVER An acute infectious disease caused by a germ. The germ can be found in the blood of a person sick with the disease. It can be passed from the bowels and contaminate the hands or food of other persons, and thus infect them. It can be spread by contaminated food and clothing, by water and milk which contain germs. The doctor who examines the patient with typhoid fever makes his diagnosis from the history of the case, the nature of the symptoms, and by careful studies of the blood using a test called the Widal test. People with typhoid fever are treated as those with other infectious diseases, but particular care is given to disinfecting their excretions.

Typhoid is prevented by the use of a vaccine against typhoid, by making sure that food is not contaminated and by detecting and isolating people who carry the germs of typhoid and excrete them. Persistent attention to water supply, to disposal of sewage, pasteurization of milk, education of the public in hygiene, and control of typhoid carriers have practically eliminated this disease. Many medical students never get to see a case.

Antibiotic drugs, particularly chloramphenicol or chloromycetin, have been found effective against typhoid. The disease is no longer the menace that it once was. (*See also* CHAPTERS XXI, XXII.)

TYPHUS An acute infectious disease in which there is a rash, serious symptoms affecting the nervous system and a high fever. This disease is transmitted to human beings by the body louse and the rat flea which are infected with an organism called *Rickettsia prowazekii*. A few days to two weeks after the person has first been infected, this disease begins, with pains in the head, back, and limbs. The fever rises rapidly to 104 or 105 degrees Fahrenheit. The symptoms affecting the nervous system are like those of typhoid fever. The eruption appears on the fourth or fifth day with rose-colored spots scattered all over the body. Because this disease occurs so often among groups of people assembled together, it used to be called camp fever, jail fever, or ship fever. A similar condition is also known as Brill's disease. In Latin America the condition is called tabardillo. Another similar condition is called scrub typhus and is known in the Orient as tsutsugamushi disease. (*See also* CHAPTER XXII.)

U

ULCER Any interruption of the continuity of the surface of the skin or of a mucous membrane with an inflammation. Ulcers are of many types, including those of the duodenum and stomach, the ulcers that form with bedsores, the ulcers that have little tendency to heal and which are called indolent ulcers. Indeed, there is one form of ulcer called kissing ulcer since it occurs where two tissues of the body touch each other. A perforating ulcer is one which bursts through the wall of the stomach or intestines. Certain carcinomas tend to destroy tissue deeply. These are called rodent ulcers. Varicose ulcers appear wherever the skin has failed to receive adequate nutrition as the result of a varicose vein.

Ulcers of the duodenum, the portion of the intestine immediately below the stomach, have been described as the commonest disease of the upper part of the intestinal system. Such ulcers are found ten times as often in the duodenum as in the stomach, four times as often in men as in women. Duodenal and stomach ulcers occur usually in people who live under stress. No single cause is known, but mental conditions are definitely related to changes in the secretion and motion of the stomach; perhaps infections occur owing to subsequent loss of resistance.

Many physicians associate the presence of stomach ulcers with an increased amount of acid in the stomach. The excess acid is responsible for the continuation of the symptoms. Most treatments are designed to decrease the excess acidity, either through action on the nervous system or directly on the acid. Many drugs are now available, called anticholinergics, like Banthine, Pamine, Prantal, and others, which act to prevent excess acid secretion. Various alkaline powders are also frequently used. Many physicians recommend the taking of milk and cream in equal proportion at frequent intervals to protect the damaged area. Most recent is a technique developed by Wangensteen which freezes the stomach for a brief period. This lowers the secretion of acid and hastens healing of the ulcer.

UMBILICUS (*See* NAVEL.)

UNDULANT FEVER An infectious disease, caused by an organism known as the Brucella, occurring in goats, sheep and cattle, and commonly transmitted to man by consumption of infected milk or milk products. Occasionally the disease results from direct contact with the flesh of infected animals. It may also spread through contamination of infected soil and water. In humans the disease occurs in acute and chronic form and leads to weakness, loss of weight and anemia. The condition is controlled nowadays principally with the antibiotics. Other names by which this condition is called are brucellosis, Malta fever, Mediterranean fever, abortus fever, and melitensis fever. (*See also* CHAPTER XXII.)

UREMIA Retention in the blood of urinary constituents. When the kidneys fail to dispose of the urine, with its waste products, the person becomes drowsy and apathetic and may pass into unconsciousness. With this is associated shortness of breath and sluggishness. Obviously this is a condition most dangerous to life. As soon as it is detected, everything possible must be done to encourage elimination of the toxic products from the body. (*See also* KIDNEY; *and also* CHAPTER VIII.)

URETER The tube that passes

from the kidneys to the bladder. (*See also* BLADDER; KIDNEY; *and also* CHAPTER VIII.)

URTICARIA (*See* HIVES; *and also* CHAPTER XXIII.)

UTERUS The womb, the organ that carries the child previous to birth. It may be subjected to various inflammations and infections. It is discussed under such terms as *Endometritis, Cervicitis* and in relationship to other infections and cancer. (*See also* PREGNANCY.)

UVULA The little tissue that hangs down from the middle of the palate into the middle of the throat. Rarely does it become infected. Practically never is it necessary to clip or cut the uvula in any way.

V

VACCINATION Inoculation with killed bodies of viruses or organisms. Today vaccines are available against infantile paralysis, typhoid fever, yellow fever, typhus, and others. (*See also* CHAPTERS XXI, XXII.)

VAGINA The canal which extends from the female outer sex organs (vulva) to the uterus.

VARICELLA (*See* CHICKEN POX; *and also* CHAPTER XXII.)

VARICOSE VEINS Dilation of the veins caused by a breakdown of

the valves which keep the column of blood returning to the heart from settling back into the veins. The veins of the legs are chiefly affected. The wearing of tight belts, such conditions as childbirth and constipation, and excessive weight, may interfere with the action of the circulation and produce varicose veins. Varicose veins in the rectum are called piles.

Varicose veins are controlled by wearing elastic bandages or stockings. They can be removed by surgery. They can be obliterated by the injection of caustic substances. If varicose veins persist and become worse, varicose ulcers may form.

VASECTOMY Cutting and tying the tubes which in man pass from the testes to the urethra, thus blocking the passing of the sperm cell. Applied to act as birth-control mechanism. In about 50 per cent of cases operation may serve to restore the opening of the ducts.

VERTIGO (*See* DIZZINESS.)

VINCENT'S ANGINA An infection of the mouth by an organism that is spread widely, sometimes by kissing, sometimes by eating from contaminated utensils or cups; also called trench mouth. When the gums bleed easily and the mouth has a foul odor, Vincent's infection should be looked for. The organism is particularly susceptible to sodium perborate, and mouth washes of this substance are used in controlling it.

VIRUS A disease-causing organism smaller than the ordinary germ, so small that it can be filtered through the pores of a clay filter. Viruses are now grown outside the body, on tissue and in fertile eggs. Among diseases caused by viruses are rabies, infantile paralysis, encephalitis, smallpox, herpes, the common cold, influenza, measles, yellow fever, and mumps. (*See also* CHAPTERS XXI, XXII.)

VITAMIN One of a group of certain substances required for normal growth and the maintenance of life in animals, including man. Sometimes these substances take part in the intricate chemical reactions of the body. They do not furnish energy, but they are required in order to carry on the chemistry of the tissues. The vitamins have been called by letters, but for most of them there are also distinctive names.

Vitamin A is known as the antixerophthalmic vitamin; it is derived from carotene. It is apparently necessary to maintain the growth of the normal cells and the ability of the eye to see. When this vitamin is deficient, bacterial infections occur; night blindness is a symptom. This vitamin is plentiful in such fish liver oils as cod liver oil, also in butter and in milk. It is now customary to enrich margarine with this vitamin.

The vitamin-B complex contains many different substances, of which some ten are already recognized and usable. These include thiamin (vitamin B_1); riboflavin (vitamin B_2); niacin (or nicotinic acid); pyridoxine (vitamin B_6), which is necessary for growth in small children, perhaps takes some part in reactions of the body—when it is absent, spasms occur; inositol. Another portion of the B complex is paraminobenzoic acid

which is sometimes believed to have something to do with gray hair but not established. This vitamin is involved in the action of the sulfonamide drugs. Biotin, adenyllic acid and folic acid are also portions of the vitamin-B complex. Folic acid is closely related to the formation of red blood cells. An antifolic acid substance called aminopterin is used in the attack on cancer. This vitamin is found in high concentration in yeast and in liver. Vitamin B_{12} is used specifically in pernicious anemia and also for such conditions as neuritis.

Vitamin C is known as ascorbic acid and cevitamic acid. it is necessary for the maintenance of the substance of teeth, bones and of the blood vessels. When it is deficient, scurvy occurs. It may be related to fragility of the capillary blood vessels. This vitamin is found particularly in citrus fruits, tomatoes, potatoes, leafy vegetables and, in some degree, in almost all raw foods.

Vitamin D is one of several different vitamins known to have the capacity to mobilize calcium and thus prevent rickets. Vitamin D is divided into vitamin D_2 (calciferol); vitamin D_3 (an irradiated cholesterol); also vitamins D_4 and D_5 which are other forms. Vitamin D_3 is most abundant in natural sources like fish-liver oils. It is also found in eggs, salmon, and may be produced artificially by the action of sunshine on the skin or by the action of ultraviolet rays on a variety of substances.

Vitamin E (tocopherol) is involved particularly in the reproductive processes of animals, but does not seem to be highly significant in the human being. Attempts have been made to relate it to certain diseases of the nervous system, but the proof is not positive.

Vitamin F is the name given to a substance found in fatty acids such as lanoleic acid.

Other vitamins are known as G and H; then comes vitamin K, which is called manadione. There are three forms of K known as K_1, K_2 and K_3. This vitamin is essential to form the substance that takes part in blood clotting. The principal dietary sources are spinach, cabbage, cauliflower, tomatoes and soy bean oil.

Vitamin L is a group of vitamins which are said to be related to production of milk by the mammary glands.

Another vitamin, M, is supposed to be a part of the vitamin-B complex. Vitamin P is found in citrus fruits, along with vitamin C. This vitamin is said to be necessary to maintain the flexibility of the capillary blood vessels and their resistance to breaking. A vitamin U is presumed to be necessary for growth of chickens. Tables of vitamins are available which show all the different ways in which they enter into human body chemistry. (*See also* CHAPTERS XIV, XV.)

VITILIGO In this condition, the pigment in the skin entirely disappears from some spots so that they appear white in contrast to the rest of the skin. The condition is rather widespread. Recently a drug was found in Egypt which seems to have the power, when taken internally or painted on and when the skin is exposed to ultraviolet rays, to bring about pigmentation. Also studies have shown that a portion of the pi-

tuitary gland seems to have the control over melanin, and thus also control over pigmentation.

VOCAL CORD (*See* LARYNGITIS, SPEECH; *and also* CHAPTER XXVI.)

VOICE (*See* LARYNGITIS, SPEECH; *and also* CHAPTER XXVI.)

VOMITING Expulsion of the contents of the stomach through the mouth. Nausea and vomiting are mentioned in connection with innumerable diseases because they may accompany the beginning of any infectious condition. The doctor treats these conditions as symptoms of disease and then tries to determine what is the cause. If vomiting occurs, something has caused the stomach to wish to be emptied. The doctor will usually recommend that the food be controlled and be not too great in amount, since much fluid may be lost through vomiting and the loss of fluid may in itself produce symptoms. The doctor sees to it that the fluids of the body are restored to normal. Often dizziness precedes vomiting. Sometimes vomiting results from reflexes, as when a finger is put down the throat. The severe pain associated with a violent blow in the abdomen may cause vomiting. (*See also* CHAPTERS II, VII.)

W

WARTS Overgrowths of portions of the skin, presumably caused by viruses. They seem to be to some extent regulated through the nervous system, since they sometimes disappear just through psychologic suggestion. They can, however, be removed by electric coagulation, by carbon dioxide snow, or by surgery. Radium and X-ray may cause a wart to degenerate and fall out. Among the most serious of the warts are those on the soles of the feet which are highly resistant to treatment. Recently a drug called euphorbia has been worked up into an application which can be applied with success to some plantar warts. Old people have a special form of warts known as senile warts. These demand prompt attention because continued irritation may cause them to develop the characteristics of cancer.

WASSERMANN TEST Blood test for the diagnosis of syphilis. Other similar tests are the Kahn test, the Eagle test and the Hinton test. These tests determine early whether or not syphilis is present. Modern treatment with penicillin and terramycin can clear up the condition and change the test to negative.

WEIGHT, OVER- AND UNDER- Most people get fat because they eat too much. Many diets have been developed which can reduce weight. These diets are low in calories and at the same time, if they are good diets, provide enough suitable protein, carbohydrate, fat, mineral salts and vitamins to maintain health.

Some people eat simply out of boredom; others have been found to eat for other psychological reasons. Some children have been found to eat vast amounts of food simply because they knew that it annoyed their mother.

Overweight may proceed to the point of being a serious menace to health. This is particularly true in cases affecting the heart, in the rheumatic diseases, in high blood pressure, and in diseases affecting the lungs. The average person may consume around 2,000 to 2,500 calories a day without gaining weight, because of his usual activities. If he takes under 1,200 calories per day he is likely to lose weight at the rate of about two pounds per week.

People who are underweight have much less trouble than those who are overweight. The life-insurance statistics indicate that underweight people live longer. People who are thin because of illness or who suffer from lack of appetite or inability to eat are a problem for both the psychologist and the nutrition expert.

In certain cases, the glands of internal secretion may be disturbed. Excess action of the thyroid tends to make people thin; insufficient action of this gland tends to make them fat. Increase in weight occurs normally with pregnancy. (*See also* CHAPTERS XIV, XV.)

WEN A sebaceous cyst. When an oil gland gets blocked at its opening the oil accumulates, and the bump can grow as large as a golf ball. If it becomes rubbed or if it comes in contact with germs, serious infections result and eventually may become abscesses. A wen should be treated to eliminate its contents of fluid and, if necessary, removed surgically.

WHOOPING COUGH An infectious inflammation of the air passages, with violent coughing. Vomiting sometimes follows the severe coughing spells. This has been known to the medical profession for many years, and is actually one of the most serious diseases of childhood. The condition is caused by an organism known as the *hemophilus pertussis*. Vaccines have been prepared which can help to prevent whooping cough. Any serious case of whooping cough should have close medical attention, perhaps in a hospital, since patients do die, from failure to eat, from exhaustion, or from secondary infections. The doctor can do much to diminish the severity of coughing spells by prescribing drugs which are sedative and relaxing. Most dangerous of complications are pneumonia, malnutrition, and prostration. The condition is also called pertussis. (*See also* CHAPTER XXII.)

WOMB (*See* UTERUS.)

WORMS Worms may be present in the bowels without causing much in the way of serious symptoms. However, some worms do cause severe symptoms and must be eliminated from the body. Among them are the hookworm (ancylostoma); the pinworm (enterobius vermicularies); the roundworm (or ascaris); the whipworm (trichuris trichurea); the tapeworm, known under such names as the beef tapeworm, the broad tapeworm, the fish tapeworm and the pork tapeworm.

By far the most common is the pinworm, also called the seat worm or thread worm. The eggs taken into the human body hatch in the small intestines, where the worms mature and mate. Females move on to the large bowel and develop the eggs. The males pass out of the body. The eggs may lodge in areas around the openings of the bowel, may get on the sleeping garments or bedclothes. They cause itching and scratching which may result in infection. In the control of pinworms, the utmost cleanliness is required. Several drugs are available which will quickly eliminate such worms, among them hexylresorcinol and other substances.

The roundworms, exceeded in frequency only by the pinworms, live in the bowel and may develop to lengths of 6 to 15 inches. They hold themselves in the bowel by a sort of springlike pressure. The female worm can discharge 200,000 eggs a day. This worm does not cause much in the way of serious symptoms, but can produce blocking of the bowel. They are controlled by giving cathartics and washing out the bowel, after which drugs are provided that destroy the worm and eliminate it.

The hookworm can produce severe anemia. It penetrates the skin, producing the condition called ground itch. It then gets into the intestines by way of the blood. The doctor establishes the presence of the condition by examining the material from the bowel. Such remedies as hexylresorcinol, oil of chenopodium and tetrachloroethylene are used. All worm remedies are poisonous if administered wrongly or in excess amounts.

The tapeworms live in the human intestine. There are thirty or forty different species. A complete tapeworm will measure one to fifteen feet long and contain as many as 2,000 parts. The presence of these worms means serious loss of appetite, secondary anemia, loss of weight, and other serious symptoms.

WOUNDS Any injury that breaks the skin or the underlying tissues. The danger lies in hemorrhage and in infection. The best treatment for small wounds is simply to wash them thoroughly and to cover them with sterile gauze. Various antiseptics are commonly applied to wounds. These include iodine, boric acid, hydrogen peroxide, mercurochrome, tinctures of metaphen and merthiolate, and many others. If a wound becomes seriously infected, it should be seen by a competent doctor or surgeon. Antibiotic drugs can be used to control infection. These are better taken internally than applied to the wound.

WRY NECK (*See* TORTICOLLIS.)

X

XANTHOMA A yellow tumor. Any tumor should be examined and diagnosed as to whether it is benign or malignant. Then the surgeon will consider how best it can be removed.

XERODERMA A skin disease with marked roughness or drying and sometimes discoloration.

X-RAY Used principally in the diagnosis and treatment of disease. X-rays are used to determine changes in the bones and in all of the soft

tissues of the body. By the use of X-ray, the size of the heart may be determined. By the internal administration of a variety of substances, either by swallowing or directly by injection into the blood, X-ray pictures may be used to show changes in the lungs, the bowel, the sinuses, the spinal fluid—in fact, changes in any portion of the body. Routine X-ray pictures of the lungs aid the early detection of tuberculosis.

Y

YAWS An infectious nonvenereal disease occurring in the hot, moist tropics. It is caused by treponema, an organism resembling that of syphilis, but the disease is not syphilis. Other names for yaws are frambesia and leishmaniasis. The condition is infrequent in the United States, but has been suffered by troops stationed in tropical countries.

YEAST Brewer's yeast is one of the richest known substances in vitamin B and is used for supplying this vitamin in some instances. (*See also* CHAPTER XV.)

YELLOW FEVER A tropical disease, which has been largely eliminated by getting rid of the mosquitoes that cause it. A vaccine has been developed which prevents yellow fever. (*See also* CHAPTERS XXII, XXIX.)

Z

ZINC Used in medicine chiefly as a component of zinc chloride, zinc oxide and the other zinc combinations used in treatment of skin diseases. In these conditions, zinc is combined with talcum powder and other substances like the petrolatum and lanolin used in ointments.

ZYGOMA A portion of the bone in the head commonly called the temple. This may be involved in fractures of the skull.

ZYME This short word taken from the Greek means ferment. From this comes the term enzyme, which is a ferment developed inside the body. The enzymes are beginning to be isolated and have a practical use in many conditions as do the hormones.

INDEX

Abscess, 259–60
Abdomen
  pain in, 259
    symptomatic, 10–11
  wounds of, 245
Abortion, 259
Abrasion, 259
Abstinence, 260
Acariasis, 260
Accidents, 260
  See also Injuries
Acetic acid, 260
Ache, 260
Achlorhydria, 260
Achondroplasia, 260
Achylia, 260–61
Acidosis, 261
Acne, 261
  vulgaris, 149–50
Acquired conditions, 261
Acrodynia, 261–62
Acromegaly, 83, 262
Acrophobia, 262
ACTH, 54–55, 262
Actinomycosis, 262
Acupuncture, 262–63
Addiction, drug, 263
Addison's disease, 263
Adenoids, 263
Adenoma, 262
Adhesions, 263
Adiposis, 263
Adjustment, 263
Adolescence, 263–64
Adrenal glands, 89
Aerophobia, 264
Afterbirth, 264
Aftereffects, 264
Aging, 42–43, 379–80
  eyesight and, 178–79
Ague, 264
Air conditioning, 264
Air pollution, 125, 368
Airsickness, 264–65
Albinos, 265
Albuminuria, 265
Alcoholism, 107–9, 251, 265
  delirium tremens in, 303–4
Alexia, 265
Alimentation, 265
Alkalosis, 265–66
Allergic disorders, 46–50, 266
  See also specific allergies
Aloes, 266

Alopecia, 266
Aluminum dust, inhalation of, 124
Amaurosis, 266
Amblyopia, 266
Amebiasis, 266–67
Amenorrhea, 267
Amnesia, 267
Amniocentesis, 267
Amphetamines, 216
Amyotrophic lateral sclerosis, 267
Analgesia, 267
Anemia, 267–68
  Cooley's, 268
  pernicious, 268
  sickle-cell, 41
Anesthesia, 269
Aneurysm, 269
Angina,
  Vincent's, 393
  pectoris, 269–70
Angioma, 270
Animal bites, 245–46
Aniseikonia, 270
Anorexia, 270
Anthrax, 270–71
Antibiotics, 128–29, 271, 363
Antihistamines, 271
Antiseptics, 221
Antitoxins, 271
Antrum, 271
Anus, 271
Anxiety, 272
Aorta, 272
Aphasia, 272
Aphonia, 272
Aphrodisiac, 272
Apoplexy, 272
Appendicitis, 272–73
Appetite, 273
Arachnodactaly, 273
Argyria, 21
Ariboflavinosis, 75–76
Arms, symptomatic pains in, 12
Arsenic poisoning, 112–13
Arteriosclerosis, 273–74
Arthritis, 53–56, 274
Artificial respiration, 247–48
Asbestosis, 123–24, 274–75
Ascites, 275
Ascorbic acid, 275
  deficiency of, 74–75
Asphyxia, 275
Asthenia, 14, 275
Asthma, 275–76
  bronchial, 47–48

400

407